Current Concepts in Genitourinary Pathology: Kidney and Testes

Guest Editor

ANIL V. PARWANI, MD, PhD

SURGICAL PATHOLOGY CLINICS

surgpath.theclinics.com

Consulting Editor
JOHN R. GOLDBLUM, MD

March 2009 • Volume 2 • Number 1

SAUNDERS an imprint of ELSEVIER, Inc.

W.B. SAUNDERS COMPANY
A Division of Elsevier Inc.

1600 John F. Kennedy Boulevard • Suite 1800 • Philadelphia, Pennsylvania 19103-2899

http://www.theclinics.com

SURGICAL PATHOLOGY CLINICS Volume 2, Number 1
March 2009 ISSN 1875-9181, ISBN-13: 978-1-4377-0578-2, ISBN-10: 1-4377-0578-2

Editor: Joanne Husovski

Surgical Pathology Clinics (ISSN 1875-9181) is published quarterly by Elsevier Inc., 360 Park Avenue South, New York, NY 10010-1710. Months of issue are March, June, September, and December. Business and Editorial Offices: 1600 John F. Kennedy Blvd., Suite 1800, Philadelphia, PA 19103-2899. Periodicals postage paid at New York, NY and additional mailing offices. Subscription prices are $159.00 per year (US individuals), $199.00 per year (US institutions), $80.00 per year (US students/residents), $199.00 per year (Canadian individuals), $225.00 per year (Canadian Institutions), $199.00 per year (foreign individuals), $225.00 per year (foreign institutions), and $99.00 per year (international & Canadian students/residents). Foreign air speed delivery is included in all *Clinics'* subscription prices. All prices are subject to change without notice. **POSTMASTER:** Send address changes to *Surgical Pathology Clinics*, Elsevier Periodicals Customer Service, 11830 Westline Industrial Drive, St. Louis, MO 63146. Customer Service: 1-800-654-2452 (US). From outside the United States, call 1-314-453-7041. Fax: 1-314-453-5170. E-mail: JournalsCustomerServiceusa@ elsevier.com (for print support) and JournalsOnlineSupport-usa@elsevier.com (for online support).

Reprints. For copies of 100 or more, of articles in this publication, please contact the Commercial Reprints Department, Elsevier Inc., 360 Park Avenue South, New York, NY 10010-1710. Tel. (212) 633-3812; Fax: (212) 462-1935; email: reprints@elsevier.com.

Printed in the United States of America.

Contributors

CONSULTING EDITOR

JOHN R. GOLDBLUM, MD
Chairman, Department of Anatomic Pathology,
Cleveland Clinic; and Professor of Pathology,
Cleveland Clinic Lerner College of Medicine,
Cleveland, Ohio

GUEST EDITOR

ANIL V. PARWANI, MD, PhD
Division Director, Pathology Informatics,
University of Pittsburgh Medical Centers;
Associate Professor, Department of Pathology;
and Staff Pathologist, Shadyside Hospital,
UPMC, Pittsburgh, Pennsylvania

AUTHORS

TEHMINA Z. ALI, MD
Assistant Professor, Department of Pathology,
University of Maryland Medical Center,
Baltimore, Maryland

ANIL V. PARWANI, MD, PhD
Division Director, Pathology Informatics,
University of Pittsburgh Medical Centers;
Associate Professor, Department of Pathology;
and Staff Pathologist, Shadyside Hospital,
UPMC, Pittsburgh, Pennsylvania

SARANGARAJAN RANGANATHAN, MD
Assistant Professor, Department of Pathology,
Children's Hospital of Pittsburgh of UPMC,
Pittsburgh, Pennsylvania

STEPHEN M. ROHAN, MD
Fellow, Surgical Oncologic Pathology,
Department of Pathology, Memorial Sloan-
Kettering Cancer Center, New York, New York

RAJAL B. SHAH, MD
Associate Professor of Pathology, Department
of Pathology; Associate Professor of Urology,
Department of Urology; and Chief, Section of
Urological Pathology, University of Michigan,
Ann Arbor, Michigan

S. JOSEPH SIRINTRAPUN, MD
Clinical Fellow, Pathology Informatics,
University of Pittsburgh Medical Center,
Pittsburgh, Pennsylvania

SATISH K. TICKOO, MD
Associate Attending Pathologist, Department
of Pathology, Memorial Sloan-Kettering
Cancer Center, New York, New York

MATTHEW J. WASCO, MD
Urologic Pathology Fellow, Department of
Pathology, University of Michigan, Ann Arbor,
Michigan

Contents

tumors aids in the choice of appropriate treatment options. This article reviews benign and malignant neoplastic entities of the testes and paratesticular tissues and illustrates the classic pathologic characteristics. The differential diagnosis, along with ancillary studies, clinical significance, and presentation are discussed also.

This article provides comprehensive review of benign diseases and neoplastic conditions of the penis. It describes and provides representative images of clinical, key pathologic features and ancillary techniques to aid in differential diagnoses. It examines these diseases from the epidemiologic standpoint, looks at environmental and genetic factors, and outlines the new histologic entities for penile neoplasms with distinct outcomes and clinical behavior that have been proposed in recent years.

With the advent of newer molecular technologies, our knowledge of cellular mechanisms with tumors of the kidney and testis has grown exponentially. Molecular technologies have led to better understanding of interplay between the von Hippel-Lindau gene and angiogenic cytokines in renal cancer and isochromosome 12p in testicular neoplasms. The result has been development of antiangiogenic-targeted therapy within recent years that has become the mainstay treatment for metastatic renal cell cancer. In the near future, classification and diagnosis of renal and testicular tumors through morphologic analysis will be supplemented by molecular information correlating to prognosis and targeted therapy. This article outlines tumor molecular pathology of the kidney and testis encompassing current genomic, epigenomic, and proteonomic findings.

Surgical Pathology Clinics

FORTHCOMING ISSUES

Current Concepts in Breast Pathology
Laura C. Collins, MD, *Guest Editor*

Current Concepts in Gastrointestinal Pathology
John Hart, MD and Amy Noffsinger, MD,
Guest Editors

Current Concepts in Gynecologic Pathology
Esther Oliva, MD, *Guest Editor*

Current Concepts in Dermatopathology
Steven Billings, MD, *Guest Editor*

THE CLINICS ARE NOW AVAILABLE ONLINE!

Access your subscription at:
www.theclinics.com

Foreword

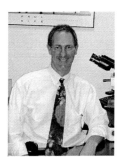

John R. Goldblum, MD
Consulting Editor

As a practicing surgical pathologist, I frequently find the need to selectively read on topics related to cases I encounter at daily sign-out. The ability to turn to a source that not only provides the essential information in a quick-hitting and efficient manner while still delving into enough detail to provide a depth of knowledge on the topic in question is a rare commodity. I believe the Surgical Pathology Clinics serves this unique purpose, and I am thrilled to serve as the series Consulting Editor.

Multi-author materials are, by their very nature, variable in terms of content and organization. Although the goal is not to obtain uniformity in style, uniformity in organization is a desired goal of this series. As such, each contribution to a given edition follows a specific format, outlining the essential gross features, microscopic features, differential diagnosis, ultimate diagnosis, and prognosis for each entity discussed. Particularly important relevant references are also provided. A special feature of this series is the inclusion of specially demarcated boxes including the "pathologic key features box," the "differential diagnosis box," and the "pitfalls box." Whenever possible, diagnostic algorithms are provided. Importantly, numerous and high-quality images are found in each contribution.

The first edition in the *Surgical Pathology Clinics* series is entitled "Current Concepts in Genitourinary Pathology" with Dr. Anil Parwani serving as Guest Editor. Dr. Parwani is a superb genitourinary

pathologist from the University of Pittsburgh Medical Center and has invited a number of outstanding and world-renowned authors to contribute to this edition of the series.

Future editions will include current concepts in breast pathology (edited by Dr. Laura Collins), gastrointestinal pathology (edited by Dr. John Hart and Dr. Amy Noffsinger), gynecologic pathology (edited by Dr. Esther Oliva), and dermatopathology (edited by Dr. Steven Billings).

The goal of this entire series is to cover the most common issues encountered by practicing surgical pathologists, and it is hoped that, in its entirety, a broad spectrum of pathologic processes is thoroughly discussed. I am confident you will enjoy this series as much as I have, and, if the current edition on genitourinary pathology is any indication, we all have a great deal to look forward to.

John R. Goldblum, MD
Chairman, Department of Anatomic Pathology
Cleveland Clinic
Professor of Pathology
Cleveland Clinic Lerner College of Medicine
9500 Euclid Avenue
Cleveland, OH 44195

E-mail address:
goldblj@ccf.org

Surgical Pathology 2 (2009) ix
doi:10.1016/j.path.2008.12.002
1875-9181/08/$ – see front matter © 2009 Elsevier Inc. All rights reserved.

surgpath.theclinics.com

Preface

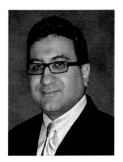

Anil V. Parwani, MD, PhD
Guest Editor

Genitourinary pathology is a complex area, with unique diseases and neoplasms not encountered in other systems and many entities that overlap with other systems. Experienced surgical pathologists, as well as trainees, often require a comprehensive and visual access to information on entities encompassing genitourinary pathology. "Current Concepts in Genitourinary Pathology" is the first edition in the *Surgical Pathology Clinics* series. This publication is intended for the practicing pathologist, as well as trainees who want to get an up-to-date and very practical overview of an entity that they might encounter in their daily practice, supplemented with high-quality images of each entity.

The topics have been carefully chosen to cover the spectrum of disease entities from genitourinary pathology and include prostate carcinoma and its mimickers, prostatic intraepilitheal neoplasia, bladder diseases and neoplasms, adult and pediatric renal neoplasms, penile diseases and tumors, and testicular neoplasms. One of the unique aspects of this issue is the comprehensive coverage of the molecular pathology of each organ from the genitourinary tract, with an up-to-date discussion of the key tumor markers and techniques. This coverage and discussion will be helpful for today's surgical pathologist, as they practice in an era where new discoveries are being made every day and new and relevant information impacting their diagnosis is becoming available at a rapid pace.

Within the issue, we have followed a specific format and have provided the reader with key gross and microscopic features, followed by differential diagnosis, diagnosis, and prognosis for each entity. Key references have been provided for each section. For all the key disease entities, we have summarized the key features, differential diagnosis, and the pitfalls in boxes. The information in this format can be rapidly available for daily sign out or even in preparation for a tumor board or teaching conference. As I have seen this issue come together over the last few months, and as I have reviewed the images and key feature boxes that the contributors have provided, I am convinced that the cumulative experience of these contributors has resulted in a rich resource of genitourinary pathology information for the practicing surgical pathologists.

One of the challenges in putting together this edition was to provide a comprehensive overview with superb illustrations, yet try to remain within a standard format and reasonable length for each of the articles while covering the broad and complex spectrum of disease entities from all the organs comprising genitourinary pathology. To do this effectively, and without compromising coverage, we decided to split this issue into two volumes in a logical manner, so that each volume is self-contained to cover prostate and bladder in one volume and kidney and testes in the other. I believe that by making this split we have provided the reader with a high quality overview of each entity that would have been more restricted and less comprehensive in a single volume. With rapid online access of the *Clinics* issues, this division will seem even more transparent to the reader who is accessing a specific disease entity.

I am grateful to the many expert genitourinary pathologists who not only succinctly provided the information but did so without compromising on the depth required to understand the disease entity. These authors have provided this issue with their collective experience and expertise in the complex subject of genitourinary pathology. The wide spectrum of illustrative cases from their

Surgical Pathology 2 (2009) xi–xii
doi:10.1016/j.path.2008.08.005

surgpath.theclinics.com

consult files has successfully highlighted the salient features of each of the entities. Their collective efforts produced this valuable resource of relevant information, including tumor subtypes, diagnostic pitfalls, and diagnostic features, leading to the generation of a more comprehensive surgical pathology report that will positively impact the care of the cancer patient.

I also want to acknowledge our clinical and pathology colleagues who have contributed consult cases to each one of the authors or have provided illustrations. Last but not the least, I am grateful to our publisher, Elsevier, and the editor of the *Clinics* series, Joanne Husovski, for her persistence, patience, and guidance throughout this effort.

Anil V. Parwani, MD, PhD
University of Pittsburgh Medical Centers
Division Director, Pathology Informatics
Staff Pathologist
Shadyside Hospital, UPMC
5230 Center Avenue, Suite WG02.10
Pittsburgh, PA 15232

E-mail address:
parwaniav@upmc.edu

Dedication

This book is dedicated to my parents, my wife Namrata, and my children, Simran, Varun, and Sanam, to whom I am grateful for their love and support, especially during the preparation of this work.

Anil

Surgical Pathology 2 (2009) xiii
doi:10.1016/j.path.2008.12.001

PATHOLOGIC FEATURES OF ADULT RENAL CORTICAL TUMORS

Satish K. Tickoo, MD*, Stephen M. Rohan, MD

KEYWORDS

• Renal cortical tumors • Renal cell carcinoma • Adults • Oncocytoma • Pathologic features

ABSTRACT

In the past few years, a much better understanding of the morphologic spectrum of renal cortical tumors has resulted in a clinically highly relevant contemporary classification system of these tumors. The current and still evolving era of targeted therapies in kidney cancer further highlights the importance of the appropriate pathologic classification. The recently gained knowledge about molecular-driven antigen expression almost certainly will have a major role to play in the characterization, development, and evaluation of targeted therapies in kidney cancer in the future.

In 1985, chromophobe renal cell carcinoma (RCC) was described for the first time as a specific entity in humans by Thoenes and colleagues.[1] One year later, the same group of investigators reported its eosinophilic variant.[2] This was instrumental in re-evaluation of the morphologic classification of renal tumors, resulting in the current, clinically more relevant classification system (**Table 1**).[3] As a result, it is now known that "granular cell carcinoma" and "sarcomatoid carcinoma" are not specific entities, as these features can be seen in a variety of renal tumors with markedly diverse clinical behavior. The current histologic classification also stands validated by several molecular studies.[4–8] One of the implications of this current classification system is that the published pre-1985 literature about clinicopathologic aspects of renal tumors may not match the current knowledge about these tumors.

The better understanding of the molecular aspects of renal tumors in the recent past has resulted in a realization that different renal tumors involve different molecular pathways. This has led to the development and usage of multiple targeted therapies, particularly for advanced clear cell RCC, with promising initial results.[9]

Challenges currently for genitourinary pathologists are to recognize the morphologic and antigenic diversities in specific tumor types so as to classify them more precisely; to learn to classify these on minimal material, such as needle biopsies and aspirates; and to understand the antigenic diversity in these tumors that may be applicable to appropriate targeted therapies.

GRADING AND STAGING OF RENAL TUMORS

The Fuhrman grading system is the most prevalent grading scheme for renal cell tumors. It uses nuclear grades based on nuclear size, nuclear membrane irregularity, and nucleolar prominence. For practical purposes, however, easily identifiable nucleoli at low power (10×) examination are characteristic of nuclear grade 3 or 4, with grade 4 nuclei also showing marked pleomorphism or multilobulation. Grade 1 or 2 nuclei generally requires examination at high magnification (40×) to identify and evaluate the level of prominence of the nucleoli. Although the usefulness of the Fuhrman grading system in clear cell RCC is well established, its value in papillary and chromophobe RCC remains controversial. Renal oncocytomas do not need grading because these are benign neoplasms.

The TNM classification of the American Joint Committee on Cancer (AJCC) and Union Internationale Contre le Cancer is the most widely used and clinically relevant staging system for renal tumors.[10] Over the years it has been modified and improved many times; the latest modifications were made in 2002. A series of publications in the

Department of Pathology, Memorial Sloan-Kettering Cancer Center, 1275 York Avenue, New York, NY 10065, USA
* Corresponding author.
E-mail address: tickoos@mskcc.org (S.K. Tickoo).

Surgical Pathology 2 (2009) 1–25
doi:10.1016/j.path.2008.07.005

Table 1
Tumors of the adult kidney

Benign	Malignant
Oncocytoma	Clear cell (conventional) RCC
Papillary adenoma	Papillary RCC
Metanephric adenoma	Chromophobe RCC
Metanephric adenofibroma	CDC
Metanephric stromal tumor	Renal medullary carcinoma
	Tubulocystic carcinoma
	Acquired cystic disease of kidney–associated RCC
	RCC, unclassified
	MTSC
	Translocation-associated carcinomas

Tumors of undetermined malignant potential
Multilocular cystic RCC

recent past have highlighted the importance of the renal sinus and sinus veins in the staging of RCC (**Fig. 1**),[11,12] factors first included in the AJCC staging system in 2002. In one such study, most patients who died of RCC with previously reported pT1 disease were retrospectively found to have renal sinus fat invasion.[13] Therefore, a careful gross examination and adequate sampling of the renal sinus-tumor interface, especially in larger tumors, is strongly recommended.

RENAL TUMORS: IMMUNOHISTOCHEMISTRY

Immunohistochemistry potentially can be used for differentiation between different subtypes of primary renal tumors or to confirm the renal origin in a metastatic site. Many antibodies have been reported to be of use in these situations.[14–22] Most of these antibodies, however, discriminate only between better-differentiated tumors, situations where immunostaining hardly ever is required. In situations where the antibodies are needed (ie, in high-grade or poorly differentiated tumors), the results tend not to be dependable. Among the more recently available antibodies, however, carbonic anhydrase IX (CA IX) shows the greatest promise in the differential diagnosis of renal cell tumors.[23,24] It exhibits diffuse and strong membranous reactivity in more than 90% of clear cell RCCs, including its

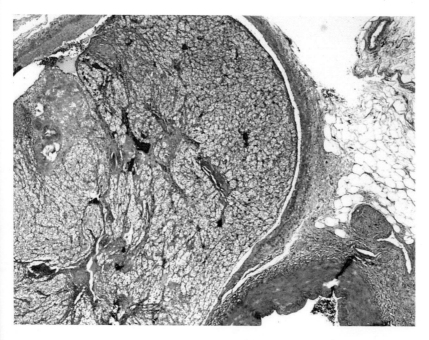

Fig. 1. Clear cell RCC involving a muscular branch of renal vein in the renal sinus. This now is considered a pT3b stage disease.

sarcomatoid components in a significant proportion of cases, compared with absent or focal, usually perinecrotic, positivity in other common subtypes of renal cell tumors.[23–25] Other antibodies found of practical use in the differential diagnosis of renal cell tumors include CD117 (c-kit), which is consistently positive in chromophobe RCC and renal oncocytoma. Diffuse positivity for cytokeratin 7 (CK7), as in a large proportion of cases of chromophobe RCCs, also is useful in their distinction from renal oncocytoma.

Multiple therapeutic options tailored to individual patients, besides surgery, now are offered for renal tumors. Some of these include in situ ablation of the tumor, targeted therapies in a neoadjuvant setting, or even watchful waiting in selected cases. In view of these developments, pathologists frequently are asked to render diagnosis on limited material, and the availability of a dependable and robust panel of immunohistochemical stains has become even more critical. Using a select panel of five antibodies—CA IX, CK7, c-kit, racemase, and CD10—the authors recently reported more than 90% diagnostic accuracy on in vivo needle core biopsies of renal cell tumors.[26] These findings indicate that if adequate biopsy samples are provided, close attention to cytomorphologic features and a judicious use of immunohistochemistry (**Table 2**) will allow pathologists to render accurate diagnose in the overwhelming majority of the cases.

CLEAR CELL (CONVENTIONAL) RENAL CELL CARCINOMA

Clear cell RCC is the most common subtype of renal cortical tumors, comprising approximately 60% to 65% of such neoplasms.[10,27]

Key Features
CLEAR CELL RENAL CELL CARCINOMA

1. The most common subtype of renal cell carcinoma

2. Most cases, hereditary or sporadic, associated with *VHL* gene abnormalities

3. Cytologic features: optically transparent clear cells, eosinophilic cells, or mixture

4. Intricate, branching, thin fibrovascular septations the most characteristic feature

5. Eosinophilic cells, generally with higher nuclear grades

6. Sarcomatoid features, marker of high-grade tumor with aggressive behavior

7. Most tumors with diffuse membranous positivity for CA IX

CLEAR CELL RENAL CELL CARCINOMA: GROSS FEATURES

Clear cell RCC typically shows a golden yellow cut surface because of the abundant intracytoplasmic lipid. The proportion of the tumor showing such gross coloration, however, is grade dependent; higher-grade tumors that usually contain less lipid have a more varied appearance. Although modern imaging techniques and early detection has brought about a considerable decrease in the median tumor size, significant numbers are 7 cm or more in size. Although not limited to such tumors, a greater proportion of larger tumors may have renal sinus fat or sinus vein invasion.[11,12]

Table 2
Results on limited and useful immunohistochemical panel among common renal tumor subtypes

	Clear Cell	Papillary	Chromophobe	Oncocytoma
CA IX	+ Diffuse membranous	–/or focal + around necrosis or papillary tips	–/or focal + around necrosis	–
CD10	+ Membranous	+ Usually luminal	–/or focal cytoplasmic	–
CK7	–	+	+	–
Racemase	–/or focal +	+ Granular cytoplasmic	–	–
c-kit	–	–	+	+, Usually not diffuse

CLEAR CELL RENAL CELL CARCINOMA: MICROSCOPIC FEATURES

In prototypic cases, tumor cells show optically transparent, clear cytoplasm (because of the abundant intracytoplasmic lipid and glycogen) and an acinar or solid-nested growth pattern. Cytoplasmic clarity, however, is more typical of lower-grade tumors, whereas pure clear cell cytology is less common in high-grade tumors. Such high-grade tumors often contain variable proportion of (or even exclusively) cells with granular/eosinophilic cytoplasm (**Fig. 2**). In the high-grade areas, a loss of the acinar growth pattern also is frequent, and they are more likely to have solid or sometimes sarcomatoid histology. Looking for areas of transition to a lower grade is important to establishing a correct diagnosis. A major diagnostic criterion of clear cell RCC is the investment of the tumor cell nests by intricate, arborizing, thin fibrovascular septae. Such delicate septations tend to be retained in most tumors, except in the very high-grade areas with solid or sarcomatoid differentiation. Sarcomatoid or spindle cell differentiation occurs in approximately 5% of these tumors and, as in other subtypes of RCC, is an indicator of high-grade tumor with generally poorer prognosis.[25] These tumors may take on a papillary or pseudopapillary appearance focally, often a result of degenerative changes rather than true papillae formation. An exception to such growth pattern in clear cell RCC is the so-called clear cell papillary RCC, recently described by the authors' group in the setting of end-stage kidneys. Such tumors occasionally also occur in non–end-stage kidneys.[28] They often are cystic, show pure clear cell cytology with prominent papillary and variable solid acinar/nested architecture, and have nuclei arranged in a linear manner away from the basement membrane (**Fig. 3**A). Unlike most clear cell RCCs, these are diffusely and strongly immunoreactive for CK7 (see **Fig. 3**B) but, like the usual clear cell RCC, show diffuse positivity for CA IX.

Clear cell RCCs are characterized by the loss of genetic material of the short arm of chromosome 3 (3p) and mutations affecting *VHL* gene.[4–8] In patients who have von Hippel-Lindau (VHL) disease, such losses and mutations are present in virtually all cases, and somatic mutations/promoter hypermethylations in the same region also are found in approximately 80% of the more common sporadic tumors.[7] In normoxemic states, the product of a normal *von Hippel-Lindau* gene, pVHL, targets hydroxylated forms of hypoxia-inducible factor (HIF), which results in its proteosomic degradation. In cells that are hypoxic or lack pVHL (as in most cases of clear cell RCC), HIF escapes degradation, is overexpressed, and activates downstream targets, including vascular endothelial growth factor, platelet-derived growth factor, glucose transporter 1, and CA IX. Many of these downstream products can be used as markers of clear cell RCC at the immunohistochemical level (see **Fig. 2**) or as targets for novel

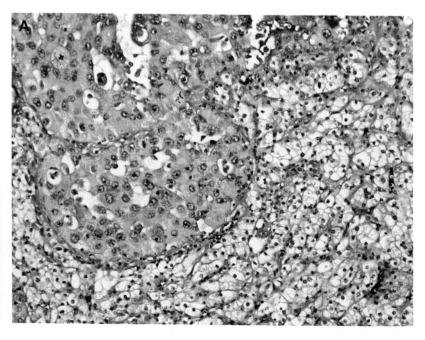

Fig. 2. Clear cell RCC. (*A*) A mixture of clear cell and granular cell features in the same tumor. Eosinophilic cytology often is associated with high Fuhrman nuclear grade.

Fig. 2. Strong and diffuse nuclear immunoreactivity for HIF-1α (*B*) and membranous positivity for CA IX (*C*) are characteristic of most clear cell RCCs.

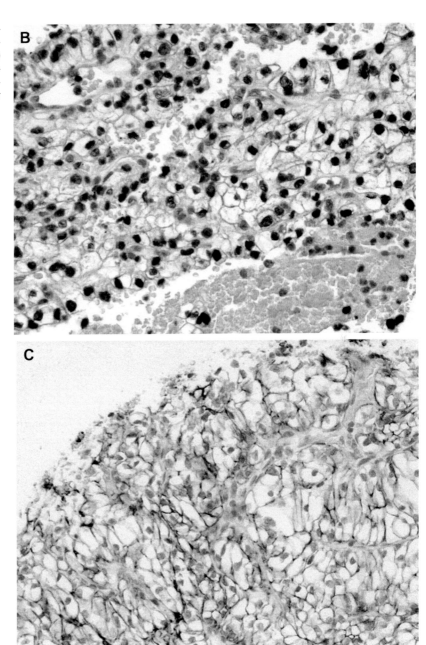

therapies.[9,23–26,29,30] CA IX and HIF-1 immunohistochemical expression also has been reported as associated with prognosis, although large prospective studies still are needed to evaluate such associations.[31–34]

CLEAR CELL RENAL CELL CARCINOMA: DIFFERENTIAL DIAGNOSIS

Adequate sampling and a good understanding of the morphologic diversity seen in clear cell RCC

△△ *Differential Diagnosis* CLEAR CELL RENAL CELL CARCINOMA

- Chromophobe renal cell carcinoma
- Papillary renal cell carcinoma with areas of cytoplasmic clarity
- Epithelioid variants of AML
- Adrenal cortical tumors

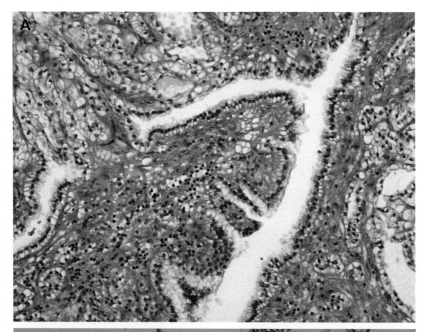

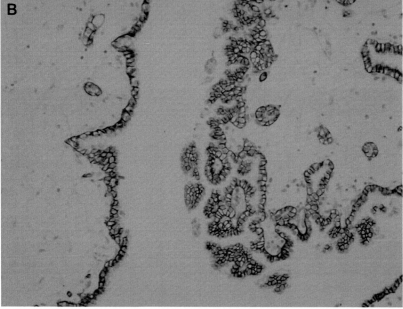

Fig. 3. Clear cell papillary RCC. (*A*) These often cystic tumors show pure clear cell cytology with prominent papillary and variable solid acinar/ nested architecture and nuclei arranged in a linear manner away from the basement membrane. They likely represent a variant of clear cell RCC. (*B*) Unlike clear cell RCC, they show diffuse and strong immunoreactivity for CK7 (as seen here).

should minimize errors in classification. Rare cases may be confused with papillary or chromophobe RCC. In most cases of clear cell RCC with papillary growth, this pattern is a result of cell drop-off away from the blood supply with resultant pseudopapillary architecture. Histiocytes are unlikely to be present within the fibrovascular stalk in these pseudopapillary areas. Unlike clear cell RCC, papillary carcinomas often show diffuse expression of CK7 and lack the diffuse expression of CA IX. Among the exceptions to such expression is the so-called clear cell papillary RCC (described previously). Unlike clear cell RCC, the clear cytoplasm of chromophobe RCC is not optically transparent but shows fine reticulations (**Fig. 4**). Other characteristic nuclear and cytoplasmic features, along with lack of intricate branching septations, should help in distinguishing it from

Fig. 4. Clear cell cytology in clear cell (*A*), chromophobe (*B*), and papillary (*C*) RCC. The clear cells in clear cell RCC usually are optically transparent; those in chromophobe RCC show fine cytoplasmic reticulations whereas they usually have fine reticulations along with granularity (hemosiderin) in the cytoplasm in papillary RCC.

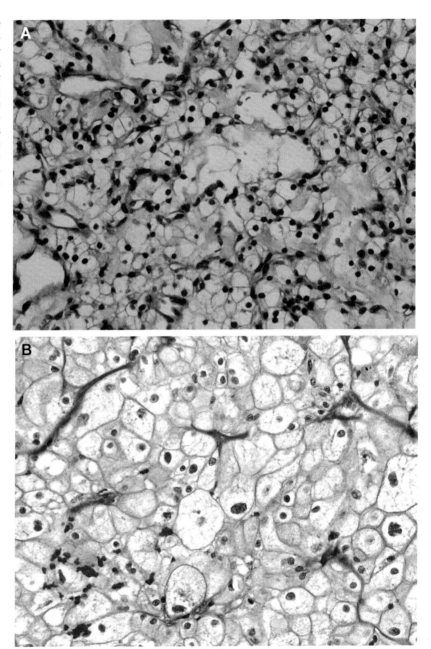

clear cell RCC in most cases. Usual diffuse positivity for c-kit, more than focal reactivity for CK7, and absence of staining for CA IX in chromophobe RCC are other differentiating features. Epithelioid variants of angiomyolipomas (AMLs) can be readily misclassified as clear cell RCC, particularly when these lack the morphologic diversity seen in classic cases. Close attention to morphologic features and immunohistochemistry can help establish the correct diagnosis. Unlike AMLs, clear cell RCC usually are immunoreactive with cytokeratins and epithelial membrane antigen (EMA) and often show diffuse membranous positivity with CD10 and CA IX, whereas AML stains for HMB-45, A103, and smooth muscle actin. Another entity to be considered in the differential diagnosis is adrenal cortical carcinoma, particularly in the case of upper pole tumors. Adrenal cortical tumors usually are negative for cytokeratins and EMA; alternatively, they express inhibin and A103.

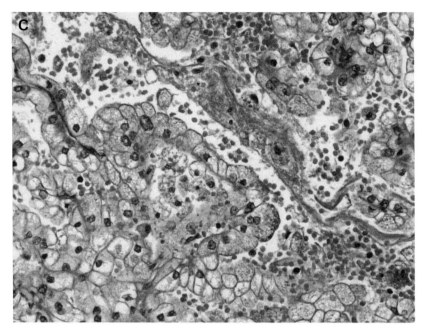

C

Fig. 4. (continued)

CLEAR CELL RENAL CELL CARCINOMA: PROGNOSIS

Clear cell RCCs are the most virulent of the common types of renal cortical carcinomas with the lowest disease-specific and progression-free 5- and 10-year survivals.[27,35,36] In general, disease-free and overall survival correlates with grade and stage. Effective systemic therapy for metastatic disease has remained elusive, making surgical resection the best chance for cure. Targeted therapies against these tumors in the recent past, however, have shown promising initial results.[9]

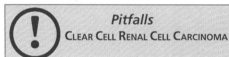

Pitfalls
CLEAR CELL RENAL CELL CARCINOMA

! Not all renal cortical tumors with clear cell cytology are clear cell renal cell carcinoma. The more important diagnostic criterion is the investment of the clear cell tumor cell nests by intricate, arborizing, thin fibrovascular septae

! In some clear cell renal cell carcinomas, clear cell cytology may be entirely lacking, raising the differential diagnostic possibility of other renal tumors with eosinophilic cytoplasm. Close attention to intricate, arborizing, thin fibrovascular septations, among other histologic features, clarifies the issue in most cases

! Clear cell cytology with prominent papillary architecture should raise the differential diagnostic considerations of translocation-associated carcinoma, clear-cell papillary variant of clear cell renal cell carcinoma, papillary renal cell carcinoma, and acquired cystic disease-associate renal cell carcinoma, among others

PAPILLARY RENAL CELL CARCINOMA

Papillary RCC constitute up to 15% of all renal cortical neoplasms.

Key Features
PAPILLARY RENAL CELL CARCINOMA

1. Most common renal cell carcinoma with a pseudocapsule, multifocality, and bilaterality

2. May have papillary, tubular, tubulopapillary, solid, or glomeruloid architecture

3. Cells may have amphophilic, eosinophilic, or focally clear cell features

4. Subtyped as type 1 and type 2

5. Use of Fuhrman nuclear grading contentious

6. Familial cases with *c-MET* or *fumarate hydratase* defects

Fig. 5. Variants of papillary RCC. (*A*) Type 1, (*B*) type 2, and (*C*) solid (glomeruloid variant), which falls into the type 1 category.

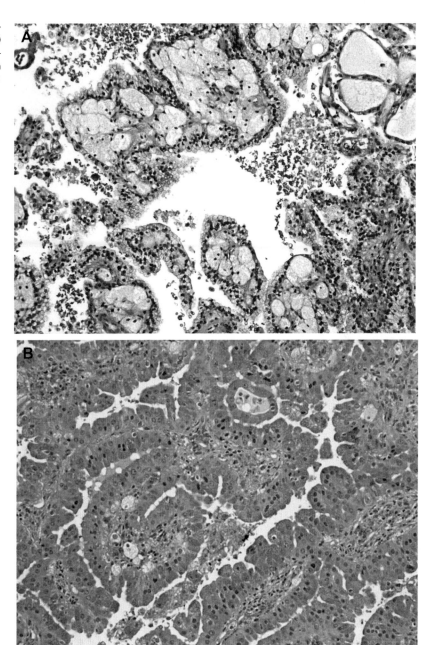

PAPILLARY RENAL CELL CARCINOMA: GROSS FEATURES

Grossly, papillary RCCs are mostly well-circumscribed tumors. Among the sporadic RCCs, papillary RCC is the most common tumor demonstrating multifocality. Most tumors exhibit a variegated appearance. Depending on the microscopic findings, tumors with abundant foamy macrophages are tan to yellow whereas those with intratumoral hemorrhage are dark tan to brown. Many lesions show large areas of necrosis.

PAPILLARY RENAL CELL CARCINOMA: MICROSCOPIC FEATURES

Architecturally, papillary RCCS have a papillary, tubular, or tubulopapillary growth pattern. Some tumors have a solid growth pattern resulting from

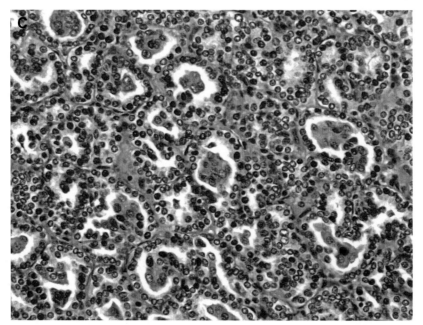

Fig. 5. (*continued*)

compression of the papillary structures, whereas other tumors show a glomeruloid (**Fig. 5**) appearance.[10,27,35,37] The cytoplasm may be amphophilic, eosinophilic, or even partially clear (see **Figs. 4** and **5**). Papillary RCCs often are multifocal, frequently associated with papillary adenomas, and the most common RCC type with bilateral disease. Classically, papillary carcinomas display abundant lipid laden, foamy macrophages within fibrovascular cores, a feature helpful in establishing the correct diagnosis.

Many experts believe that the Fuhrman grading scheme is well suited for papillary RCC but others disagree.[10,27,36,38,39] To date, whether or not these tumors should be graded and, if so, which system to use remains controversial.[40] Delahunt and Eble[41] proposed subtyping of papillary RCC into types 1 and 2 (see **Fig. 5**A, B) based on nuclear features and growth pattern characteristics, and this was accepted in the 2004 World Health Organization classification system.[10]

The majority of sporadic PRCCs are characterized by trisomy of chromosomes 7 and 17 (type 1 tumors) and loss of chromosome Y.[5,6,8,42] Some investigators have suggested that tumors exhibiting trisomy 7/17 only are likely to be benign, whereas those tumors exhibiting additional genetic abnormalities will behave aggressively, a hypothesis not confirmed in the literature. Approximately 10% of the sporadic PRCC also are reported to show somatic mutations in *c-MET*

gene, a genetic abnormality commonly seen as a germline mutation in familial cases.[43] Recently, hereditary leiomyomatosis and RCC syndrome (HLRCC) with mutations in the *fumarate hydratase* gene has been shown to be associated with RCCs showing type 2 papillary RCC features.[44]

PAPILLARY RENAL CELL CARCINOMA: DIFFERENTIAL DIAGNOSIS

Papillary RCC may be confused principally with clear cell RCC, exhibiting a papillary or pseudopapillary growth, and with collecting duct carcinoma (CDC). Papillary RCC may focally

---

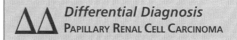

Differential Diagnosis
PAPILLARY RENAL CELL CARCINOMA

1. Clear cell renal cell carcinoma with focal papillations/psuedopapillations

2. Clear cell papillary renal cell carcinoma

3. Collecting duct carcinoma

4. Translocation-associated carcinoma

5. Acquired cystic disease of kidney–associated renal cell carcinoma

Pitfalls
PAPILLARY RENAL CELL CARCINOMA

! Papillary architecture alone is not definitive for the diagnosis of papillary renal cell carcinoma. Other gross and microscopic features need to be taken into consideration before making this diagnosis

! Tumors with prominent papillary architecture but more than focal desmoplasia, particularly when associated with solid, glandular, cribriform, or cystic areas, most likely represent collecting duct carcinoma, rather than papillary RCC

! Prominent papillary architecture with variable clear cell cytology may be seen in papillary RCC, clear cell papillary variant of clear cell RCC, translocation-associated carcinomas, and acquired cystic disease–associated carcinoma

contain tumor cells with clear cytoplasm (but often with fine cytoplasmic granules) (see **Fig. 4**C), especially in areas with a solid growth pattern. Similarly, clear cell RCC may be focally papillary, although this usually is the result of cell drop-off in areas away from feeding vessels, which creates a pseudopapillary appearance. Adequate sampling should clarify the issue in most cases. Psammoma bodies, hemosiderin deposition within tumor cells, and fibrovascular cores containing foamy macrophages are more likely to be seen in papillary RCC. CK7 immunoreactivity is present at least focally in many papillary RCCs and usually is negative in clear cell RCCs. CA IX at the most shows only patchy positivity (usually perinecrotic and in the papillary tips) in papillary RCC. If needed, molecular genetics can be used to solve difficult cases. CDC may have a papillary growth pattern and resemble papillary RCC. Nevertheless, they are centered in the medulla, virtually always have features of a high-grade adenocarcinoma, and are associated with a desmoplastic stroma. In the authors' opinion, tumors with prominent papillary architecture but more than focal desmoplasia, particularly when associated with solid, glandular, cribriform, or cystic areas, most likely represent CDC, rather than papillary RCC. Reactivity for carcinoembryonic antigen, peanut and soybean agglutinins, Ulex europaeus, and high molecular weight cytokeratin 34bE12 is common in CDC. CK7 may be expressed in both tumors. Again, cytogenetic studies can be used to solve

difficult diagnostic problems. Translocation-associated RCCs may have prominent papillary growth pattern.[45,46] They are more common, however, in young patients, rarely multifocal, and usually have a high nuclear grade and abundant (sometimes voluminous) cytoplasm. In general they are negative or only focally positive for cytokeratins and characteristically exhibit nuclear immunoreactivity for TFE3 or TFEB, depending on the translocation.

PAPILLARY RENAL CELL CARCINOMA: PROGNOSIS

In most large, well-studied series, papillary RCC is a less aggressive tumor than clear cell RCC, with reported 5-year survival rates of 80% to 85%.[10,35,36,38,39]

CHROMOPHOBE RENAL CELL CARCINOMA

Chromophobe RCCs, first described in 1985 by Thöenes and colleagues,[1] constitute approximately 6% of renal cortical neoplasms.

CHROMOPHOBE RENAL CELL CARCINOMA: GROSS FEATURES

Characteristically, chromophobe RCCs are well circumscribed but not encapsulated tumors. Depending on the microscopic findings (ie, relative proportion of clear or eosinophilic cells in the tumor), the tumors may show a homogeneous pale tan or beige/brown cut surface. A central scar is present in approximately 15% of cases.

Key Features
CHROMOPHOBE RENAL CELL CARCINOMA

1. Solid sheet-like architecture with incomplete septations; may have nested, tubular, or focal microcystic architecture

2. Clear cell or eosinophilic cytology; clear cells usually not optically transparent but have fine cytoplasmic reticulations

3. Characteristically, hyperchromatic and wrinkled nuclei with perinuclear halos

4. Fuhrman nuclear grading not useful

5. Ultrastructural presence of microvesicles and mitochondria with tubulocystic cristae

6. Prognosis better than clear cell or papillary RCC

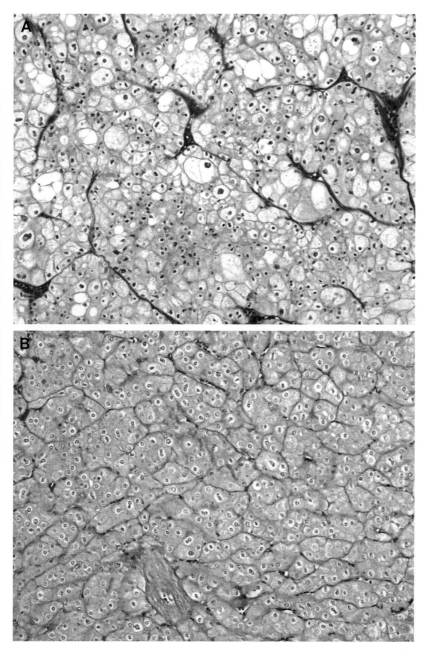

Fig. 6. Chromophobe RCC. (*A*) Classical type with a combination of clear and eosinophilic cells, a finding that is common in most tumors. Note the incomplete septations that are quite characteristic. (*B*) Eosinophilic variant. Such tumors need to be differentiated from oncocytoma. Perinuclear halos and nuclear irregularities, at least focal, as seen here are helpful in the distinction.

CHROMOPHOBE RENAL CELL CARCINOMA: MICROSCOPIC FEATURES

Because of their cytoplasmic features, many chromophobe RCCs may have been previously classified as clear cell RCC, granular cell RCC, or even renal oncocytoma. The morphologic features include a solid growth pattern with sheets of cells separated by incomplete fibrovascular septations (**Fig. 6**A). Occasionally, tubular, nested, or cord-like growth may be present. The cells may be predominantly clear (usually with finely reticulated cytoplasm) or eosinophilic or most often show a mixture of clear and eosinophilic cell features. Nuclei often are hyperchromatic with nuclear membrane irregularity (raisinoid), but such nuclear features sometimes may be only focal. Classically, perinuclear cytoplasmic clearing (perinuclear halo) is seen, corresponding to the predominant localization of microvesicles. The microvesicles are a distinctive ultrastructural feature of chromophobe RCC. Thöenes and colleagues[2] also described an eosinophilic variant (see **Fig. 6B**) that may be confused with oncocytoma. As in other RCC types, chromophobe RCC with sarcomatoid features is a highly aggressive variant.

Chromophobe RCCs are characterized genetically by multiple chromosomal losses, usually affecting chromosomes 1, Y, 6, 10, 13, 17, and 21, and by resultant hypodiploidy.[47–50]

CHROMOPHOBE RENAL CELL CARCINOMA: DIFFERENTIAL DIAGNOSIS

Many tumors designated in the past as granular cell RCC actually are chromophobe RCC whereas others are clear cell RCC, RCC unclassified, papillary RCC, epithelioid AML, or oncocytoma. Given the differing clinical behavior among these tumors, distinction between them is mandatory and can be performed easily in most cases by adequate sampling and paying close attention to the growth pattern and cytologic characteristics of the tumor. Immunohistochemistry, electron microscopy, and cytogenetics may be useful in difficult cases.

CHROMOPHOBE RENAL CELL CARCINOMA: PROGNOSIS

Chromophobe RCCs have a much better prognosis than clear cell and papillary RCC, with 5-year disease-free survivals greater than 90%.[10,27,35] Even in metastatic settings, chromophobe carcinomas tend to progress more indolently than other non–clear cell RCCs.[51]

Pitfalls
CHROMOPHOBE RENAL CELL CARCINOMA

! Solid nested growth pattern, similar to that of renal oncocytoma, does not exclude the diagnosis of chromophobe RCC. Examination at higher magnification revealing at least focal nuclear irregularities with perinuclear halos is diagnostic of eosinophilic variant of chromophobe RCC

! Prominent clear cell cytology, again, does not exclude the diagnosis of chromophobe RCC in favor of clear cell RCC. Attention to the vascular pattern and cytologic features is helpful in the differentiation in most cases

! CK7 positivity in chromophobe RCC and diffuse membranous staining for CA IX in clear cell RCC clinches these differential diagnostic possibilities in overwhelming majority of the cases

RENAL ONCOCYTOMA

Renal oncocytomas constitute approximately 6% to 9% of renal cortical neoplasms.[10,27,35]

RENAL ONCOCYTOMA: GROSS FEATURES

Renal oncocytomas are well-circumscribed, non-encapsulated neoplasms that are classically mahogany brown and less often tan to pale yellow. The presence of a central, stellate, radiating scar is seen in approximately 33% of cases and usually is associated with larger tumor size. However, low-grade clear cell RCC and chromophobe RCC also may contain a central scar. Gross hemorrhage is

Key Features
RENAL ONCOCYTOMA

1. Solid nested, tubular, microcystic architectural patterns

2. Cells with uniform round nuclei; no perinuclear halos

3. Clusters or single cells with marked nuclear hyperchromasia, multilobulation, and degenerative, smudgy appearance quite common

4. Gross central scar in a third of the tumors; characteristic but not specific

5. A benign neoplasm

Differential Diagnosis
CHROMOPHOBE RENAL CELL CARCINOMA

• Renal oncocytoma (for eosinophilic variant)

• Clear cell RCC (for classic and eosinophilic variants)

• RCC, unclassified (oncocytic, low-grade type)

• Epithelioid AML

present in 20% of cases but necrosis is rare. Cysts and gross extension into perinephric adipose tissue are seen occasionally. Multifocality is seen in up to 17% of cases and bilateral tumors in 4%.

RENAL ONCOCYTOMA: MICROSCOPIC FEATURES

Renal oncocytomas are benign neoplasms that require distinction from several malignant renal epithelial neoplasms with eosinophilic cytoplasm. Histologically, oncocytomas are characterized by cells with deeply eosinophilic cytoplasm arranged in nests, cords, tubules, or cysts and with uniform round, vesicular nuclei often with prominent central nucleoli (**Fig. 7**A).[52–55] Uniformity of nuclear features is the rule, although occasional isolated or groups of cells may exhibit marked degenerative-appearing hyperchromasia and pleomorphism (see **Fig. 7**B). Prominent papillary growth and extensive tumor necrosis are not the features of renal oncocytoma. Similarly, mitotic activity rarely is noted. A central, stellate scar has been considered characteristic of this neoplasm; however, it also can be seen in other low-grade renal cortical neoplasms. Occasionally, focal cytoplasmic clarity may be observed around the areas of scarring. Otherwise, clear cells are not a feature of renal oncocytoma. Tumor cells may infiltrate perirenal soft tissue and occasionally may be present within small and even the larger vessels. None of these features, however, affect its benign clinical behavior. Electron microscopy reveals cytoplasm loaded with mitochondria, which is responsible for the cytoplasmic eosinophilia and a mahogany brown gross appearance.[56,57]

Oncocytomas do not exhibit 3p, trisomy 7/17, or multiple combined chromosomal losses. They often exhibit loss of chromosomes Y and 1, and a few cases have been described with translocations involving chromosome 5 or 11.[10]

RENAL ONCOCYTOMA: DIFFERENTIAL DIAGNOSIS

Although the differential diagnosis includes any renal neoplasm with granular eosinophilic cytoplasm, tumors most likely to be confused with oncocytoma are the eosinophilic variant of chromophobe RCC, eosinophilic RCC, unclassified, and, rarely, epithelioid oncocytoma-like AML.[58] Unlike oncocytoma, eosinophilic chromophobe RCC shows at least some areas with nuclear irregularities and perinuclear halos. In the vast majority of cases, careful attention to the morphologic features allows correct classification on routine hematoxylin-eosin–stained sections. A subset of cases may require ancillary studies to confirm the diagnosis, however. Diffuse CK7 positivity supports the diagnosis of

Differential Diagnosis
RENAL ONCOCYTOMA

- Chromophobe RCC (eosinophilic variant)
- Clear cell RCC (eosinophilic variant)
- RCC, unclassified (oncocytic, low-grade type)
- Epithelioid oncocytoma-like AML

chromophobe RCC over oncocytoma. By ultrastructural examination, chromophobe RCC shows presence of variable number, usually abundant, cytoplasmic microvesicles and mitochondria with tubulocystic cristae, whereas renal oncocytoma is characterized by cells with numerous mitochondria, the majority of which with lamellar cristae, and absence of microvesicles.[56,57] In the classic examples of oncocytoma, Hale's colloidal iron stain is negative or shows focal staining in a luminal distribution in contrast to the diffuse cytoplasmic staining found in the classic examples of chromophobe RCC.[59] In contrast to renal oncocytoma, the vast majority of AMLs are immunoreactive to HMB-45 and A103 (Mart-1).

RENAL ONCOCYTOMA: PROGNOSIS

If properly classified using the strict diagnostic criteria (described previously), renal oncocytoma is a benign tumor and no reported patient has died of disease.

Recently the authors described a group of patients who had multiple oncocytic lesions (oncocytosis). Among several characteristic morphologic

Pitfalls
RENAL ONCOCYTOMA

! Both eosinophilic variant of chromophobe RCC and RCC, unclassified, with low-grade eosinophilic features can have the architectural features typical of renal oncocytoma

! At low magnification, eosinophilic variant of chromophobe RCC or RCC unclassified may appear to have uniform, round nuclei, similar to those in renal oncocytoma. Tumors with perinuclear halos and those with diffuse nuclear irregularities on higher magnification evaluation, however, should not to be considered renal oncocytoma and should be classified as chromophobe or unclassified RCCs, respectively

Fig. 7. Renal oncocytoma. (*A*) Uniform, round nuclei are a requirement for the diagnosis. (*B*) Focal single cells or foci of markedly pleomorphic, degenerate-looking nuclei are common, however.

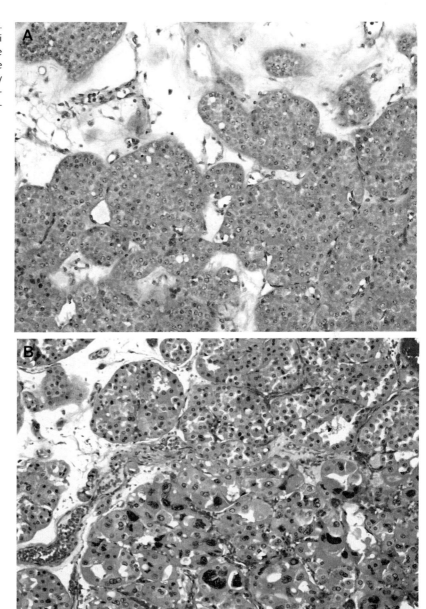

features, some had hybrid morphology between oncocytomas and chromophobe RCC, suggesting that these tumors may be related genetically or causally.[60] There is a hypothesis that chromophobe tumors may represent a genetic/morphologic progression from oncocytoma. It is likely that many if not all of those patients belonged to Birt-Hogg-Dubé syndrome (BHD) families.

COLLECTING DUCT CARCINOMA AND RENAL MEDULLARY CARCINOMA

CDC (Bellini duct) constitutes approximately 1% of renal epithelial tumors. In general, the tumors are centered in the renal medulla, particularly when small, and show features of a high-grade adenocarcinoma, with marked multinodular growth

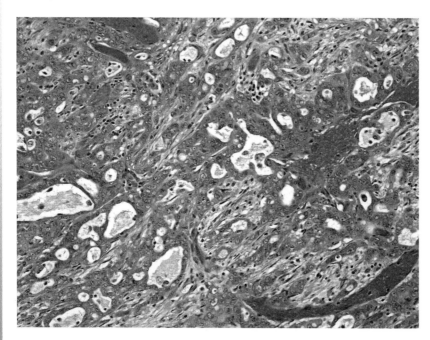

Fig. 8. CDC. High-grade cytology, glandular/tubular/cribriform architecture, stromal desmoplasia, and intratumoral inflammation are the characteristic features. Some tumors may show variable proportions of papillary architecture.

pattern and desmoplasia, highly atypical cytology, and tubular, papillary, solid, or microcystic architecture (**Fig. 8**).[61–63] The papillae rarely, if ever, contain foamy macrophages, but acute or chronic inflammatory cells usually are abundant within the tumor. Characteristically, dysplastic or neoplastic cells may be present within adjacent renal tubules. Cytoplasmic and luminal mucin is frequent. Most show immunoreactivity for carcinoembryonic antigen, peanut lectin agglutinin, and Ulex europaeus agglutinin.[10] Cytokeratins 34bE12 and CK 7 also may be positive.

CDC may present at any age although it tends to occur in younger patients.[10,27,61–63] More than 50% of the patients present with metastatic disease. In a recent series of 81 cases from Japan, regional lymph node metastasis was detected in 44%, and distant metastasis in another 32%.[64] Most patients die of disease within 3 years of diagnosis.

Another tumor that some investigators believe to be a particularly virulent variant of CDC is the medullary carcinoma.[10,65,66] This highly aggressive tumor develops preferentially in young patients who have sickle cell trait, hemoglobin SC disease, or, rarely, sickle cell disease. They may show some morphologic overlaps with CDC and high-grade urothelial tumors and in some instances have features reminiscent of yolk sac tumor or adenoid cystic carcinoma. Sickled and deformed red blood cells are easily identified within the vessels. Most reported cases

had metastatic disease at the time of presentation. The reported mean survivals in the two largest series to date have been 15 weeks[65] and 4 months.[66]

TUBULOCYSTIC CARCINOMA

In the past, some tumors characterized by a tubulocystic pattern of growth, tumor cells with low-grade nuclei, and mucin production were considered low-grade CDC.[67] More recently, the term, *tubulocystic carcinoma of the kidney*, has been proposed for these tumors.[68] They are grossly well circumscribed. Microscopically, besides the tubulocystic growth pattern, the tumor cells show abundant eosinophilic cytoplasm and usually round nuclei with prominent nucleoli (**Fig. 9**). The authors believe, however, that not only do tumors with such exclusive morphology exist but also other tumors showing similar histology admixed with otherwise high-grade CDC-like areas can be observed. Therefore, their relationship to CDC remains to be evaluated further.

RENAL CELL CARCINOMA, UNCLASSIFIED

RCCs, unclassified, form up to 6% of all renal epithelial tumors.[10,27,35,37] By definition, they include tumors of unrecognizable cell or architectural types or those with apparent composites of the recognized cell types, tumors that do not fit into any of the usual

Fig. 9. Tubulocystic carcinoma. Similar morphology may be seen focally in some tumors that otherwise look like typical CDC.

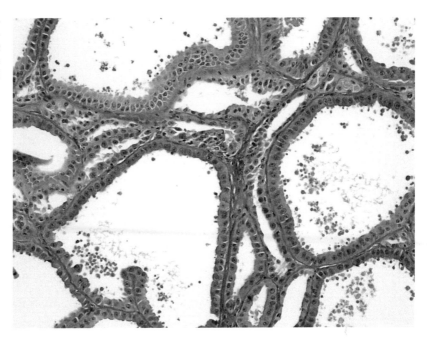

subtypes of renal cortical tumors.[3] Although many of the tumors are of high cytomorphologic grade (**Fig. 10A**) and aggressive clinical behavior, they are not a pure entity and include many other low-grade (see **Fig. 10B**), less-aggressive tumors.

One of the purposes of placing tumors into this category is to prevent forcing of nonconforming tumors into specific types that may dilute the actual clinicopathologic features of those specific entities. Also, it is expected that with accumulation of tumors in the unclassified category, and gaining more experience with them, tumors with similar features from this group will be better recognized. This should enable extracting tumors from the unclassified category and reclassifying them as distinct entities, as exemplified by the few tumor types described here.

MUCINOUS TUBULAR AND SPINDLE CELL CARCINOMA

This recently described entity, mucinous tubular and spindle cell carcinoma (MTSC), is unique among renal tumors; in spite of showing a spindle cell (low-grade sarcomatoid) component, it usually does not behave in an aggressive manner.[69–71] Of the close to 100 reported cases in the literature, only one has been reported to metastasize to regional lymph node. They occur predominantly in women, ranging in age from 17 to 78 years (average 53 years). Grossly, it is a well-circumscribed tumor usually located in the renal medulla. Histologically, the tumor is composed of elongated,

interconnected tubules, many with slit-like lumina, solid compressed cords, and prominent low-grade spindle cell areas (**Fig. 11**). The nonspindled cells are low cuboidal, showing small amount of amphophilic to eosinophilic cytoplasm, with low-grade, bland-appearing nuclei. Myxoid stroma is present in virtually all cases.[71] The closest differential diagnostic possibility is papillary RCC, and immunohistochemical staining usually is not useful in this differentiation.

Ultrastructural evaluation done in a few cases shows close resemblance to the normal loop of Henle.[69,70] Comparative genomic hybridization data available from a few cases show frequent losses at chromosomes 1, 4q, 6, 8p, 11q, 13, 14, and 15, with gains at 11q, 16q, 17, and 20q. No evidence of VHL deletions or trisomy 7 and 17 was found by fluorescence in situ hybridization (FISH) analysis.[70] Although some investigators have suggested that MTSC may be a variant of papillary RCC with spindle cell features,[72] Argani and colleagues[73] recently further confirmed that FISH for trisomies 7/17 distinguishes MTSC from its very close morphologic mimic—papillary RCC with low-grade spindle cell areas.

ACQUIRED CYSTIC DISEASE OF KIDNEY–ASSOCIATED RENAL CELL CARCINOMA

This recently described RCC is associated with end-stage kidneys with acquired cystic disease.[28] Most, but not all, cases occur in patients on dialysis.

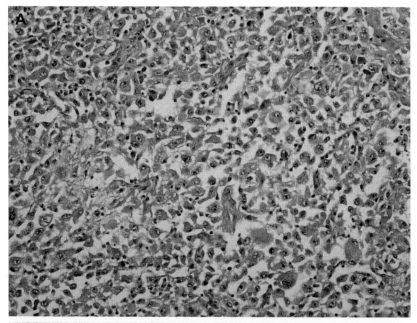

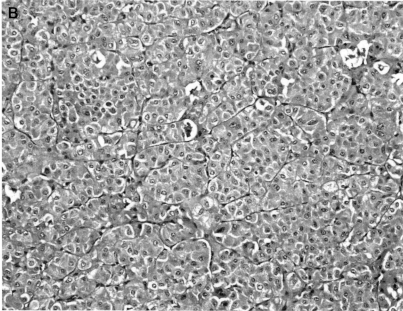

Fig. 10. RCC, unclassified. (*A*) Example of a high-grade carcinoma with rhabdoid features but no clue as to its cell of origin. (*B*) In this low-grade tumor the differential diagnosis includes an eosinophilic variant of chromophobe RCC and oncocytoma. Nuclear atypia and the absence of perinuclear halos, however, preclude of these two designations.

The tumors are characteristically composed of large eosinophilic cells with prominent nucleoli and inter- and intracellular vacuoles (holes), imparting a vaguely cribriform architecture, and intratumoral oxalate crystals (**Fig. 12**). Architecture is variable with papillary, acinar, tubular, and sheet-like areas in variable proportions. Such architectural features may have led in the past to many of these being considered papillary, clear cell, or even un-classified RCC.[74] Immunohistochemical staining for AMACR is strongly positive, whereas CK7 is mostly negative.[28] Rarely, these tumors may behave aggressively, metastasize, and cause death.

TRANSLOCATION-ASSOCIATED RENAL CELL CARCINOMA

Translocation-associated RCCs constitute a small group of RCC that may exhibit papillary features,

Fig. 11. MTSC with typical tubular and spindle cell areas with low-grade cytology and myxoid stroma.

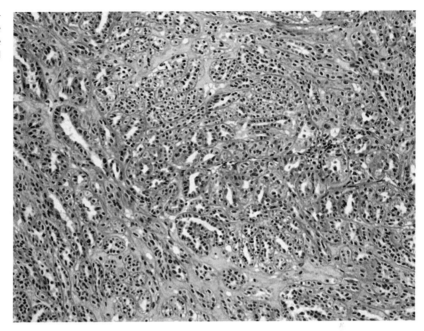

with clear cell or mixed clear and eosinophilic cell cytology, or even solid alveolar growth pattern (**Fig. 13A**), and are genetically and clinically distinct.[45,46] In general they tend to present in younger patients, although a series of cases in adults recently was described.[75] Association with prior chemotherapy for other malignant tumors or nontumorous conditions also has been reported.[76]

These often are associated with aggressive behavior, more so in adults. A subgroup is associated with t(X;1)(p11;q21), a translocation that results in the fusion of the *TFE3* gene on chromosome X to a novel gene, *PRCC*, on chromosome 1. Another subgroup shows the translocation of *TFE3* gene at Xp11.2 with fusion to the *ASPL* gene at 17q25, a translocation also seen in alveolar soft

Fig. 12. Acquired cystic disease–associated RCC. Notice the tubular, cribriform, and papillary architecture and abundant intratumoral oxalate crystals. Because of the variable proportions of the tumors showing papillary architecture, many of these tumors may have been considered papillary RCC in the past.

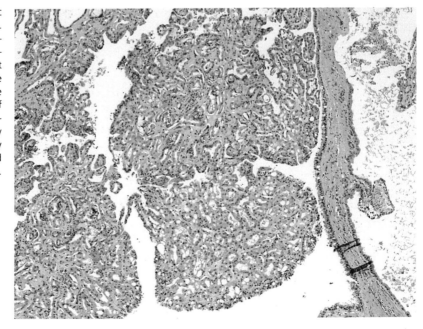

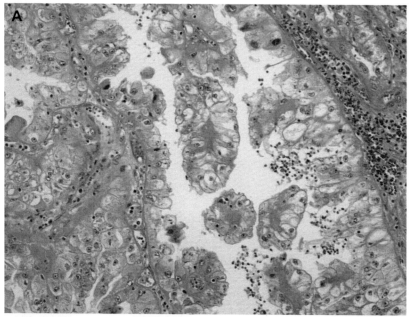

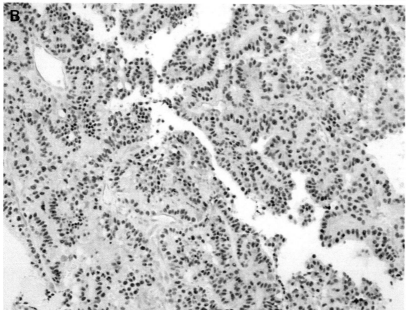

Fig. 13. Xp11 translocation–associated RCC. (*A*)
The tumors usually show
high-grade nuclei, and
often, although not al-
ways, have a prominent
papillary architecture
and clear cell cytology.
(*B*) Immunostain for
TFE3 in one such tumor
showing diffuse nuclear
immunoreactivity.

part sarcoma. Another variant seen in children and young adults is characterized by t(6;11)(p21;q12). On immunohistochemical staining, these tumors tend to be negative or at the most only focally positive for cytokeratins and EMA. Strong and diffuse nuclear immunoreactivity for TFE3 (in Xp11 tumors) (see **Fig. 13**B) or TFEB (in t(6;11) tumors) is considered highly sensitive and a specific marker for these. It is likely that translocation-associated

carcinomas have been incorrectly classified in the past as unusual variants of clear cell carcinoma, PRCC, or even RCC, unclassified type.

ANGIOMYOLIPOMA

AMLs are distinctive neoplasms composed of variable combinations of smooth muscle, adipose tissue, and vasculature. Although found most

Fig. 14. Epithelioid angiomyolipoma with pleomorphic and clear cell features.

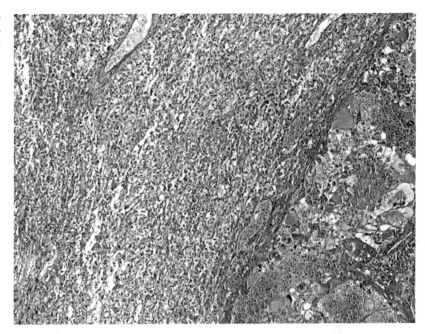

commonly within the kidneys, they may occur at extrarenal sites, including liver, lungs, lymph nodes, and retroperitoneal soft tissues. More than half of all cases occur in patients without tuberous sclerosis; however, approximately 80% of patients who have tuberous sclerosis develop AML.[77,78] More than 90% of tumors contain at least focal areas of mature adipose tissue.[79] The smooth muscle component ranges from elongated spindle cells to sheets of epithelioid cells with abundant eosinophilic granular cytoplasm. The smooth muscle cells often appear to originate and radiate from vessel walls. Thickened and hyalinized vessels with eccentric lumina are seen in most cases. Some tumors may show marked predominance of only one component. Muscle- or fat-predominant tumors need to be differentiated from smooth muscle or adipocytic tumors. Close attention to morphologic features, searching specifically for the focal presence of other tumor components, is helpful in the differential diagnosis in most cases, although immunostaining for HMB-45 and A103 also is needed in some cases. In general, from 5% to 10% of tumor cells are immunoreactive with these antibodies. The epithelioid smooth muscle cell components are positive most often with these antibodies, although the spindled smooth muscle and adipose tissue components also may show focal staining.

The epithelioid variant of AML is composed exclusively or predominantly of polygonal cells with densely eosinophilic cytoplasm. Variable degrees of nuclear atypia are seen, including cells with multilobulated nuclei and multinucleated forms. Focal to extensive clear cell cytology may be present, which may lead to a mistaken diagnosis of clear cell RCC (**Fig. 14**).[80,81] Although some investigators have considered epithelioid AML as a malignant neoplasm, such inferences are based primarily on case reports and may not necessarily represent the true biologic behavior of these tumors as a group.[82]

Recently, a group of AMLs with epithelial cysts lined by cuboidal to hobnail type cells, and presenting as cystic mass, also have been described.[83]

HEREDITARY FORMS OF RENAL TUMORS

The majority of renal neoplasms are sporadic, although a small percentage may be hereditary.[8,10,43,44,84–90] In all forms of inherited renal neoplasms, tumors are more likely to be diagnosed at an earlier age and often are multifocal and bilateral.[87] The most common form of hereditary clear cell RCC occurs in VHL disease, an autosomal dominant syndrome characterized by retinal hemangiomas, clear cell (conventional) RCCs and multiple renal cysts, cerebellar and spinal hemangioblastomas, pheochromocytomas, endocrine pancreatic tumors, and epididymal cystadenomas. The tumor-suppressor *VHL* gene is located at chromosome 3p25 and can be inactivated by various mutations, loss of heterozygosity, promoter hypermethylation, or alterations in VHL modifier genes. Lack of normal VHL protein increases the HIF-1α levels, with the resultant overexpression of endothelial growth factors culminating in a hypervascular state seen in most VHL-related tumors and possible tumorigenesis. Other familial non-VHL clear cell RCCs are reported, most of which involve translocations of chromosome 3, including 3p14 (fragile histidine triad), 3q13.3, and 3q21 genes, whereas a few others do not involve chromosome 3.[10,87]

Hereditary forms of papillary RCC sometimes are associated with tumors of the breast, pancreas, lung, skin, and stomach. The syndrome is associated with activating mutations of c-MET proto-oncogene at chromosome 7q34.[88] Up-regulation of the gene results in the activation of a tyrosine kinase that is a receptor for hepatocyte growth factor/scatter factor and is involved in angiogenesis, cellular motility, growth, invasion, and cellular differentiation. The papillary RCCs associated with syndromic c-MET mutations all are described as type 1. HLRCC is an autosomal dominant familial syndrome with mutation in the fumarate hydratase (1q42.3-q43) gene and is characterized by the development of cutaneous and uterine leiomyomas and renal tumors. Most renal tumors in this syndrome show a high-grade papillary phenotype, but tubular, solid, cribriform, and mixed architectural patterns also may be present.[44]

BHD is another syndrome recently recognized as related to multifocal and bilateral renal tumors. This autosomal dominant syndrome is characterized by cutaneous lesions (fibrofolliculomas, trichodiscomas, and acrochordons), spontaneous pneumothorax, bronchiectasis, bronchospasm, colonic neoplasms, lipomas, and renal tumors.[89–91] The renal tumors are predominantly oncocytic neoplasms displaying hybrid features of chromophobe RCC and oncocytoma, pure chromophobe RCC, renal oncocytoma, or tumors with some unusual morphologic features.[91] The BHD gene has been mapped to chromosome 17p12-q11.2, and the exact mode of tumorigenesis is not yet completely elucidated. Of the families identified with familial renal oncocytoma, several subsequently have been found to have BHD.[89,90] Rarely, a constitutional reciprocal translocation between 8q24.1 and 9q34.3 has been reported in cases of bilateral, multifocal renal oncocytoma.[92]

In summary, recent advances in the study of renal neoplasms have allowed modifying the classification and more accurately correlating morphologic phenotyps to their genotypes. It has allowed doing away with nonspecific entities, such as "granular cell" and "sarcomatoid" RCC. Antigen expression, as detected by some newly available antibodies within different subtypes, is allowing classification of the tumors more accurately. At the same time, this antigenic expression also potentially may be of great use in evaluating targeted therapy.

REFERENCES

1. Thoenes W, Störkel S, Rumpelt HJ. Human chromophobe cell renal carcinoma. Virchows Arch B Cell Pathol Incl Mol Pathol 1985;48:207–17.

2. Thoenes W, Störkel S, Rumpelt HJ. Histopathology and classification of renal cell tumors (adenomas, oncocytomas and carcinomas). The basic cytological and histopathological elements and their use for diagnostics. Pathol Res Pract 1986;181:125–43.

3. Störkel S, Eble JN, Adlakha K, et al. Classification of renal cell carcinoma: Workgroup No. 1. Union Internationale Contre le Cancer (UICC) and the American Joint Committee on Cancer (AJCC). Cancer 1997; 80(5):987–9.

4. Kovacs G, Erlandsson R, Boldog F, et al. Consistent chromosome 3p deletion and loss of heterozygosity in renal cell carcinoma. Proc Natl Acad Sci U S A 1988;85:1571–5.

5. Walter TA, Berger CS, Sandberg AA. The cytogenetics of renal tumors. Where do we stand, where do we go? Cancer Genet Cytogenet 1989;43:15–34.

6. Presti JC Jr, Rao PH, Chen Q, et al. Histopathological, cytogenetic, and molecular characterization of renal cortical tumors. Cancer Res 1991;51:1544–52.

7. Zbar B. Von Hippel-Lindau disease and sporadic renal cell carcinoma. Cancer Surv 1995;25:219–32.

8. Linehan WM, Walther MM, Zbar B. The genetic basis of cancer of the kidney. J Urol 2003;170:2163–72.

9. Motzer RJ, Hutson TE, Tomczak P, et al. Sunitinib versus interferon alfa in metastatic renal-cell carcinoma. N Engl J Med 2007;356:115–24.

10. Eble JN, Sauter G, Epstein JI, et al. Tumours of the kidney World Health Organization classification of tumours; pathology and genetics; tumours of the urinary system and male genital organs. Lyon (France): IARC Press; 2004.

11. Bonsib SM. The renal sinus is the principal invasive pathway: a prospective study of 100 renal cell carcinomas. Am J Surg Pathol 2004;28(12):1594–600.

12. Bonsib SM. T2 clear cell renal cell carcinoma is a rare entity: a study of 120 clear cell renal cell carcinomas. J Urol 2005;174(4 Pt 1):1199–202.

13. Thompson RH, Blute ML, Krambeck AE, et al. Patients with pT1 renal cell carcinoma who die from disease after nephrectomy may have unrecognized renal sinus fat invasion. Am J Surg Pathol 2007;31:1089–93.

14. Avery AK, Beckstead J, Renshaw AA, et al. Use of antibodies to RCC and CD10 in the differential

diagnosis of renal neoplasms. Am J Surg Pathol 2000;24:203–10.

15. McGregor DK, Khurana KK, Cao C, et al. Diagnosing primary and metastatic renal cell carcinoma: the use of the monoclonal antibody 'Renal Cell Carcinoma Marker'. Am J Surg Pathol 2001;25:1485–92.

16. Martignoni G, Pea M, Chilosi M, et al. Parvalbumin is constantly expressed in chromophobe renal carcinoma. Mod Pathol 2001;14:760–7.

17. Mathers ME, Pollock AM, Marsh C, et al. Cytokeratin 7: a useful adjunct in the diagnosis of chromophobe renal cell carcinoma. Histopathology 2002;40:563–7.

18. Kuroda N, Guo L, Toi M, et al. Paxillin: application of immunohistochemistry to the diagnosis of chromophobe renal cell carcinoma and oncocytoma. Appl Immunohistochem Mol Morphol 2001;9:315–8.

19. Kuroda N, Naruse K, Miyazaki E, et al. Vinculin: its possible use as a marker of normal collecting ducts and renal neoplasms with collecting duct system phenotype. Mod Pathol 2000;13:1109–14.

20. Daniel L, Lechevallier E, Giorgi R, et al. Pax-2 expression in adult renal tumors. Hum Pathol 2001; 32:282–7.

21. Eyzaguirre EJ, Miettinen M, Norris BA, et al. Different immunohistochemical patterns of Fhit protein expression in renal neoplasms. Mod Pathol 1999;12: 979–83.

22. Tickoo SK, Amin MB, Linden MD, et al. Antimitochondrial antibody (113-1) in the differential diagnosis of granular renal cell tumors. Am J Surg Pathol 1997;21:922–30.

23. Al-Ahmadie HA, Alden D, Qin L-X, et al. Carbonic anhydrase IX expression in clear cell renal cell carcinoma: an immunohistochemical study comparing two antibodies. Am J Surg Pathol 2008;32:377–82.

24. Tu JJ, Chen Y-T, Hyjek E, Tickoo SK. Carbonic anhydrase IX as a highly sensitive and specific marker of clear cell renal cell carcinoma: a comparative immuno-histochemical study using a panel of commonly utilized antibodies in the differential diagnosis of renal cell tumors. Mod Pathol 2005;18:169A.

25. Tickoo SK, Alden D, Olgac S, et al. Immunohistochemical expression of hypoxia inducible factor-1 alpha and its downstream molecules in sarcomatoid renal cell carcinoma. J Urol 2007;177:1258–63.

26. Al-Ahmadie HA, Alden D, Olgac S, et al. The role of immunohistochemical evaluation of adult renal cortical tumors on core biopsy: an ex-vivo study. Mod Pathol 2007;20:134A.

27. Reuter VE, Tickoo SK. Adult renal tumors. In: Mills SE, Carter D, Greenson JK, et al, editors. Sternberg's diagnostic surgical pathology. 4th edition. Philadelphia: Lippincott Williams & Wilkins; 2004. p. 1955–99.

28. Tickoo SK, dePeralta-Venturina MN, Harik LR, et al. Spectrum of epithelial neoplasms in end-stage renal disease: an experience from 66 tumor-bearing kidneys with emphasis on histologic patterns distinct from those in sporadic adult renal neoplasia. Am J Surg Pathol 2006;30:141–53.

29. Linehan WM. Molecular targeting of VHL gene pathway in clear cell kidney cancer. J Urol 2003;170:593–4.

30. Pantuck AJ, Zeng G, Belldegrun AS, et al. Pathobiology, prognosis, and targeted therapy for renal cell carcinoma: exploiting the hypoxia-induced pathway. Clin Cancer Res 2003;9:4641–52.

31. Kim HL, Seligson D, Liu X, et al. Using protein expressions to predict survival in clear cell renal carcinoma. Clin Cancer Res 2004;10:5464–71.

32. Bui MH, Seligson D, Han KR, et al. Carbonic anhydrase IX is an independent predictor of survival in advanced renal clear cell carcinoma: implications for prognosis and therapy. Clin Cancer Res 2003; 9:802–11.

33. Klatte T, Seligson DB, Riggs SB, et al. Hypoxia-inducible factor 1 alpha in clear cell renal cell carcinoma. Clin Cancer Res 2007;13:7388–93.

34. Leibovich BC, Sheinin Y, Lohse CM, et al. Carbonic anhydrase IX is not an independent predictor of outcome for patients with clear cell renal cell carcinoma. J Clin Oncol 2007;25:4757–64.

35. Amin MB, Tamboli P, Javidan J, et al. Prognostic impact of histologic subtyping of adult renal epithelial neoplasms: an experience of 405 cases. Am J Surg Pathol 2002;26:281–91.

36. Cheville JC, Lohse CM, Zincke H, et al. Comparisons of outcome and prognostic features among histologic subtypes of renal cell carcinoma. Am J Surg Pathol 2003;27:612–24.

37. Reuter VE, Presti JC Jr. Contemporary approach to the classification of renal epithelial tumors. Semin Oncol 2000;27:124–37.

38. Amin MB, Corless CL, Renshaw AA, et al. Papillary (chromophil) renal cell carcinoma: histomorphologic characteristics and evaluation of conventional pathologic prognostic parameters in 62 cases. Am J Surg Pathol 1997;21(6):621–35.

39. Tickoo S, Reuter V. Subtyping papillary renal cell carcinoma: a clinicopathologic study of 103 cases. Mod Pathol 2001;14:124A.

40. Sika-Paotonu D, Bethwaite PB, McCredie MR, et al. Nucleolar grade but not Fuhrman grade is applicable to papillary renal cell carcinoma. Am J Surg Pathol 2006;30(9):1091–6.

41. Delahunt B, Eble JN. Papillary renal cell carcinoma: a clinicopathologic and immunohistochemical study of 105 tumors. Mod Pathol 1997;10(6):537–44.

42. van den Berg E, van der Hout AH, Oosterhuis JW, et al. Cytogenetic analysis of epithelial renal-cell tumors: relationship with a new histopathological classification. Int J Cancer 1993;55:223–7.

43. Schmidt L, Junker K, Nakaigawa N, et al. Novel mutations of the MET proto-oncogene in papillary renal carcinomas. Oncogene 1999;18:2343–50.

44. Merino MJ, Torres-Cabala C, Pinto P, et al. The morphologic spectrum of kidney tumors in hereditary leiomyomatosis and renal cell carcinoma (HLRCC) syndrome. Am J Surg Pathol 2007; 31(10):1578–85.

45. Argani P. The evolving story of renal translocation carcinomas. Am J Clin Pathol 2006;126:332–4.

46. Argani P, Lae M, Hutchinson B, et al. Renal carcinomas with the t(6;11)(p21;q12): clinicopathologic features and demonstration of the specific alpha-TFEB gene fusion by immunohistochemistry, RT-PCR, and DNA PCR. Am J Surg Pathol 2005;29:230–40.

47. Bugert P, Gaul C, Weber K, et al. Specific genetic changes of diagnostic importance in chromophobe renal cell carcinomas. Lab Invest 1997;76: 203–8.

48. Schwerdtle RF, Störkel S, Neuhaus C, et al. Allelic losses at chromosomes 1p, 2p, 6p, 10p, 13q, 17p, and 21q significantly correlate with the chromophobe subtype of renal cell carcinoma. Cancer Res 1996;56:2927–30.

49. Kovacs A, Kovacs G. Low chromosome number in chromophobe renal cell carcinomas. Genes Chromosomes Cancer 1992;4:267–8.

50. Akhtar M, Al-Sohaibani MO, Haleem A, et al. Flow cytometric DNA analysis of chromophobe cell carcinoma of the kidney. J Urologic Pathology 1996;4:15–23.

51. Motzer RJ, Bacik J, Mariani T, et al. Treatment outcome and survival associated with metastatic renal cell carcinoma of non-clear-cell histology. J Clin Oncol 2002;20:2376–81.

52. Lieber MM, Tomera KM, Farrow GM. Renal oncocytoma. J Urol 1981;125(4):481–5.

53. Amin MB, Crotty TB, Tickoo SK, et al. Renal oncocytoma: a reappraisal of morphologic features with clinicopathologic findings in 80 cases. Am J Surg Pathol 1997;21(1):1–12.

54. Perez-Ordonez B, Hamed G, Campbell S, et al. Renal oncocytoma: a clinicopathologic study of 70 cases. Am J Surg Pathol 1997;21(8):871–83.

55. Davis CJ Jr, Mostofi FK, Sesterhenn I, et al. Renal oncocytoma. Clinicopathological study of 166 patients. J Urogenital Pathology 1991;1:41–52.

56. Tickoo SK, Lee MW, Eble JN, et al. Ultrastructural observations on mitochondria and microvesicles in renal oncocytoma, chromophobe renal cell carcinoma, and eosinophilic variant of conventional (clear cell) renal cell carcinoma. Am J Surg Pathol 2000;24(9):1247–56.

57. Erlandson RA, Shek TW, Reuter VE. Diagnostic significance of mitochondria in four types of renal epithelial neoplasms: an ultrastructural study of 60 tumors. Ultrastruct Pathol 1997;21(5):409–17.

58. Martignoni G, Pea M, Bonetti F, et al. Oncocytoma-like angiomyolipoma. A clinicopathologic and immunohistochemical study of 2 cases. Arch Pathol Lab Med 2002;126(5):610–2.

59. Tickoo SK, Amin MB, Zarbo RJ. Colloidal iron staining in renal epithelial neoplasms, including chromophobe renal cell carcinoma: emphasis on technique and patterns of staining. Am J Surg Pathol 1998; 22(4):419–24.

60. Tickoo SK, Reuter VE, Amin MB, et al. Renal oncocytosis: a morphologic study of fourteen cases. Am J Surg Pathol 1999;23(9):1094–101.

61. Fleming S, Lewi HJ. Collecting duct carcinoma of the kidney. Histopathology 1986;10(11):1131–41.

62. Amin MB, Varma MD, Tickoo SK, et al. Collecting duct carcinoma of the kidney. Adv Anat Pathol 1997;4:85–94.

63. Srigley JR, Eble JN. Collecting duct carcinoma of kidney. Semin Diagn Pathol 1998;15(1):54–67.

64. Tokuda N, Naito S, Matsuzaki O, et al. Collecting duct (Bellini duct) renal cell carcinoma: a nationwide survey in Japan. J Urol 2006;176(1):40–3.

65. Davis CJ, Mostofi FK, Sesterhenn IA. Renal medullary carcinoma. The seventh sickle cell nephropathy. Am J Surg Pathol 1995;19:1–11.

66. Swartz MA, Karth J, Schneider DT, et al. Renal medullary carcinoma: clinical, pathologic, immunohistochemical, and genetic analysis with pathogenetic implications. Urology 2002;60:1083–9.

67. MacLennan GT, Farrow GM, Bostwick DG. Low-grade collecting duct carcinoma of the kidney: report of 13 cases of low-grade mucinous tubulocystic renal carcinoma of possible collecting duct origin. Urology 1997;50(5):679–84.

68. Azoulay S, Vieillefond A, Paraf F, et al. Tubulocystic carcinoma of the kidney: a new entity among renal tumors. Virchows Arch 2007;451(5):905–9.

69. Parwani AV, Husain AN, Epstein JI, et al. Low-grade myxoid renal epithelial neoplasms with distal nephron differentiation. Hum Pathol 2001;32(5): 506–12.

70. Srigley JR, Reuter V, Amin M, et al. Phenotypic, molecular and ultrastructural studies of a novel low grade renal epithelial neoplasm possibly related to the loop of Henle. Mod Pathol 2002;12:182A.

71. Fine SW, Argani P, DeMarzo AM, et al. Expanding the histologic spectrum of mucinous tubular and spindle cell carcinoma of the kidney. Am J Surg Pathol 2006;30(12):1554–60.

72. Shen SS, Ro JY, Tamboli P, et al. Mucinous tubular and spindle cell carcinoma of kidney is probably a variant of papillary renal cell carcinoma with spindle cell features. Ann Diagn Pathol 2007;11(1):13–21.

73. Argani P, Netto GJ, Parwani AV. Papillary renal cell carcinoma with low-grade spindle cell foci: a mimic of mucinous tubular and spindle cell carcinoma. Am J Surg Pathol 2008;32:1353–9.

74. Sule N, Yakupoglu U, Shen SS, et al. Calcium oxalate deposition in renal cell carcinoma associated with acquired cystic kidney disease: a comprehensive study. Am J Surg Pathol 2005;29(4): 443–51.

75. Argani P, Olgac S, Tickoo SK, et al. Xp11 translocation renal cell carcinoma in adults: expanded clinical, pathologic, and genetic spectrum. Am J Surg Pathol 2007;31(8):1149–60.

76. Argani P, Lae M, Ballard ET, et al. Translocation carcinomas of the kidney after chemotherapy in childhood. J Clin Oncol 2006;24:1529–34.

77. Bernstein J, Robbins TO. Renal involvement in tuberous sclerosis. Ann N Y Acad Sci 1991;615: 36–49.

78. Stillwell TJ, Gomez MR, Kelalis PP. Renal lesions in tuberous sclerosis. J Urol 1987;138:477–81.

79. Bryant DA, Gaudin PB, Hutchinson B, et al. Angiomyolipoma of the kidney: ahistologic and immunohistochemical study of 39 cases. Mod Pathol 1998; 11:77A.

80. Eble JN, Amin MB, Young RH. Epithelioid angiomyolipoma of the kidney: a report of five cases with a prominent and diagnostically confusing epithelioid smoothmuscle component. Am J Surg Pathol 1997; 21(10):1123–30.

81. Cibas ES, Goss GA, Kulke MH, et al. Malignant epithelioid angiomyolipoma ('sarcoma ex angiomyolipoma') of the kidney: a case report and review of the literature. Am J Surg Pathol 2001;25(1):121–6.

82. Aydin H, Lane B, Sercia L, et al. Renal angiomyolipomas: clinicopathologicalstudy of 202 cases with emphasis on the epithelioid variant. Mod Pathol 2008;21:147A.

83. Fine SW, Reuter VE, Epstein JI, et al. Angiomyolipoma with epithelial cysts (AMLEC): a distinct cystic variant of angiomyolipoma. Am J Surg Pathol 2006; 30:593–9.

84. Zbar B, Glenn G, Lubensky I, et al. Hereditary papillary renal cell carcinoma: clinical studies in 10 families. J Urol 1995;153:907–12.

85. King CR, Schimke RN, Arthur T, et al. Proximal 3p deletion in renal cell carcinoma cells from a patient with von Hippel-Lindau disease. Cancer Genet Cytogenet 1987;27:345–8.

86. Goodman MD, Goodman BK, Lubin MB, et al. Cytogenetic characterization of renal cell carcinoma in von Hippel-Lindau syndrome. Cancer 1990;65: 1150–4.

87. Bodmer D, van den Hurk W, van Groningen JJ, et al. Understanding familial and non-familial renal cell cancer. Hum Mol Genet 2002;11:2489–98.

88. Schmidt L, Duh FM, Chen F, et al. Germline and somatic mutations in the tyrosine kinase domain of the MET proto-oncogene in papillary renal carcinomas. Nat Genet 1997;16:68–73.

89. Zbar B, Alvord WG, Glenn G, et al. Risk of renal and colonic neoplasms and spontaneous pneumothorax in the Birt-Hogg-Dube syndrome. Cancer Epidemiol Biomarkers Prev 2002;11:393–400.

90. Khoo SK, Giraud S, Kahnoski K, et al. Clinical and genetic studies of Birt-Hogg-Dube syndrome. J Med Genet 2002;39:906–12.

91. Pavlovich CP, Walther MM, Eyler RA, et al. Renal tumors in the Birt-Hogg-Dube syndrome. Am J Surg Pathol 2002;26:1542–52.

92. Teh BT, Blennow E, Giraud S, et al. Bilateral multiple renal oncocytomas and cysts associated with a constitutional translocation (8;9)(q24.1;q34.3) and a rare constitutional VHL missense substitution. Genes Chromosomes Cancer 1998;21:260–4.

Fig. 1. Morphologic features of WT. (*A*) Gross image showing an eccentric, large fleshy, hemorrhagic mass that is well encapsulated and distorts the parenchyma. (*B*) Photomicrograph showing broad sperpiginous nests and nodules of blastemal pattern separated by a loose pale fibrous stroma (hematoxylin-eosin stain [HE] ×100).

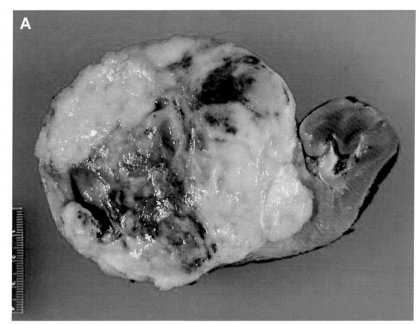

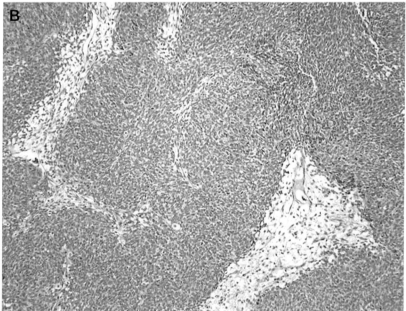

metastasis of the tumor at the gross bench. A synopsis of gross handling technique for renal tumors in general and specifically for WT is shown in **Box 2**.[9–11] There is a variable degree of hemorrhage and necrosis and the tumor usually is separated from the adjacent kidney by a distinct pseudocapsule. They are usually unicentric but can be multicentric in the same kidney or may be associated with perilobar NR (discussed later). Cysts are common and occasionally may be a dominant feature of this tumor. The tumor frequently projects into the pelvicaliceal system and

also infiltrates into the soft tissues surrounding the renal pelvis. This is the area of the renal sinus and is an important area to sample adequately for staging of the tumor. The tumor sometimes may extend into the renal vein.

WILMS' TUMOR: MICROSCOPIC FEATURES

A typical nephroblastoma is a triphasic tumor with an admixture of primitive round to oval cells that constitute the renal blastema, immature epithelial elements that compose the tubules and stroma

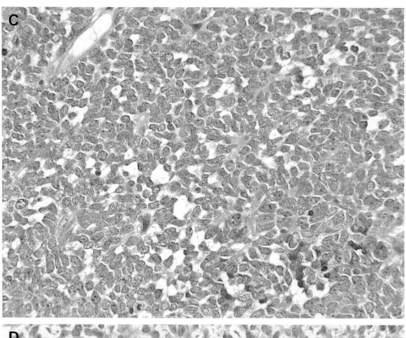

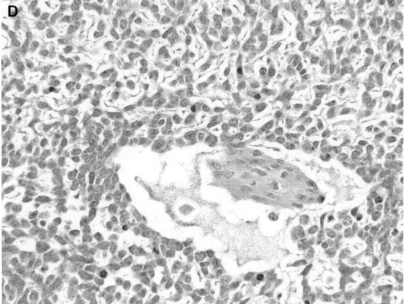

Fig. 1. (*C*) Higher magnification showing an area of pure blastemal WT composed of small round to ovoid cells with scant cytoplasm and hyperchromatic nucleus (HE ×400). (*D*) Another area showing blastemal cells separated by a loose myxoid stroma with rich vascularity that can mimic a CCSK pattern (HE ×200).

that range from the primitive mesenchyme to differentiated smooth and striated muscle.[2–4,9,12]

The metanephric blastema is the most primitive element of the tumor and is characterized by diffuse, densely packed small round to oval cells that are noncohesive and lack any features of epithelial differentiation (see **Fig.** 1B, C). Several patterns of blastemal arrangement are recognized. The diffuse pattern is represented by diffuse sheets of small blue undifferentiated cells that have infiltrative margins and are associated with an aggressive behavior and are frequently beyond stage I according to data from the NWTS. The organoid pattern is represented by aggregates of blastemal cells that are separated by a myxoid stroma and are more well defined in their margins and can be arranged as serpentine blastemal islands that are characterized by undulating cords of tumor cells separated by stroma. The nodular blastemal pattern has rounded nests

Fig. 1. (*E*) Epithelial differentiation with tubular profiles lined by cells with abundant cytoplasm and basal angulated nuclei that are arranged in a parallel fashion around the central lumen. Primitive blastemal cells frequently are seen surrounding the tubules (HE ×400). (*F*) This photograph highlights an area of anaplasia with nuclear pleomorphism, large cells, and large atypical mitoses (HE ×400).

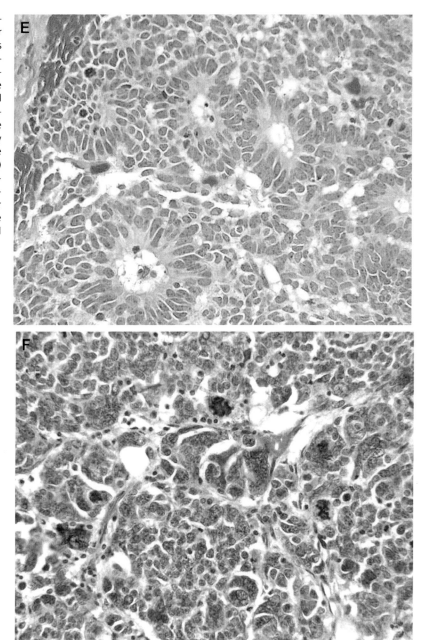

and the basaloid pattern has nests or cords lined by more columnar cells. Sometimes sheets of cells separated by loose myxoid stroma may be seen (see **Fig. 1**D).

The epithelial pattern (see **Fig. 1**E) is divided into the nephrogenic epithelial pattern, where the tumor elements recapitulate the developing kidney with tubular and glomeruloid elements, and heterologous epithelial elements, such as mucinous epithelium, squamous epithelium, and neuroepithelium.

The stromal pattern usually is in the form of undifferentiated myxoid spindle cells that may show fibrous or smooth muscle differentiation and may have some trapped adipose tissue. Other heterologous elements, such as striated muscle, bone, and cartilage, may also be seen. Tumors with

---

Box 2
Precautions in handling pediatric renal tumor cases

1. Discourage frozen section diagnosis

2. Encourage surgeons to submit specimen intact

3. Weigh specimen and ink external surface

4. Identify any capsular breaks

5. Make a clean slice through center of kidney/tumor.

6. Wash knife blade between each cut to prevent knife metastasis

7. Take photographs before and after overnight fixation

8. Freeze tumor and normal kidney for Children's Oncology Group (COG) protocols (biology studies). Submit for cytogenetics and fluorescence in situ hybridization (FISH)/molecular studies where indicated

9. Submit multiple sections with most from tumor-kidney interface to evaluate renal sinus

10. Submit resection margins of renal vein, artery, and ureter

11. Map the sections submitted on the photograph or on paper for orientation

12. Evaluate all unusual areas of tumor

13. Submit sections of nontumoral kidney and any NR if present

14. In cases of resection after chemotherapy, map the sections to assess response to chemotherapy

---

heterologous elements have been called teratoid WT in the past.

Anaplasia in Nephroblastoma

It is important to recognize anaplastic foci in WT as the prognosis and chemotherapy response is determined by their presence or absence. Anaplasia as defined by Beckwith has enlarged nuclei that are three or more times as large as adjacent nuclei together with the presence of large abnormal mitoses that may be tripolar or quadripolar and are characterized by an increase in chromosomal content as revealed by their size in relation to adjacent typical mitotic cells.[9,13] There are two types: focal anaplasia is defined by one or more foci that is characterized by a well-demarcated periphery of nonanaplastic tumor that results in a small well-defined focus. Anaplasia may be in the blastemal, epithelial, or stromal components. Another important criterion of focal anaplasia is the lack of nuclear unrest in the remaining tumor, defined as increased mitosis and karyorrhexis.[14]

As opposed to focal anaplasia, diffuse anaplasia is characterized by random ill-defined foci of anaplasia that may involve the entire tumor or portion of the tumor (see **Fig. 1**F). These foci are not surrounded by nonanaplastic tumor and any focal anaplasia with nuclear unrest in the remaining

tumor is now classified as diffuse anaplasia. By definition, the presence of any anaplasia in a needle biopsy, metastatic focus, or extrarenal site, automatically categorizes the primary tumor as having diffuse anaplasia.

Nephrogenic Rests and Nephroblastomatosis

NR are precursor lesions that are believed to represent developmental events that result in primitive renal tissue persisting in the developed kidney.[1,2,15–19] They are categorized broadly as perilobar or intralobar NR depending on their location in the kidney. The perilobar NR usually are at the periphery of the developmental renal unit and ovoid in shape, well demarcated, numerous, and epithelial or blastemal by morphology (**Fig. 2**A, B). They sometimes are so large as to form a rind of rests at the periphery of the kidney that enlarge the kidney. Extensive perilobar nephroblastomatosis is seen in cases of bilateral tumors in patients who have Beckwith-Wiedemann syndrome. The intralobar NR, alternatively, can occur anywhere deep in the cortex or medulla and also involve the renal sinus and pelvicaliceal system (see **Fig. 2**C). They usually are single or few in number and show tubular or glomerular elements surrounded by blastema. NR also are divided into dormant

Fig. 2. Morphologic features of NR and nephroblastomatosis. (*A*) Composite gross image showing three slices of the same kidney with nodular masses of tan brown color that have an ovoid shape and merge with each other with a round mass arising from the upper pole that represents a WT. The tumor shows areas of hemorrhage and necrosis whereas the NR show a uniform cut surface. The arrow points to a perilobar NR. (*B*) Low-magnification image of a perilobar NR that is made up predominantly of blastemal elements located at the periphery of the kidney beneath the capsule and extending along the columns of Bertini (HE ×40).

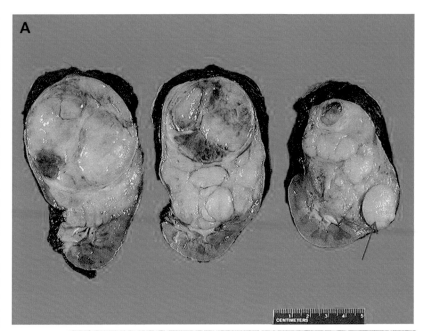

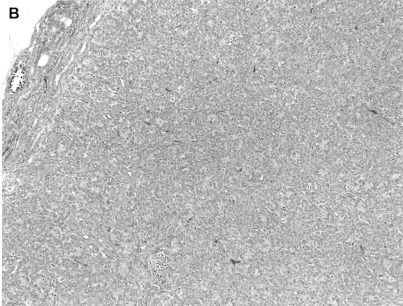

or incipient NR, regressing or sclerosing NR, and hyperplastic and neoplastic NR. The hyperplastic rests are most likely to be mistaken for WT.

Multifocal WT almost always arise from NR (98%) whereas a solitary WT is more variable in its association with NR, especially because minute foci of NR may not be recognized or sampled because of the dominant tumor.

NEPHROBLASTOMA / WILMS' TUMOR: DIFFERENTIAL DIAGNOSIS

WTs are an easy group of tumors to diagnose, especially when they have the characteristic triphasic morphology with epithelial, blastemal, and stromal components. No other tumor has this characteristic triphasic feature. WT, however, needs to be differentiated from other tumors that

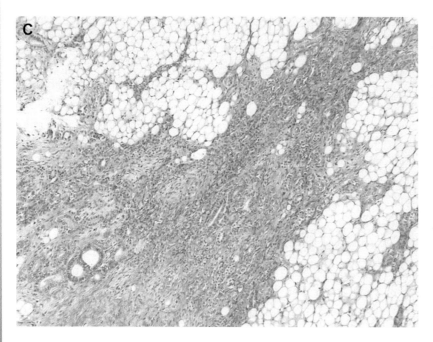

Fig. 2. (*C*) Low-magnification picture of an intralobar NR composed predominantly of tubular and stromal elements that infiltrate the fat of the renal hilum and sinus (HE × 40).

involve the kidney especially when one or the other component predominates.

Lymphomas come into the differential of diffuse blastema-predominant WT and can be differentiated by the presence of extrarenal nodal involvement and by immunohistochemical stains for leukocyte common antigen (LCA) and B- and T-cell markers. They also have characteristic cytogenetic alteration, especially Burkitt's lymphoma and diffuse large cell lymphoma, that show t(8;14) translocation.

Intrarenal neuroblastomas have been reported but often they are extension of tumor from the adjacent adrenal gland. An undifferentiated tumor is most likely to be mistaken for WT and can be differentiated by immunohistochemical stains for NSE, PGP9.5, NB84, and WT1.

Primary renal PNETs are reported and need to be differentiated from blastema-predominant WT. Immunohistochemistry is helpful in these cases, as PNETs are positive for CD99 and some neural markers and show the EWS translocation by FISH analysis and variant translocations by cytogenetics. Reverse transcriptase–polymerase chain reaction (RT-PCR) techniques for the fusion proteins also are helpful.

Synovial sarcoma can have varied morphology and also occur in the kidney. They need to be differentiated from blastema-predominant WT by immunohistochemistry for cytokeratin, epithelial membrane antigen (EMA), CD99, and bcl2 that are often positive in these tumors. These markers are negative in WTs. Cytogenetics for t(X;18) also confirms the diagnosis of synovial sarcoma.

CCSK also is mistaken for WT and is discussed later.

The epithelial component of WT needs to be differentiated from NR (discussed previously). NR usually merge with the adjacent renal parenchyma as opposed to WT that have a pseudocapsule around the tumor. The cellular components of the two lesions, however, can be similar although the blastema of WT are more mitotically active and show areas of hemorrhage and necrosis.

△△ *Differential Diagnosis*
WILMS' TUMOR

- Perilobar and intralobar NR
- MA
- CMN
- CCSK
- Malignant rhabdoid tumor
- PNET
- Synovial sarcoma
- Desmoplastic small round cell tumor

A papillary WT needs to be differentiated from a papillary RCC (PRCC) and can be difficult morphologically in some cases. Staining for cytokeratin 7 (CK7) is helpful because PRCC are diffusely positive as opposed to WT that may be negative or more focal. Rarely, the two tumors can co-exist.

The stromal component of WT can be extremely cellular and needs to be differentiated in cases where it predominates from mesoblastic nephromas (discussed later). Cellular mesoblastic nephromas now have been identified to have the classic ETV6-NTRK3 fusion gene product corresponding to the t(12;15)(p13;q25) translocation.

Areas of WT also may have cells with pseudo-rhabdoid morphology (see **Fig.** 1D) that mimics rhabdoid tumor. Classic areas of WT and staining of nuclei for INI1 help in this differential.

Rhabdomyosarcomas (RMS) and other rare spindle cell sarcomas involve the kidney. Detailed search for more typical areas of blastema and epithelial components usually helps in diagnosing WT. Almost all rhabdomyosarcomas are believed to arise from WT and isolated primary RMS of the kidney is unusual.

NEPHROBLASTOMA/WILMS' TUMOR: DIAGNOSIS

Any abdominal mass in a child in the first decade of life must include WT in the differential diagnosis. Most tumors occur in children in the second and third year of life and 90% of children are under 5 years of age. It is unusual for a WT to be diagnosed in the first year of life and other renal tumors are higher on the list in this age group.[1–3] Imaging studies are critical in diagnosing these tumors. Ultrasound screening usually identifies a renal mass and CT scan confirms the diagnosis of a renal tumor. Imaging also is useful in determining if a tumor is unicentric or multicentric and if it is bilateral. CT scans also may help in identifying perilobar NR as these tend to appear as oval masses occupying the cortex and may show a more rounded WT arising in these. Biopsy is seldom used for diagnosis and only in those cases that are high stage at presentation. Biopsy should be discouraged in cases of bilateral tumors where the question of nephroblastomatosis may arise. There are no specific gross features of WT other than a variegated hemorrhagic and necrotic tumor. The histologic

Table 1
Genetic defects in pediatric renal tumors and their associated syndromes

Renal Tumor	Associated Genetic Defect	Any Known Syndromes
Wilms' tumor	11p13/WT1; also PAX6 gene	WAGR
	11p13/WT1	Denys-Drash, Frasier
	11p15	Beckwith-Wiedemann
	Xp26/GPC3	Simpson-Golabi-Behmel
	5q35/NSD1	Sotos
	17q12-21	Familial WT1
	19q13.4	Familial WT2
	Unknown	Perlman
Cellular CMN	t(12;15)(p13;q25)–ETV6-NTRK3 fusion	
	Trisomy 8, 11, 17	
Malignant rhabdoid tumor	22q deletion, mutation or loss of hSNFS/INI1 gene	Rhabdoid predisposition syndrome
Renal PNET	t(11;22)(q24;q12) (EWS-FLI1)	
	t(21;22)(q22;q12) (EWS-ERG)	
	t(7;22)(p22;q11.2) (EWS-ETV1)	
	t(17;22)(q12;q12) (EWS-E1AF)	
	t(2;22)(q33;q12) (EWS-FEV)	
	t(X;22)(q27;q11) (EWS-?)	
Synovial sarcoma	t(X;18)(p11;q11) (SYT-SSX)	
RCCs		
Xp11.2 translocation	t(X;17)(p11.2;q25) (ASPL-TFE3)	
	t(X;1)(p11.2;q21) (PRCC-TFE3)	
	t(X;1)(p11.2;p34) (PSF;TFE3)	
	t(X;17)(p11.2;q23) (CLTC-TFE3)	
t(6;11) carcinomas	t(6;11)(p21;q12) (Alpha-TFEB)	
PRCC	Chromosome 7, 17 gains	
Adult-type RCC	VHL locus	

diagnosis of WT usually is straightforward when all three components of blastema, epithelia, and stroma are identified in the same tumor. Immuno-histochemistry is of limited value in diagnosis of WT and is more helpful in eliminating the mimickers of WT. Stains for WT1 are variably positive with the blastemal and primitive epithelial component of WT showing strong nuclear staining pattern, whereas the more differentiated epithelial elements show more variable staining and the stromal elements are negative. The epithelial elements are positive for cytokeratins and react variably with CK7. The mesenchymal elements may stain for smooth muscle actin and if striated muscle is present these can stain for desmin and even myogenin and myoD1 when they appear rhabdomyoblastic. The blastema is vimentin positive and shows some desmin staining but no staining for cytokeratins. Electron microscopy is not necessary for diagnosis of most WT. Recent molecular studies have shown several genetic events in WT that can be demonstrated by molecular techniques. These can be seen especially in familial syndromes with increased risk for WT and show specific point mutations in many instances (**Table 1**).[20–21]

Pitfalls in Diagnosis
WILMS' TUMOR

! Diagnosis of WT on a biopsy may be difficult in cases of radiologic evidence of multiple lesions, as differentiation from NR may be impossible.

! Post chemotherapy, it may be impossible to differentiate a treated WT from areas of NR.

! Biopsy diagnosis of blastema-predominant WT has a differential of small round cell tumors in the absence of foci of tubular or stromal differentiation.

! A pure stromal WT easily can be mistaken for mesoblastic nephroma.

! Frozen section diagnosis of WT is discouraged for the above reasons.

! Differentiation from neuroblastoma involving the kidney may be difficult and may require stains for PGP9.5 and WT1 to aid the diagnosis.

NEPHROBLASTOMA / WILMS' TUMOR: PROGNOSIS

The prognostic factors identified from the NWTS studies include the following.

Age

Patients who develop WT at an earlier age (<2 years) tend to have more disease-free survival and frequently present with low-stage disease.

Weight of Tumor

Prior NWTS studies show that a weight cutoff of 550 g is important for prognosis of children who have WT. Tumors less than 550 g in young children under age 2 do well with surgery alone and need no further adjuvant therapy if the disease is localized to the kidney. Tumors above 550 g usually are treated with adjuvant chemotherapy or radiotherapy depending on stage of the tumor.

Histology

The single most important criterion for response to therapy is the presence or absence of anaplasia. Tumors without anaplasia are classified as favorable histology tumors and as a group do better at all stages of disease. The overall 4-year disease free survival for favorable histology tumors is approximately 90%, with stage I tumors having

a survival rate of almost 96%. Presence of any anaplasia classifies the tumor as unfavorable histology and is associated with a lower disease-free survival that ranges from 70% for low-stage disease to 17% for stage IV disease.

Stage

The staging of WT is shown in **Box 3** and is applicable to all pediatric renal tumors except the carcinomas. As discussed previously, stage I tumors usually are associated with high disease-free survival rates whereas higher-stage disease decreases survival. WT shows a propensity to invade the blood vessels; hence, gross and microscopic examination is important to stage the tumor. Invasion of the renal sinus or extension to local hilar lymph nodes upstages the tumor to stage II whereas invasion and extension along the renal vein or capsular rupture makes it a stage III tumor. Extension to intra-abdominal distant nodes also upstages the tumor to stage III whereas distant metastasis to the lungs, liver, bone, and other sites, such as the brain, make it a stage IV tumor. Bilateral tumors traditionally have been classified as stage V, adding to the confusion because they are not truly a higher-stage disease but instead each tumor is staged individually as a single primary and the prognosis

Box 3
Staging of pediatric renal tumors[11]

Stage I

Tumor limited to the kidney and completely resected

Intact renal capsule

No previous rupture or biopsy

Renal sinus vessels not involved

No evidence of tumor at or beyond margins of resection

Stage II

Tumor completely resected

No evidence of tumor at or beyond the margins of resection

Tumor extends beyond the kidney, as evidenced by one of the following:

   Penetration through the renal capsule

   Extensive invasion of the soft tissue of the renal sinus

   Blood vessels within the nephrectomy specimen outside the renal parenchyma,

   including those of the renal sinus, contain tumor

Stage III

Residual nonhematogenous tumor confined to the abdomen is present after surgery as evidence by any one of the following:

   Involvement of lymph nodes within the abdomen or pelvis

   Penetration through the peritoneal surface

   Tumor implants on the peritoneal surface

   Tumor present at the margin of surgical resection

   Tumor not resectable because of local infiltration into vital structures

   Biopsy of tumor before removal of kidney

   Tumor spillage of any degree or localization occurring before or during surgery

   Tumor removed in greater than one piece

Stage IV

Hematogenous metastases (lung, liver, bone, brain, etc.)

Lymph-node metastases outside the abdomino-pelvic region

Stage V

Bilateral renal involvement at diagnosis

Each side should be staged individually according to the criteria above

is determined by the highest-stage tumor in a patient.

LOSS OF HETEROZYGOSITY STUDIES

Recently, LOH for 1p and 16q have been associated with decreased recurrence-free interval especially in favorable histology WT and are treated with adjuvant chemotherapy besides surgery.[2,11,22] The exception to this is all stage I tumors with favorable histology, with tumor weight less than 550 g in children under age 2, LOH is not a frequent finding and does not decrease the survival. These children are treated with surgery alone. Anaplastic tumors show a higher rate of LOH and are always treated aggressively irrespective of LOH studies. Bilateral WT also is shown to have a low incidence of LOH for 1p or 16q. Currently in the United States, all LOH studies are performed as part of biology studies by COG centers.

CYSTIC NEPHROMA AND CYSTIC PARTIALLY DIFFERENTIATED NEPHROBLASTOMA

Cystic nephroma and CPDN are considered benign tumors and are part of the spectrum of nephroblastoma.[23–25] They probably represent early lesions that subsequently develop into nephroblastomas with large cysts. They occur primarily in young children and the tumors referred to as cystic nephromas in adults are believed to be unrelated tumors. They are unusual tumors occurring in children younger than age 4 and have a male predominance. The tumors are identified on radiologic studies and surgical resection is the usual treatment for this cystic mass of the kidney. They may be unilocular or multilocular. When pure stromal elements are present in the cyst wall, they are referred to as cystic nephromas whereas presence of any embryonal elements, such as blastema, tubules, and glomeruli, make them a CPDN. No solid nodules of these elements should be noted. Cystic nephroma and CPDN differ from a nephroblastoma with cysts by the absence of a capsule around the lesion, lack of NR, lack of any anaplasia (which automatically classifies them as nephroblastomas), and lack of any mitoses and atypia. They have an excellent prognosis and only rare cases of recurrence of CPDN are reported due to incomplete resection.

METANEPHRIC TUMORS

Metanephric tumors arise from the primitive metanephric blastema. They range from the purely epithelial MA to the intermediate mixed epithelial and stromal MAF to the predominantly stromal MST. They all are benign tumors and are believed to be related to the WT family of lesions and to arise from NR.

MA is a benign tumor of the kidney that can be seen in children and adults, with an age range from 3 years to 83 years.[2,26,27] They vary in size from 0.3 to 15.0 cm in diameter. Polycythemia as an associated finding is more common in MA than in other renal tumors. They are well-circumscribed, unencapsulated tumors that consist of small epithelial cells arranged in acinar and tubular profiles with scant acellular stroma in-between (**Fig. 3**A, B). Glomeruloid and papillary configurations also may be seen and calcospherites frequently are present. Blastema is absent and helps in differentiating this tumor from WT and NR. Mitoses usually are absent or scant. No

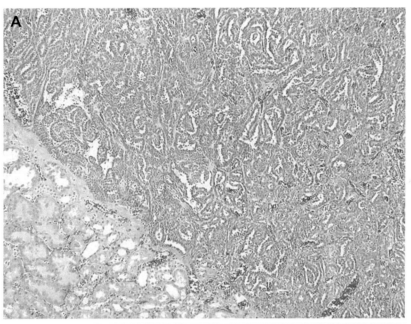

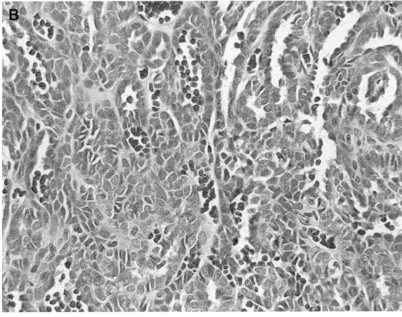

Fig. 3. Morphology of MA and MST. (*A*) Low-magnification image showing the interface between the kidney and a MA made up of back-to-back embryonic tubules (HE ×40). (*B*) Higher magnification of a MA showing the tubular profiles that show no atypia and are lined by cells with hyperchromatic nuclei and scant cytoplasm. Some glomeruloid profiles also are seen. There is no atypia or mitoses in the lesion (HE × 400).

Fig. 3. (*C*) Low magnification showing an interface between normal parenchyma and a MST. The interface is similar to that seen with CMN (HE ×40). (*D*) Higher magnification showing a primitive tubule surrounded by a concentric ring of spindle cells resembling the collarettes seen in dysplastic kidneys (HE ×200).

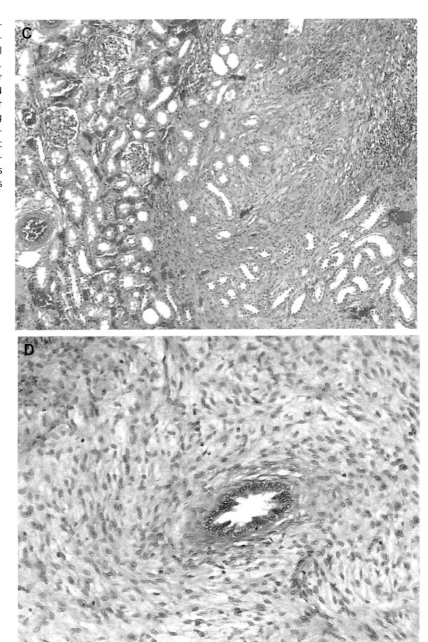

anaplasia is noted. The tumors usually are localized to the medulla and central portions of the kidney and do not invade vessels. They are believed closely related to PRCC and epithelial nephroblastoma but lack a capsule and atypia usually associated with the latter two tumors. They usually are negative for EMA and cytokeratin AE1/AE3 and show only weak focal staining for CK7 as opposed to PRCC.

MAF is a tumor in the middle of the spectrum of metanephric tumors. Originally it was described as nephrogenic adenofibroma but later revised to the present name.[2] MAF is now believed to be in the spectrum of differentiated WTs and cases of a transition from MA to WT have been described.[28,29] They occur in children and adults, with an age range from 5 months to 30 years. They have a slight male predominance with a male to female ratio of 2:1. They can be asymptomatic or symptomatic and can present with polycythemia. Grossly, they are solitary tumors varying in size with a tan-yellow cut surface that may show cysts. Foci of

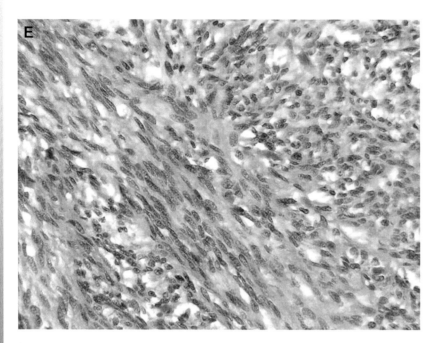

Fig. 3. (*E*) Other areas of a MST may have a fascicular arrangement of spindle cells resembling a CMN. Atypia and mitoses are uncommon (HE ×400).

hemorrhage and necrosis also may be noted. Histologically they are made up of two major components. The stromal component is made up of spindle to stellate cells with tapered, hyperchromatic nuclei and narrow cytoplasmic processes. The stroma vary from minimal with only bands of stroma around a predominantly epithelial tumor to those made up of predominantly stroma with few entrapped areas of epithelium. Areas with onionskin appearance of stroma surrounding normal entrapped tubules also can be seen. The stroma usually show inconspicuous mitoses but a few cases of more prominent mitoses are reported. Heterologous elements also are reported and include glial tissue, fat, and cartilage. The vessels in the stroma have been described to show angiodysplasia with epithelioid change of the smooth muscle media.

The epithelial component of MAF resembles MA in that it is made up of unencapsulated, tightly packed tubules and blunt, short papillae resembling glomeruli. Psammoma bodies are frequent. The tubules are lined by a low cuboidal epithelium that is basophilic and has a hyperchromatic nucleus with inconspicuous nucleolus. Mitoses are usually inapparent and the cases where epithelial component shows greater than 5 mitoses per 20 high-power fields are called MAF with mitoses. Rare cases of transition from MAF to WT and to PRCC were also reported by Arroyo and colleagues.[28] The stroma of MAF resembles that of CMN but is negative for desmin and smooth

muscle actin while being positive for CD34. The epithelial component is variable in its staining for CK7 with only small tubules staining whereas others are negative. This helps in their differentiation from PRCC, which is diffusely CK7 positive. The treatment for these tumors is usually surgical resection with nephrectomy as the main surgical option, especially because they mimic a malignancy clinically and radiologically. No recurrences are reported in the NWTS series.[2,28]

MST is the stroma-dominant end of the spectrum of metanephric tumors. This previously was believed to represent a form of CMN but its association with the metanephric tumors subsequently was identified. The largest series is from the NWTS collection and included 31 cases.[30] The mean age of presentation is 2 years. Grossly they are large fleshy nodular tumors located in the renal medulla and merge imperceptibly with the renal parenchyma (see **Fig. 3C**). They are unencapsulated and histologically they frequently entrap tubules from the adjacent renal parenchyma. The histologic hallmark of this lesion is the onionskin concentric arrangement of spindle cells around the entrapped tubules (see **Fig. 3D**). The stromal cells have a similar appearance to that seen in MAF and show no atypia or significant mitotic activity (see **Fig. 3E**). They stain for CD34 and not for actins or desmin. No embryonal tubules are identified in these lesions. Presence of any embryonal tubules classifies a lesion as MAF. The stroma can show heterologous differentiation similar to MAF. They

Fig. 4. Morphology of CMN. (*A*) Gross image of a classic CMN showing a large mass occupying one pole of the kidney with a tan, whorled, homogeneous cut surface without hemorrhages or necrosis. (*B*) Interface of kidney with tumor showing entrapment of occasional tubules at the edges. The tumor is made up of fascicles of spindle cells with abundant eosinophilic cytoplasm (HE × 40).

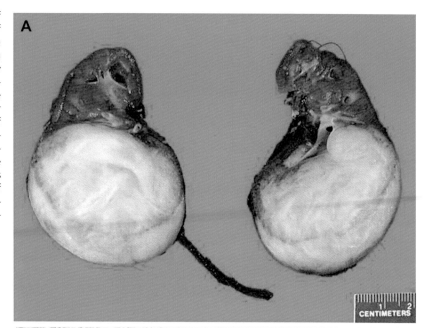

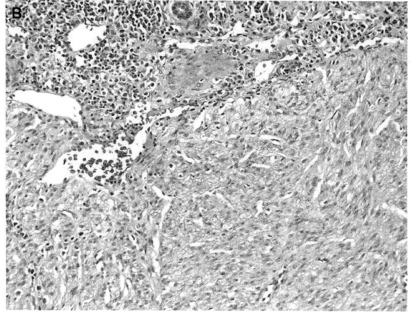

are important to recognize because unlike the CMN they do not require any adjuvant therapy and surgery is curative.[2]

MESENCHYMAL TUMORS OF THE KIDNEY

CONGENITAL MESOBLASTIC NEPHROMA

CMN is a tumor described by Bolande and colleagues.[31] It is seen almost exclusively in the first year of life and is not reported beyond age 2. It is the most common congenital tumor of the kidney and accounts for 2% of all pediatric renal tumors. CMN frequently is detected by prenatal ultrasound. Although most CMNs behave in a benign fashion, the cellular variants are aggressive and patients can die of metastatic disease. There is a male predominance. They are not associated with WT or NR although occasional cases can occur in the Beckwith-Wiedemann syndrome. A specific translocation has been described in the cellular variant of CMN. It presents with an

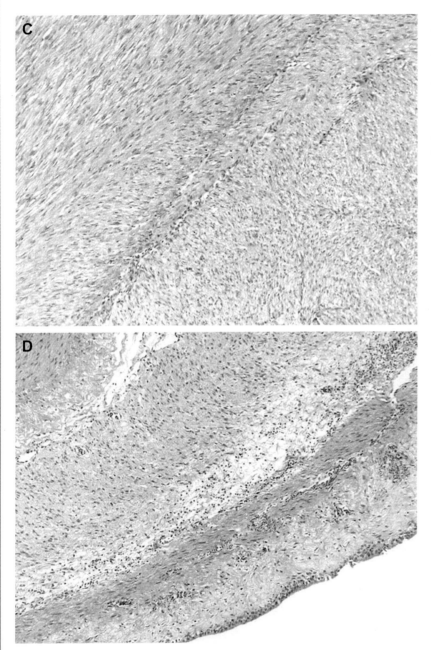

Fig. 4. (C) Low magnification showing the fascicular arrangement of cells with abundant cytoplasm and an ovoid to spindle, vesicular nucleus with inconspicuous nucleolus, and no atypia (HE × 40). *(D)* Tumor invades the soft tissues of the renal sinus frequently as shown in this photomicrograph (HE × 40).

abdominal mass and can be associated with hypertension, hydrops, and polyhydramnios, the latter two resulting in premature delivery.

Congenital Mesoblastic Nephroma: Gross Features

CMNs usually are solitary, large, gray-white to tan tumors that have a whorled appearance (**Fig. 4**A). They have a soft, bulging cut surface and cysts are frequently seen. They are ill defined and permeate the adjacent renal parenchyma and extensively infiltrate into the soft tissues of the hilum of the kidney. Sections from this portion of the tumor should be submitted because the outcome is determined by the completeness of resection of the tumor.

Congenital Mesoblastic Nephroma: Microscopic Features

CMN usually are classified into three major categories: classic, cellular, and mixed. The classic

Fig. 4. (*E*) Low magnification of a cellular tumor with primitive mesenchymal cells with scanty cytoplasm and hyperchromatic nucleus with cyst formation due to entrapment of tubules that undergo cystic transformation (HE × 40). (*F*) High magnification of the cellular CMN shown in **Fig.** 3E. The cells are ovoid and have scant eccentric cytoplasm and an ovoid nucleus with stippled chromatin that is pushed to the periphery giving some of the nuclei a clear appearance. An inconspicuous nucleolus is also noted (HE × 400).

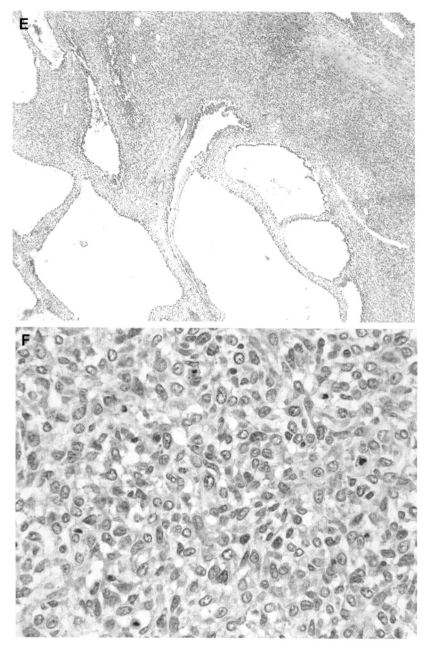

pattern of CMN is characterized by fascicles of spindle cells that resemble fibroblasts and myofibroblasts, with variable collagen in-between (see **Fig.** 4B, C). The mitotic activity is low. A hemangiopericytomatous vascular pattern may be seen. The cells are characterized by abundant cytoplasm with tapered ends with indistinct cellular borders and a spindled nucleus with inconspicuous nucleolus. The edges of the tumor are irregular and frequently tongues of cells extend beyond the gross limits of the tumor (see **Fig.** 4D). The tumor frequently surrounds areas of renal parenchyma and the entrapped tubules can become cystic and undergo metaplastic change. Skeletal muscle differentiation has not been reported in a CMN and its presence warrants a diagnosis of stroma-predominant WT. The cellular variant is characterized by crowding of cells that have similar morphology but higher mitotic activity (see **Fig.** 4E). The fascicles sometimes can be composed of immature

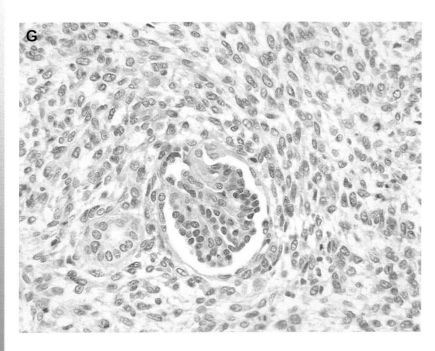

Fig. 4. (*G*) A cellular CMN frequently infiltrates and surrounds normal glomeruli and tubules as seen in this photograph (HE × 200).

Key Features
CONGENITAL MESOBLASTIC NEPHROMA

1. Congenital tumor—most common

2. Frequently cystic with a soft, whorled, pale leiomyomatous cut surface

3. Indistinct borders with normal kidney

4. Classic pattern with fascicles of spindle cells with abundant eosinophilic cytoplasm and vesicular nuclei, resembling fibromatosis

5. Cellular pattern with primitive ovoid to spindle cells with scant cytoplasm and frequent mitoses, resembling infantile fibrosarcoma with which it shares the translocation t(12;15)(p13;q25)

6. Frequent invasion of soft tissues of renal sinus and cellular variant can metastasize

spindled cells that are compactly arranged resembling an infantile fibrosarcoma (see **Fig. 4**F). More often, the cells are plump and show large vesicular nuclei with nucleoli. Necrosis is common. Cells also can have a rhabdoid appearance and a myxoid variant also is present. They frequently entrap adjacent renal parenchyma (see **Fig. 4**G). Mixed CMN is characterized by an admixture of classic and cellular variants. The classic foci may be seen at the periphery of the cellular component

or may be seen as the dominant component. Immunohistochemistry is positive for vimentin, muscle actins, and desmin in the spindle cells, confirming their fibroblastic/myofibroblastic nature. They are negative for WT1 and epithelial markers.

Congenital Mesoblastic Nephroma: Differential Diagnosis

The main differential diagnosis for CMN includes a stroma-predominant WT, a CCSK, synovial sarcoma, and the malignant rhabdoid tumor. The salient differentiating features of the common pediatric tumors are highlighted in **Table 2**.

CMNs differ from WTs in that they occur earlier in life and almost never are seen beyond 2 years, whereas many of the WTs appear in the second and third year of life. They have indistinct borders and grossly have a whorled appearance in contrast to WT, which are more variegated and show a pseudocapsule around the tumor. Histologically, skeletal muscle differentiation can be seen in WT although it never is seen in a CMN. NR are associated with WT and not CMN. The only caveat to this distinction is in patients who have been treated with chemotherapy before nephrectomy. In those cases a treated WT mimics a CMN; hence, the latter diagnosis never should be entertained under those circumstances.

Cellular CMN can mimic CCSK but again the age of presentation, the ill-defined borders with infiltration of adjacent parenchyma, the characteristic

Table 2
Differentiating features between common pediatric renal tumors

Features	WT	CMN	CCSK	RTK
Age in years (range)	Usually 3–4 (1–10)	First year (0–2), congenital	2–3 (1–adult)	1–2 (0–4)
Gross features				
Capsule	+	−	−	−
Variegated cut surface	+	±	±	+
Vascular invasion	+	± Cellular	±	+
Microscopy pattern	Triphasic, blastemal, or epithelial	Fascicular spindle cells	Sheets with arborizing vessels	Cells in sheets with extensive necrosis
Cytoplasm	Scant in blastema, more in epithelial and mesenchymal	Abundant (classic), less in cellular	Variable with vacuolation	Abundant with eosinophilic hyaline inclusion
Nucleus	Hyperchromatic	Stippled chromatin	Pale chromatin to clear	Chromatin pushed to periphery
Nucleolus	−	±	−	+
Anaplasia	+	−	+	+
Nephrogenic rests	+	−	−	−
IHC	Vimentin+, CK7+ epithelial, WT1+, desmin + stroma	SMA+, Vim+, MSA+, desmin usually focal	Vim+, CD99 cytoplasmic	Vim+, CK+, desmin ±, INI1-, WT1 -, MSA±, CD99+ membranous
Cytogenetics	WT1, WT2	t(12;15)(p13;q25)	Unknown	22q loss or mutation

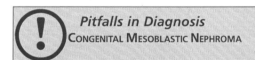

△△ Differential Diagnosis
CONGENITAL MESOBLASTIC NEPHROMA

- Classic CMN
- Stroma-predominant WT
- Spindle cell variant of CCSK rarely
- Myofibromatosis involving the kidney
- MST
- MAF
- Cellular CMN
- CCSK
- Stroma-predominant WT
- Monophasic synovial sarcoma
- Malignant rhabdoid tumor

trapping of islands of renal tissue in CMN as opposed to single tubules and nephrons in CCSK, the high cell density, and the presence of actin staining by immunohistochemistry help in the differentiation.

The rhabdoid variant can mimic a rhabdoid tumor of the kidney (RTK) but the latter frequently are aggressive tumors with vascular invasion and distant metastasis at presentation, show distinct cytoplasmic inclusions and prominent nucleoli uniformly, and may be associated with intracranial tumor. Immunohistochemistry for INI1 also is helpful in this distinction as rhabdoid tumors show universal loss of INI1 staining of nuclei of tumor cells.

The spindle areas of cellular CMN also can mimic synovial sarcoma and can be differentiated by their staining for cytokeratins and EMA that highlight the epithelial elements in synovial sarcoma and by CD99 and bcl2 that are positive in synovial sarcoma and not in CMN. Cytogenetics, including FISH for t(X;18) for synovial sarcoma and t(12;15) for cellular CMN, can assist in making this distinction.

Congenital Mesoblastic Nephroma: Diagnosis

The diagnosis of CMN is based on the clinical setting of a congenital tumor of the kidney that is detected often on routine prenatal screening. Morphologically, it has a fleshy, whorled, bulging cut surface and histology has been described previously. The clue to the diagnosis lies in the tumor tending to entrap islands of renal parenchyma at the periphery.

Immunohistochemistry is helpful in some cases as the spindle cells show a myofibroblastic phenotype with staining for vimentin, actins, and desmin, but this is variable. The cellular variant may not show any markers besides vimentin and resembles the infantile fibrosarcoma. The cytogenetics of CMN has been unraveled in the past decade and although the classic CMN has no specific genetic abnormality, the cellular CMN has been shown to be aneuploid with extra copies of chromosomes 8, 11, and 17. They also show the characteristic t(12;15)(p13;q25) translocation in greater than 90% of cases. This translocation fuses the ETV6 gene on chromosome 12p13 with the neurotrophin-3 receptor gene NTRK3 on 15q25.[32–34] The same translocation and aneuploidy also may be demonstrated in the cellular areas of mixed CMN that leads to the proposal that the three variants may be transitions of the same tumor with the classic preceding the mixed and cellular variants. This unique translocation also has led to the understanding that cellular CMN and congenital fibrosarcoma are related tumors and the former may represent an intrarenal variant of the latter. More recent studies of gene expression analysis have shown a high degree of expression of insulin-like growth factor 2 in CMN and low to no expression of WT1, which helps in the differentiation from WT. It has been shown that CMN and WT tend to cluster close to each other on gene expression analysis but have distinct molecular signatures.

Congenital Mesoblastic Nephroma: Prognosis

The two major prognostic determinants of CMN are the completeness of surgical resection and the subtype with the cellular CMN behaving in

! Pitfalls in Diagnosis
CONGENITAL MESOBLASTIC NEPHROMA

! The cellular variant of CMN can be mistaken for a clear cell sarcoma and rhabdoid tumor or primitive sarcoma and needs cytogenetics or molecular tests for diagnosis

! WT is always in the differential, and a stain for smooth muscle actin and finding blastema is helpful. Also the interface between the kidney and tumor is indistinct in CMN.

! A MST can be difficult to differentiate from CMN and the finding of tubules surrounded by concentric spindle cells confirms the diagnosis of MST.

! Cellular CMN can metastasize and be difficult to diagnose at metastatic sites and needs confirmation of the genetic defect for diagnosis.

a more aggressive manner than classic CMN.[35,36] The importance of surgical margin evaluation already has been stressed but to reiterate, because of the location of the tumor in the medulla, it is of utmost importance to ink the medial aspect of the kidney, including the hilum, before cutting open the tumor at the grossing bench. Correlation with the surgeon's observation is also important to assess whether or not there was gross tumor left behind. Adjuvant chemotherapy similar to that of congenital infantile fibrosarcoma is now advocated for tumors that are not completely excised although observation is all that is needed for completely excised tumors. Recurrence is known in patients who have incomplete resection and chemotherapeutic response of recurrences are reported. The recurrences usually are confined to the retroperitoneum or peritoneal cavity. Most recurrences occur within 1 year; hence, the average recommended period of surveillance is 1 year for CMN. The overall survival rates for CMN are high with almost 98% long-term survival. Metastasis is known with the cellular variant and the sites of metastases include the lungs, heart, liver, bone, and brain. They are more common in older infants and can be evident at presentation and progress rapidly.

CLEAR CELL SARCOMA OF THE KIDNEY

Clear cell sarcoma is a high-grade sarcoma of infants and young children and constitutes approximately 3.5% of renal tumors in the NWTS.[37] It was recognized as a distinct entity by Kidd and colleagues in 1970. It also was recognized early on to have a propensity for metastasis to the bone and has been called the bone-metastasizing tumor of infancy.[38] The peak incidence of CCSK is in the second year of life but the age range varies from as early as age 2 months to 14 years although occasional cases have been reported in adults. There is a male preponderance with a male to female ratio of 2:1 but no differences in geographic distribution are noted. There is no genetic or syndromic association noted for CCSK. Only one case was associated with perilobar NR in the largest series published from the NWTS. A large proportion of patients present with high-stage disease with evidence of lymph node and distant metastasis at presentation.

Clear Cell Sarcoma of the Kidney: Gross Features

CCSK usually present as large, unicentric masses that replace the kidney or may be localized to the medulla. They vary in size from approximately

> ## Key Features
> ### CLEAR CELL SARCOMA OF THE KIDNEY
>
> 1. Frequent mimic of other pediatric renal tumors
> 2. Well-circumscribed, unencapsulated, usually solid appearance with areas of necrosis and hemorrhage and occasional cysts
> 3. Entrapment of renal tissue, mainly nephrons at the periphery with cystic change
> 4. Classic pattern of cells with pale cytoplasm, ovoid to spindle nucleus with pale chromatin "clear" cell appearance
> 5. Myxoid stroma with typical arborizing vessels
> 6. Variant forms—epithelioid, spindle, rhabdoid, sclerosing pattern
> 7. Anaplasia may be seen
> 8. Bone metastasis presentation common
> 9. Vimentin-only positive, INI1 positive
> 10. Aggressive behavior

2.3 cm to 24 cm. They are well circumscribed but do not show a definite capsule or pseudocapsule and merge with the renal parenchyma (**Fig. 5**A). Cysts may be seen grossly. Areas of necrosis and hemorrhage also may be seen in the background of a fleshy gray-white to tan-colored mass. The tumor may extend into the renal vein in some cases.

Clear Cell Sarcoma of the Kidney: Microscopic Features

The classic pattern of CCSK is made up of sheets or broad nests and cords of plump ovoid to round cells with scant cytoplasm and indistinct cell borders separated by an arborizing network of vascular septa (see **Fig. 5**B, C). The nuclei of tumor cells have fine stippled chromatin with no chromatin clumping or nucleoli. The nucleus may appear empty, or clear, and this helps in the diagnosis. The cytoplasm may be vacuolated or scant. Spindle cell areas also may be noted. The fibrovascular septa are composed of thin delicate vessels surrounded by spindled fibroblasts that constitute the septal cells. There is abundant Alcian blue–positive matrix in the tumor that is responsible for the pale appearance of the tumor and its name. The abundant matrix also results in the less dense cellularity of the tumor. The mitotic

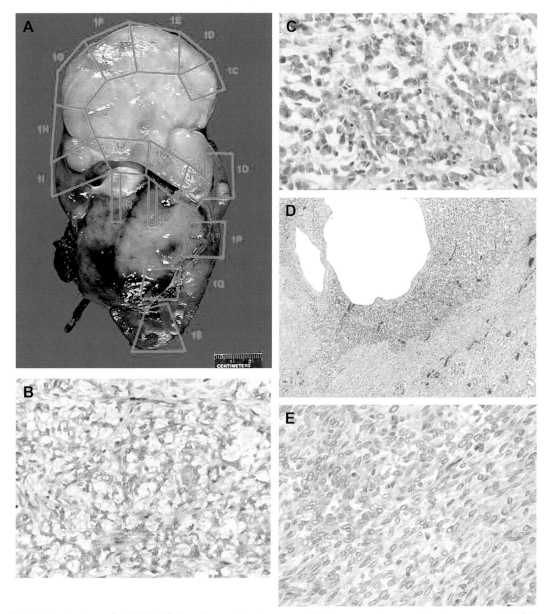

Fig. 5. Morphology of a CCSK. (*A*) Gross image showing a tan, fleshy tumor that occupies the upper pole of the kidney. It has a nodular, homogeneous appearance. The tumor grossly appears to be well demarcated. The photograph also shows how to map various sections that are submitted for histology for reference. (*B*) The classic pattern of CCSK with ovoid cells separated by a loose myxoid stroma with rich arborizing vasculature and a vesicular nucleus (HE × 200). (*C*) A cellular area of the tumor where the cells now have eccentric nuclei with an eosinophilic cytoplasm that is prominent in places mimicking a rhabdoid tumor (HE × 400). (*D*) Another case showing the indistinct edges of the tumor where it entraps tubules that show cystic change (HE × 40). (*E*) A more spindled area of a CCSK that still retains the cellular feature of CCSK but shows scant myxoid stroma in between and can resemble a CMN (HE × 400).

rate is variable but low in most cases. There is frequent entrapment of tubules and glomeruli at the periphery and there may be cystic dilatation of the entrapped tubules (see **Fig. 5**D), resulting in the gross cystic appearance of CCSK. There is

no pseudocapsule noted separating the tumor from adjacent normal kidney.

Several histologic variants of CCSK are recognized.[2,39] It is this variegated morphology that results in frequent misdiagnosis of this tumor. The classic pattern of CCSK, however, is found in most of these tumors on detailed search. The various patterns are shown in the table and include the spindle cell variant (see **Fig. 5E**), epithelioid variant, sclerosing variant, myxoid variant, cystic variant, pericytomatous variant, neural variant, and monstrocellular variant. The last variant also is referred to the anaplastic variant and is characterized by large bizarre cells with atypical mitoses.

Clear Cell Sarcoma of the Kidney: Differential Diagnosis

The multifaceted morphology of CCSK creates difficulty in diagnosing the tumor. Because of the variant patterns, almost all tumors that occur in the kidney enter into the differential diagnosis. Only the more common ones are discussed.

Wilms' Tumor
One of the clues to the differences is the gross appearance, especially the presence of a pseudocapsule in WT as opposed to the well-circumscribed but nonencapsulated appearance of CCSK. Histologically, the vascular pattern seen in CCSK may be noted in WT but the blastema is more densely cellular as opposed to the CCSK and the cells are hyperchromatic as opposed to the vesicular and clear nuclei in CCSK in most cases. Also, CCSK tends to trap isolated tubules and glomeruli at the periphery with cystic change of these tubules as opposed to WT, which shows clear demarcation from adjacent parenchyma and tends to merge only when arising from a NR. Immunohistochemistry may not be helpful as CCSK is reactive only for vimentin and WT1 is too variable in its staining of WT to help differentiate the two.

Congenital Mesoblastic Nephroma
The spindle cell variant of CCSK can be mistaken for CMN. The age group, however, is distinct in that most CMNs occur in the first year of life whereas the peak incidence of CCSK is in the second year. Also, CMN tends to trap large islands of renal tissue at the periphery as opposed to CCSK, which traps only individual nephrons. The nuclear characteristics also help in the differential. In difficult cases, cytogenetics for the t(12;15) translocations in cellular CMN clinch the diagnosis.

Rhabdoid Tumor
The epithelioid variant of CCSK can be misdiagnosed as a rhabdoid tumor and can be distinguished by the presence of the classic prominent nucleolus and cytoplasmic inclusions in MRT as opposed to the vesicular nucleus and clear to scant cytoplasm of CCSK. Immunohistochemistry for cytokeratin, EMA, vimentin, and loss of INI1 confirm the diagnosis of MRT. Cytogenetics also confirm the presence of chromosome 22 alterations in MRT.

Primitive Neuroectodermal Tumor and Synovial Sarcoma
Renal PNET typically is a small round tumor similar to its extrarenal counterparts and can be a source of confusion especially because isolated cases of CCSK are known to be focally positive for CD99. The dense cellularity, high turnover of cells, and high mitoses in PNET, however, together with the strong diffuse membranous positivity for CD99 as opposed to the cytoplasmic staining in CCSK should help in the diagnosis. The characteristic EWS translocations also can be looked for in difficult cases by FISH or other techniques. Synovial sarcoma usually is biphasic and has epithelial markers, such as CK and EMA, besides CD99, they are bcl2 positive and show the t(X;18) translocation.

Clear Cell Sarcoma of the Kidney: Diagnosis

The diagnosis of CCSK is based on its characteristic light microscopic features that give the tumor its name. The presence of ovoid cells with pale vacuolated cytoplasm and vesicular to clear nuclei in a loose myxoid stroma with an arborizing vascular pattern and staining only for vimentin provides clues to the diagnosis. It is important, however, to recognize the variants of CCSK as these cause the problems in diagnosis. A careful search for the presence of typical areas helps in the diagnosis. Immunohistochemistry has a limited role but can help in excluding its mimics, such as WT, CMN, RTK, and PNET. Vimentin is the only marker that is uniformly positive in CCSK and they do not stain for cytokeratins, actins, desmin, or diffusely for CD99. The current belief is that any tumor with strong CD99 staining in the kidney should be

Differential Diagnosis
CLEAR CELL SARCOMA
OF THE KIDNEY

- Blastema-predominant WT—classic pattern
- CMN—spindle cell pattern
- Malignant rhabdoid tumor—rhabdoid/epithelioid variant of CCSK
- PNET
- Synovial sarcoma

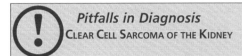

Pitfalls in Diagnosis
CLEAR CELL SARCOMA OF THE KIDNEY

! Mimicking almost every tumor that can occur in the kidney

! Rare occurence in older children

! Having no specific immunohistochemical marker to date

! An undifferentiated sarcoma in a bone in a young child should always have CCSK in the differential especially if it has no specific lineage markers

! Variant histology difficult to diagnose in the absence of typical areas

considered a renal PNET. No cytogenetic abnormalities have been shown present in CCSK. Recent gene expression analysis of renal tumors has shown presence of several neuroectodermal genes that are over-expressed in CCSK leading to the current belief that these tumors have a neural/neuroectodermal origin. Nerve growth factor receptor has been shown to be strongly expressed in CCSK in these expression analyses and may be used as an immunohistochemical marker in the future.[40,41]

Clear Cell Sarcoma of the Kidney: Prognosis

The prognosis of CCSK is dependent on the stage of the disease, and a staging system similar to WT is used. All patients irrespective of stage are treated with adjuvant chemotherapy although the number of drugs may vary. Stage I disease has an excellent survival with no recurrences reported in those cases treated with adjuvant chemotherapy alone and no radiation. Higher-stage diseases usually are treated with a combination of chemotherapy and radiation. The disease-free survival is least for stage IV disease and the survival rates decreased from 98% for stage I disease to 50% 6-year survival for stage IV patients in the largest NWTS series. Significant prognostic factors besides stage included age of the patients, with patients in the 2- to 4-year age group surviving more than those younger or older, and presence of anaplasia. The most common sites of metastasis were the lymph nodes; hence, adequate sampling of lymph nodes was necessary for staging of patients. Nonavailability of lymph nodes for examination at surgery automatically stages the patients as stage II disease. The distant sites of metastasis include the bone, brain, and

unusual sites, such as muscle, orbit, and spine.[2,10,11,39]

MALIGNANT RHABDOID TUMOR OF THE KIDNEY

MRT is a highly malignant tumor of the kidney first recognized by Beckwith in 1981.[2,3,42,43] Since its first description, similar tumors have since been recognized in the brain, where they are called atypical rhabdoid teratoid tumor (ATRT) and cutaneous lesions in the disseminated form of the disease.[44,45] Recent molecular developments have resulted in the discovery of the specific genetic defect in these tumors and patients, and the occurrence of a familial form of this tumor called the rhabdoid predisposition syndrome has been recognized to have the same genetic defect. Most of the tumors occur in the first 2 years of life and may be associated synchronously or asynchronously by the ATRT. They are highly aggressive tumors and have a high mortality rate with rare cases of long-term survival in patients. It also now is recognized that there are several tumors in the body that can take on a rhabdoid phenotype and these are now termed, *pseudorhabdoid*, to differentiate them from true RT.[46] The mimics do not share the genetic defect seen in RTK. Extrarenal sites of true rhabdoid tumors also are reported, including the soft tissues.[47]

Malignant Rhabdoid Tumor: Gross Features

Malignant rhabdoid tumors usually are spherical with a pale tan cut surface and a soft consistency

Key Features
MALIGNANT RHABDOID TUMOR

1. Highly aggressive tumor of infancy

2. Classic cytologic features of large cells with eccentric nucleus that shows a prominent nucleolus and eccentric cytoplasmic globular eosinophilic inclusion.

3. Characteristic immunohistochemical profile of CK-positive, vimentin-positive, EMA-positive, desmin-negative, myogenin-negative cells

4. Characteristic loss of INI1 staining of tumor cell nuclei corresponding to the chromosome 22 mutation.

5. May be associated with extrarenal and intracranial counterparts

6. Vascular invasion common

7. Poor prognosis currently

Fig. 6. Morphology of a RTK. (*A*) Microscopic image showing the characteristic appearance of a rhabdoid tumor with cells with abundant eosinophilic cytoplasm and a nucleus with prominent nucleolus (HE × 400). (*B*) A focus of tumor seen invading blood vessels consistent with the aggressive behavior of RTK (HE × 40).

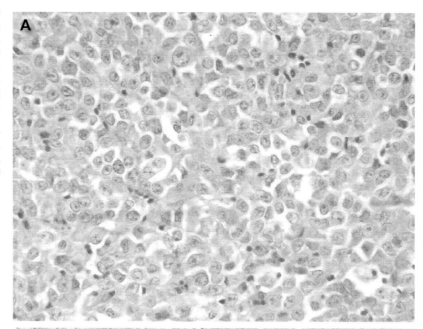

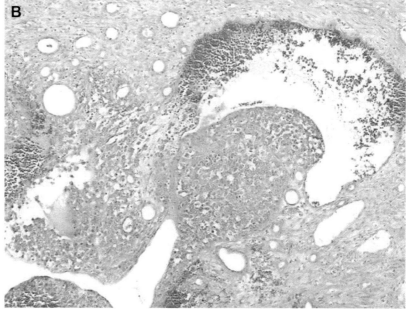

and are located in the central portion of the kidney. They frequently extend beyond the kidney and more often than not are associated with extrarenal metastatic disease at diagnosis. Areas of hemorrhage and necrosis may be seen.

Malignant Rhabdoid Tumor: Microscopic Features

The histology of MRT is characteristic and made up of large ovoid to epithelioid cells that have abundant eosinophilic cytoplasm with the characteristic cytoplasmic dense hyaline inclusion and a large vesicular nucleus with prominent nucleolus (**Fig. 6**A). The dense cytoplasmic inclusion is responsible for its name because they resemble developing muscle cells or rhabdomyoblasts. They can, however, be an acquired change and are seen in all tumors that exhibit the pseudorhabdoid phenotype. Vascular invasion is a common feature (see **Fig. 6**B). The tumor is usually ill defined and may entrap

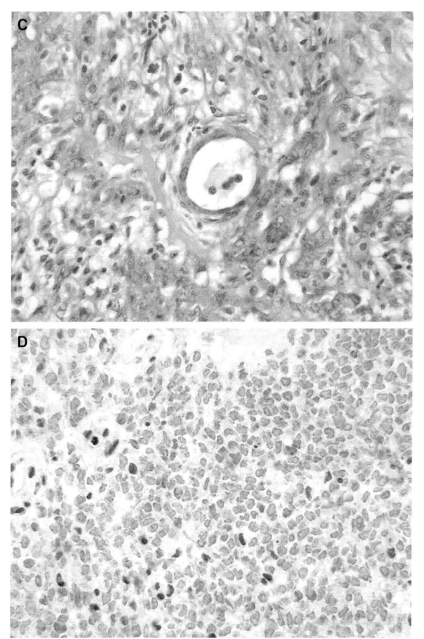

Fig. 6. (*C*) The tumor infiltrates into adjacent renal parenchyma and entraps tubules (HE × 400). (*D*) An INI1 stain shows loss of INI1 staining of nuclei of tumor cells. The background stromal and endothelial cells retain the INI1 (PAP × 200).

adjacent nephrons similar to CCSK (see **Fig.** 6C). Cystic changes in entrapped tubules may be seen. They are not associated with NR or with any associated underlying renal disease. Areas of necrosis and hemorrhage are common and indicate the high cell turnover of this turnover. The cytoplasmic inclusions are PAS positive. Several histologic subtypes exist similar to the CCSK and coexist with the classic areas. The variant patterns include spindle cells, small blue cells, and sclerosing, hemangiopericytomatous, pseudopapillary, and cystic patterns. The stroma may show myxoid change in some cases and have the appearance of osteoid in rare cases.

Malignant Rhabdoid Tumor: Differential Diagnosis

The differential diagnosis for RTK is extensive because of its diverse morphologic patterns.[46,47] They need to be differentiated from renal medullary carcinoma, WT, CCSK, CMN, renal PNET, synovial sarcoma, rhabdomyosarcoma, and other renal tumors that can have a rhabdoid phenotype and from metastasis of tumors that have a rhabdoid phenotype (pseudorhabdoid tumors). (Differences from WT, CCSK, and CMN are described previously.) Renal medullary carcinoma is the most likely mimic of this tumor, but has a characteristic clinical setting of sickle cell trait and occurs in older individuals compared with RTK. They also do not show the INI1 defect. They differ from rhabdomyosarcomas in that RTKs do not express by definition any myogenic markers and are negative for myogenin and myoD1. They also demonstrate loss of INI1, which is not seen in rhabdomyosarcomas. Their differentiation from renal PNET may be more difficult because of the small round cell appearance of some rhabdoid tumors and their expression of CD99, but loss of INI1 stain is diagnostic of RTK. Cytogenetics may be used for differentiation in some cases. Synovial sarcoma is another tumor that may mimic rhabdoid tumors and absence of staining for cytokeratin, EMA, and vimentin in the same cell and preservation of INI1 stain in the nucleus and the characteristic t(X;18) translocation help in the differential. Synovial sarcomas also are uniformly positive for bcl2. Loss of INI1 stain in the nuclei of rhabdoid tumors help in its differentiation from the pseudorhabdoid tumors that do not show the chromosome 22 deletion and may show the specific genetic alterations of the original tumor.

Malignant Rhabdoid Tumor: Diagnosis

MRT has a characteristic histologic appearance that helps in the diagnosis with its large pale nucleus with characteristic prominent nucleolus and the cytoplasmic hyaline inclusions. The cytoplasmic inclusions are aggregates of microfilaments that can be seen by ultrastructure and stain for cytokeratins, epithelial membrane, and vimentin. There may be some expression for actins and sometimes desmin but other myogenic markers, such as myogenin, myoD1, and myoglobin, are never expressed in MRT. They are positive for CD99 stain and may show a diffuse membranous pattern of expression but are negative for bcl2 and CD34. They may express neural markers, such as synaptophysin, NSE, and S100.

Recently, the molecular signature of rhabdoid tumors has been elucidated and it has been shown to have biallelic inactivation of the hSNF5/INI1/SMARCB1/BAF47 tumor suppressor gene on chromosome 22q11-12.[48,49] Similar mutations have been detected in the CNS rhabdoid (ATRT) tumors leading to the understanding that these are related tumors. It also has been shown that hSNF5/INI1 modulates cell cycle control and cytoskeletal organization through the regulation of the retinoblastoma protein E2F and Rho pathways. Up to 20% of rhabdoid tumors have been shown to not demonstrate the mutations for the INI1 gene. An immunohistochemical marker for INI1 (see **Fig. 6**D) is now available and shown to be

---

Differential Diagnosis
MALIGNANT RHABDOID TUMOR

- Blastemal WT
- CCSK, rhabdoid, and epithelioid variants
- CMN
- RCC with rhabdoid phenotype
- Metastatic or intrarenal neuroblastoma, undifferentiated
- Rhabdomyosarcoma
- Synovial sarcoma

! Pitfalls in Diagnosis
MALIGNANT RHABDOID TUMOR

! Rhabdoid phenotype is seen in many primary renal and metastatic tumors—so-called pseudo-rhabdoid tumors.

! Diagnosis may be difficult in biopsies, especially if there is extrarenal extension of tumor.

! May be mistaken for rhabdomyosarcoma, but RTK never expresses muscle markers, especially desmin and myogenin.

! Sclerosing pattern may resemble desmoplastic small cell tumor.

! INI1 stain is retained in all pseudo-rhabdoid tumors and this is the most useful differentiating feature to separate these entities from RTK but difficult to standardize.

lost only in true rhabdoid tumors irrespective of site and retained in all tumors that enter into its differential or exhibit rhabdoid phenotype.[50] There was some variability, however, in the expression of INI1 in synovial sarcomas and epithelioid sarcomas.

Malignant Rhabdoid Tumor: Prognosis

The prognosis for MRT is uniformly poor, most cases behave in an aggressive fashion, and survival beyond a year is unusual according to the largest series published from the NWTS. The therapy includes a combination of high-dose chemotherapy and radiation. More recent data suggest some improvement in survival with a combination of high-dose chemotherapy and stem cell transplant.[2,3]

SARCOMAS OF THE KIDNEY

Sarcomas are an uncommon group of tumors (discussed briefly previously). They include common pediatric sarcomas affecting the sift tissues that rarely may manifest as a primary renal tumor and are causes of diagnostic pitfalls. The most common ones include PNET,[51] synovial sarcoma,[52] rhabdomyosarcoma, and, more rarely, desmoplastic small round cell tumor. They have the same histologic, immunohistochemical, and cytogenetic/molecular defects as seen in the soft tissue counterparts with no expression of WT1 in most except desmoplastic small round cell tumor and staining for CD34 and bcl-2.[53] A primary anaplastic sarcoma of the kidney has been reported more recently and is characterized by a polyphenotypic expression of vimentin, desmin, and variable neural markers.[54]

RENAL CELL CARCINOMAS IN CHILDHOOD

RCCs were believed mainly tumors of adults and the only form that was recognized as distinct to the pediatric age group was the PRCC believed related to WT and metanephric tumors. The classic adult RCC was reported in older children. The past decade has seen an entire transformation in the field of pediatric RCC and several variants have been described based on cytogenetic abnormalities in these tumors that have generated a whole group of translocation-associated RCC in children and young adults. Currently, pediatric RCC are believed to represent 5% to 6% of all tumors in this age group.[2,55] They are staged using the TNM classification. Only the major subtypes, with brief descriptions, are discussed.

CLEAR CELL Xp11.2 RENAL CELL CARCINOMAS

Clear cell RCC of the adult type with LOH for the von Hippel-Lindau gene is not typically seen in the pediatric age group (**Fig. 7**A, B, C). Instead the majority of the pediatric clear cell tumors show areas of papillary or pseudopapillary configuration. A subgroup of these tumors shows voluminous cytoplasm and they show a characteristic Xp11.2 translocation involving the TFE3 gene (**Fig. 7**D, E). The common translocations include the t(X;1)(p11.2;q21), resulting in fusion of the PRCC and TFE3 genes; t(X;1)(p11.2;p34), fusing the PSF and TFE3 genes; and t(X;17)(p11.2; q25), resulting in fusion of the TFE3 gene with the novel ASPL on 17q25, a translocation that is typical of alveolar soft part sarcoma.[56–58] The last group with the ASPL-TFE3 fusion shows large cells with clear to pale eosinophilic cytoplasm with distinct cell borders, vesicular nuclear chromatin, and prominent nucleoli with arrangement in nests. Tumor cells are discohesive leading to their alveolar and pseudopapillary pattern of arrangement. Psammoma bodies frequently are noted. Immunohistochemically, they only occasionally express cytokeratins and EMA and vimentin staining is also patchy. They show staining for the RCC marker and CD10 and the characteristic nuclear staining for TFE3 antibody, which helps differentiate this subgroup of tumors. Clear cell RCC is highly aggressive and is usually advanced stage at presentation; however, it has an indolent course.

t(6;11)(p21;Q12) TRANSLOCATION CARCINOMAS

The t(6;11) RCC is an uncommon variant occurring in late childhood and in young adults and is characterized by nests and tubules of polygonal epithelial cells separated by thin capillary network.[55,59–61] The cells have abundant clear to granular eosinophilic cytoplasm and well-defined cell borders. A second population of small epithelioid cells aggregating around basement membrane–like material also is a feature. The tumor cells are negative for cytokeratins and stain more often for melanocytic markers, such as HMB45 and Melan A, and are negative for the RCC marker. They show the characteristic translocation that involves the TFEB gene and immunohistochemistry for TFEB delineates this group.

PAPILLARY RENAL CELL CARCINOMA

PRCC is the most frequent carcinoma seen in children and shows similar cytogenetic features as the adult RCC with gains of chromosome 7 and 17.[2,3,55,62,63]

Fig. 7. Morphology of RCC. (*A*) Gross image of a RCC showing a partly solid, partly cystic tumor with extensive areas of hemorrhage and necrosis. (*B*) Cysts that are lined by cuboidal cells with central nuclei and a pale to clear cytoplasm (HE × 100).

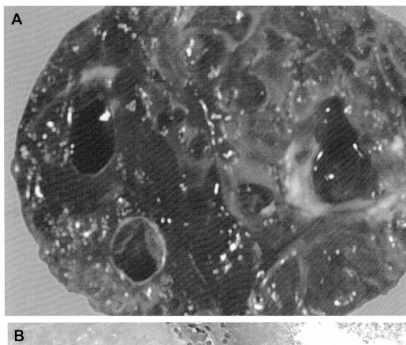

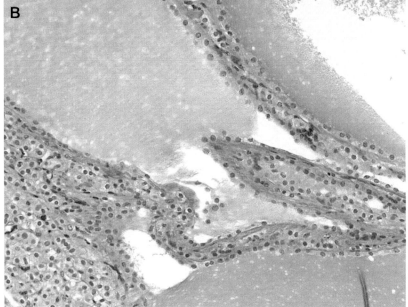

Grossly, PRCCs have a papillary architecture with a pale yellow appearance and can be cystic. They are well circumscribed and eccentric in location. They are made up of a single layer or pseudostratified lining of cells on a fibrovascular stalk with many foamy cells in the papillary cores. Psammomatous calcification is common.

There are two types of cells: type 1 are small cells with scanty, pale, usually basophilic cytoplasm; small nuclei; inconspicuous nucleoli; nuclear grooves; and a single layer; and type 2 are large cells with voluminous cytoplasm and prominent nucleoli with little pleomorphism and rare mitotic activity.

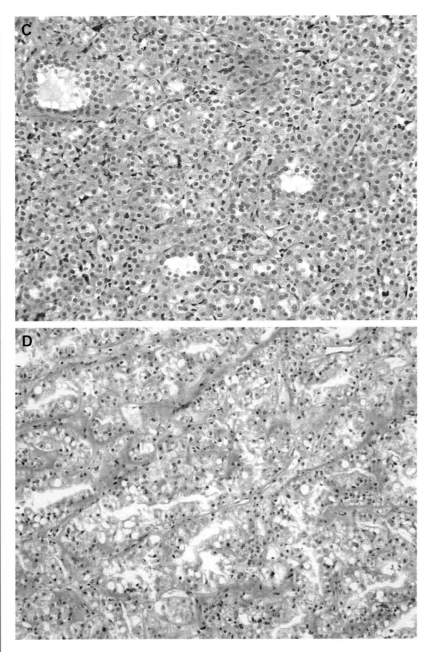

Fig. 7. (*C*) A more typical solid area with mixed clear and granular cells that make up the classic RCC (HE × 200). (*D*) Another example that shows cells with voluminous cytoplasm arranged in an alveolar pattern with clear cytoplasm and central small round nucleus without significant atypia (HE × 400). (*Courtesy of* P. Argani, MD, Baltimore, MD.)

The tumor cells uniformly stain for CK7, a stain that can be useful in the differential diagnosis that includes an epithelial nephroblastoma and MA.[64] They have a pseudocapsule similar to a nephroblastoma but unlike an adenoma. Some are reported to have Xp11.2 translocation.

RENAL MEDULLARY CARCINOMAS

These are rare tumors that affect mainly young individuals who have sickle cell trait and only rarely those who have sickle cell disease.[65,66] The age range for presentation ranges from 5 to 32 years. Patients present with flank pain, hematuria, and a palpable mass. They are poorly circumscribed and involve the medulla. There may be evidence of intrarenal hematogenous spread. They have a cribriform architecture with microcystic, solid, and sarcomatous areas. Stromal desmoplasia is common. There may be a striking inflammatory infiltrate. The cells have large nuclei with vesicular

Fig. 7. (*E*) A RCC stained with TFE3 that shows nuclear staining of the tumor cells confirming the diagnosis of a translocation associated carcinoma (TFE3 × 400, PAP). (*Courtesy of* P. Argani, MD, Baltimore, MD.)

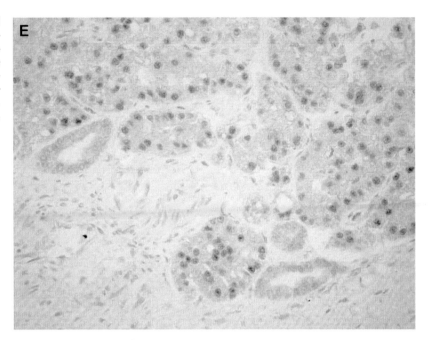

chromatin pattern with prominent nucleoli and abundant acidophilic cytoplasm and, hence, are mistaken for rhabdoid tumor. They are positive for epithelial markers, CAM5.2 and EMA, and for vimentin. They carry a poor prognosis because of their poor response to therapy. The survival ranges from 2 weeks to 15 months.

Rare cases of postneuroblastoma RCCs have been reported in older children and young adults.[67] They usually have an oncocytoid appearance with solid and papillary architecture. There is no association with chemotherapy. Cases of RCC are also reported in association with tuberous sclerosis.[55]

PEDIATRIC KIDNEY NEOPLASMS: SUMMARY

Pediatric renal tumors constitute a diverse group of embryonal tumors that are unique to the pediatric age group and constitute the majority of tumors in children. Eighty percent of pediatric tumors are WTs. They present with diverse presentations and although some are restricted to distinct age groups of children, they show a wide overlap in morphology, resulting in difficulty in diagnosis in occasional cases. Recent advances in molecular techniques and gene array analysis have been shown to separate distinct categories of pediatric renal tumors and may provide specific markers that can be used to separate these tumors at the cellular level. The RCCs that were initially pooled together with their adult counterparts now are recognized as a distinct group with specific molecular and cytogenetic

differences, the biology of which is slowly being discerned as more cases are recognized and reported.

REFERENCES

1. Beckwith JB. Nephrogenic rests and the pathogenesis of Wilms tumor: developmental and clinical considerations. Am J Med Genet 1998;79(4):268–73.
2. Murphy WM, Grignon DJ, Perlman EJ, editors. Kidney tumors in children, Tumors of the kidney, bladder and related urinary structures, Series 4, AFIP Atlas of tumor pathology. Washington, DC: ARP; 2004. p. 1–100.
3. Eble JN, Sauter G, Epstein JL, et al, editors. Tumors of the kidney. In WHO Classification of tumors: tumors of the urinary system and male genital organs. Lyon, France: IARC Press; 2004.
4. Beckwith JB, Palmer NF. Histopathology and prognosis of Wilms tumors: results from the First National Wilms' Tumor Study. Cancer 1978;41(5):1937–48.
5. Beckwith JB. Wilms' tumor and other renal tumors of childhood: a selective review from the National Wilms' Tumor Study Pathology Center. Hum Pathol 1983;14(6):481–92.
6. Beckwith JB. Vignettes from the history of overgrowth and related syndromes. Am J Med Genet 1998;79:238–48.
7. Breslow NE, Beckwith JB. Epidemiological features of Wilms' tumor: results of the National Wilms' Tumor Study. J Natl Cancer Inst 1982;68(3):429–36.
8. Fukuzawa R, Breslow NE, Morrison IM, et al. Epigenetic differences between Wilms' tumours in white and east-Asian children. Lancet 2004;363:446–51.

9. Beckwith JB. National Wilms Tumor Study: an update for pathologists. Pediatr Dev Pathol 1998;1:79–84.

10. Qualman SJ, Bowen J, Amin MB, et al. Protocol for the examination of specimens from patients with Wilms tumor (nephroblastoma) or other renal tumors of childhood. Arch Pathol Lab Med 2003;127:1280–9.

11. Perlman EJ. Pediatric renal tumors: practical updates for the pathologist. Pediatr Dev Pathol 2005; 8:320–38.

12. Schmidt D, Beckwith JB. Histopathology of childhood renal tumors. Hematol Oncol Clin North Am 1995;9:1179–200.

13. Faria P, Beckwith JB, Mishra K, et al. Focal versus diffuse anaplasia in Wilms tumor—new definitions with prognostic significance: a report from the National Wilms Tumor Study Group. Am J Surg Pathol 1996;20:909–20.

14. Hill DA, Sheer TD, Liu T, et al. Clinical and biologic significance of nuclear unrest in Wilms tumor. Cancer 2003;97:2318–26.

15. Beckwith JB. Precursor lesions of Wilms Tumor: clinical and biologic implications. Med Pediatr Oncol 1993;21:158–68.

16. Beckwith JB, Kiviat NB, Bonadio JF. Nephrogenic rests, nephroblastomatosis and the pathogenesis of Wilms' tumor. Pediatr Pathol 1990;10:1–36.

17. Bove KE, McAdams AJ. The nephroblastomatosis complex and its relationship to Wilms' tumor: a clinicopathologic treatise. Perspect Pediatr Pathol 1976; 3:185–223.

18. Hennigar RA, O'Shea PA, Grattan-Smith D. Clinicopathologic features of nephrogenic rests and nephroblastomatosis. Adv Anat Pathol 2001;8:276–89.

19. Perlman EJ, Faria PA, Soares A, et al. Hyperplastic perilobar nephroblastomatosis: long-term survival of 52 patients. Pediatr Blood Cancer 2006;46:203–21.

20. Rivera MN, Haber DA. Wilms' tumor: connecting tumorigenesis and organ development in the kidney. Nat Rev Cancer 2005;5:699–712.

21. Berry PJ. Microdissecting the genetic events in nephrogenic rests and Wilms tumor development. Am J Pathol 1998;153:991–1000.

22. Grundy PE, Breslow NE, Li S, et al. Loss of heterozygosity for chromosomes 1p and 16q is an adverse prognostic factor in favorable-histology Wilms tumor: a report from the National Wilms Tumor Study Group. J Clin Oncol 2005;23:7312–21.

23. Beckwith JB, Kiviat NB. Multilocular renal cysts and cystic renal tumors. AJR Am J Roentgenol 1981;136: 435–6.

24. Joshi VV. Cystic partially differentiated nephroblastoma: an entity in the spectrum of infantile renal neoplasia. Perspect Pediatr Pathol 1979;5:217–35.

25. Joshi VV, Beckwith JB. Multilocular cyst of the kidney (cystic nephroma) and cystic, partially differentiated nephroblastoma. Terminology and criteria for diagnosis. Cancer 1989;64:466–79.

26. Davis CJ Jr, Barton JH, Sesterhenn IA, et al. Metanephric adenoma. Clinicopathologic study of fifty patients. Am J Surg Pathol 1995;19:1101–14.

27. Muir TE, Cheville JC, Lager DJ. Metanephric adenoma, nephrogenic rests and Wilms tumor: a histologic and immunophenotypic comparison. Am J Surg Pathol 2001;25:1290–6.

28. Arroyo MR, Green DM, Perlman EJ, et al. The spectrum of metanephric adenofibroma and related lesions: clinicopathologic study of 25 cases from the National Wilms Tumor Study Group Pathology Center. Am J Surg Pathol 2001;25:433–44.

29. Hennigar RA, Beckwith JB. Nephrogenic adenofibromas. A novel kidney tumor of young people. Am J Surg Pathol 1992;16:325–34.

30. Argani P, Beckwith JB. Metanephric stromal tumor: report of 31 cases of a distinctive pediatric renal neoplasm. Am J Surg Pathol 2000;24:917–26.

31. Bolande RP. Congenital mesoblastic nephroma of infancy. Perspect Pediatr Pathol 1973;1: 227–50.

32. Argani P, Fritsch M, Kadkol SS, et al. Detection of the ETV6-NTRK3 chimeric RNA of infantile fibrosarcoma/cellular congenital mesoblastic nephroma in paraffin-embedded tissue: application to challenging pediatric renal stromal tumors. Mod Pathol 2000;13:29–36.

33. Knezevich SR, Garnett MJ, Pysher TJ, et al. ETV6-NTRK3 gene fusions and trisomy 11 establish a histogenetic link between mesoblastic nephroma and congenital fibrosarcoma. Cancer Res 1998;58: 5046–8.

34. Sandberg AA, Bridge JA. Updates on the cytogenetics and molecular genetics of bone and soft tissue tumors: congenital (infantile) fibrosarcoma and mesoblastic nephroma. Cancer Genet Cytogenet 2002;132:1–13.

35. Beckwith JB, Weeks DA. Congenital mesoblastic nephroma. When should we worry? Arch Pathol Lab Med 1986;110:98–9.

36. Howell CG, Othersen HB, Kiviat NE. Therapy and outcome in 51 children with mesoblastic nephroma: a report of the National Wilms' Tumor Study. J Pediatr Surg 1982;17:826–31.

37. Haas JE, Bonadio JF, Beckwith JB. Clear cell sarcoma of the kidney with emphasis on ultrastructural studies. Cancer 1984;54:2978–87.

38. Schmidt D, Harms D, Evers KG, et al. Bone metastasizing renal tumor (clear cell sarcoma) of childhood with epithelioid elements. Cancer 1985;56: 609–13.

39. Argani P, Perlman EJ, Breslow NE, et al. Clear cell sarcoma of the kidney: a review of 351 cases from the National Wilms Tumor Study Group Pathology Center. Am J Surg Pathol 2000;24:4–18.

40. Schuster AE, Schneider DT, Fritsch MK, et al. Genetic and genetic expression analysis of clear

cell sarcoma of the kidney. Lab Invest 2003;83:1293–9.

41. Cutcliffe C, Kersey D, Huang CC, et al. Clear cell sarcoma of the kidney: up-regulation of neural markers with activation of the sonic hedgehog and Akt pathways. Clin Cancer Res 2005;11: 7986–94.

42. Weeks DA, Beckwith JB, Mierau GW, et al. Rhabdoid tumor of kidney. A report of 111 cases from the National Wilms' Tumor Study Pathology Center. Am J Surg Pathol 1989;13:439–58.

43. Weeks DA, Beckwith JB, Mierau GW. Rhabdoid tumor. An entity or a phenotype? Arch Pathol Lab Med 1989;113:113–4.

44. White FV, Dehner LP, Belchis DA, et al. Congenital disseminated malignant rhabdoid tumor: a distinct clinicopathologic entity demonstrating abnormalities of chromosome 22q11. Am J Surg Pathol 1999;23: 249–56.

45. Burger PC, Yu IT, Tihan T, et al. Atypical teratoid/rhabdoid tumor of the central nervous system: a highly malignant tumor of infancy and childhood frequently mistaken for medulloblastoma: a Pediatric Oncology Group study. Am J Surg Pathol 1998;22: 1083–92.

46. Weeks DA, Beckwith JB, Mierau GW, et al. Renal neoplasms mimicking rhabdoid tumor of kidney. A report from the National Wilms' Tumor Study Pathology Center. Am J Surg Pathol 1991;15: 1042–54.

47. Parham DM, Weeks DA, Beckwith JB. The clinicopathologic spectrum of putative extrarenal rhabdoid tumors. An analysis of 42 cases studied with immuno-histochemistry or electron microscopy. Am J Surg Pathol 1994;18:1010–29.

48. Biegel JA, Zhou JY, Rorke LB, et al. Germ-line and acquired mutations of INI1 in atypical teratoid and rhabdoid tumors. Cancer Res 1999;59: 74–9.

49. Schofield DE, Beckwith JB, Sklar J. Loss of heterozygosity at chromosome regions 22q11-12 and 11p15.5 in renal rhabdoid tumors. Genes Chromosomes Cancer 1996;15:10–7.

50. Hoot AC, Russo P, Judkins AR, et al. Immunohistochemical analysis of hSNF5/INI1 distinguishes renal and extra-renal malignant rhabdoid tumors from other pediatric soft tissue tumors. Am J Surg Pathol 2004;28:1485–91.

51. Parham DM, Roloson GJ, Feely M. Primary malignant neuroepithelial tumors of the kidney: a clinicopathologic analysis of 146 adult and pediatric cases from the National Wilms' Tumor Study Group Pathology Center. Am J Surg Pathol 2001;25: 133–46.

52. Argani P, Faria PA, Epstein JL, et al. Primary renal synovial sarcoma: molecular and morphologic delineation of an entity previously included among

53. Shao L, Hill DA, Perlman EJ. Expression of WT-1, Bcl-2 and CD34 by primary renal spindle cell tumors in children. Pediatr Dev Pathol 2004;7: 577–82.

54. Vujanic GM, Kelsey A, Perlman EJ, et al. Anaplastic sarcoma of the kidney. A clinicopathologic study of 20 cases of a new entity with polyphenotypic features. Am J Surg Pathol 2007;31:1459–68.

55. Bruder E, Passera O, Harms D, et al. Morphologic and molecular characterization of renal cell carcinoma in children and young adults. Am J Surg Pathol 2004;28:1117–32.

56. Argani P, Antonescu CR, Couturier J, et al. PRCC-TFE3 renal carcinomas: morphologic, immunohistochemical, ultrastructural, and molecular analysis of an entity associated with the t(X;1)(p11.2;q21). Am J Surg Pathol 2002;26:1553–66.

57. Argani P, Lal P, Huchinson B, et al. Aberrant nuclear immunoreactivity for TFE3 in neoplasms with TFE3 gene fusions: a sensitive and specific immunohistochemical assay. Am J Surg Pathol 2003;27: 750–61.

58. Argani P, Lui MY, Couturier J, et al. Cloning of a novel CLTC-TFE3 gene fusion in pediatric renal adenocarcinoma with t(X;17)(p11.2;q23). Oncogene 2003;22: 5374–8.

59. Argani P, Lae M, Hutchinson B, et al. Renal carcinomas with the t(6;11)(p21;q12): clinicopathologic features and demonstration of the specific alpha-TFEB gene fusion by immunohistochemistry, RT-PCR, and DNA PCR. Am J Surg Pathol 2005;29: 230–40.

60. Argani P, Hawkins A, Griffin CA, et al. A distinctive pediatric renal neoplasm characterized by epithelioid morphology, basement membrane production, focal HMB45 immunoreactivity, and t(6;11)(p21.1;q12) chromosome translocation. Am J Pathol 2001;158:2089–96.

61. Argani P, Antonescu CR, Illei PB, et al. Primary renal neoplasms with the ASPL-TFE3 gene fusion of alveolar soft part sarcoma: a distinctive tumor entity previously included among renal cell carcinomas of children and adolescents. Am J Pathol 2001;159: 179–92.

62. Delahunt B, Eble JN. Papillary renal cell carcinoma: a clinicopathologic and Immunohistochemical study of 105 tumors. Mod Pathol 1997;10:537–44.

63. Amin MB, Corless CL, Renshaw AA, et al. Papillary (chromophil) renal cell carcinomas: histomorphologic characteristics and evaluation of conventional pathologic prognostic parameters in 62 cases. Am J Surg Pathol 1997;21:621–35.

64. Skinnider BF, Folpe AL, Hennigar RA, et al. Distribution of cytokeratins and vimentin in adult renal cell neoplasms and normal renal tissue. Potential utility of

a cytokeratin antibody panel in the differential diagnosis of renal tumors. Am J Surg Pathol 2005;29:747–54.

65. Davis CJJ, Mostofi FK, Sesterhenn IA. Renal medullary carcinoma. The seventh sickle cell nephropathy. Am J Surg Pathol 1995;19:1–11.

66. Swartz MA, Karth J, Schneider DT, et al. Renal medullary carcinoma: clinical pathologic, Immunohistochemical, and genetic analysis with pathogenetic implications. Urology 2002;60:1083–9.

67. Medeiros LJ, Palmedo G, Krigmann HR, et al. Oncocytoid renal cell carcinoma after neuroblastoma: a report of four cases of a distinct clinicopathologic entity. Am J Surg Pathol 1999;23:772–80.

BENIGN AND MALIGNANT NEOPLASMS OF THE TESTIS AND PARATESTICULAR TISSUE

Tehmina Z. Ali, MD[a],*, Anil V. Parwani, MD, PhD[b]

KEYWORDS

• Testis • Testicular tumors • Paratesticular tissues • Paratesticular neoplasms • Testicular cancer

ABSTRACT

Benign and malignant tumors of the testes and paratesticular tissues present an interesting spectrum of diagnostic entities often encountered in routine surgical pathology practice. Germ cell tumors are the most common tumors of the testes and, despite a rising incidence, have excellent prognosis because of their radiosensitivity and/or effective chemotherapeutic agents. The proper classification of these tumors aids in the choice of appropriate treatment options. This article reviews benign and malignant neoplastic entities of the testes and paratesticular tissues and illustrates the classic pathologic characteristics. The differential diagnosis, ancillary studies, clinical significance, and presentation are discussed also.

BENIGN AND MALIGNANT NEOPLASMS OF THE TESTIS AND PARATESTICULAR TISSUE

OVERVIEW

Although the unique location of the testis allows even a small mass to be palpated, the painless nature of most testicular lesions often leads to a delay in diagnosis. Tumors that occur predominantly in the testes comprise a unique group of entities, although a few occur elsewhere in the body as well (**Box 1**). The incidence of testicular germ cell tumors increases shortly after puberty and peaks in the third and fourth decades of life.

Testicular germ cell tumors and sex cord–stromal tumors have counterparts that occur in the ovary. Testicular carcinoma is the most common malignancy in boys and young men age 15 to 34 years. More than 90% of all testicular tumors are malignant, and a mass or swelling in the testis is the most common presenting symptom. Testicular tumors can be categorized further as germ cell and non–germ cell tumors.

Germ cell tumors arise from spermatogenic cells, comprise more than 95% of testicular tumors, and account for most of the deaths caused by testicular tumors. Germ cell tumors can be divided into seminomatous and non-seminomatous tumors. Non-seminomatous germ cell tumors (NSGCTs) are composed of embryonal carcinoma, yolk sac tumor, immature or mature teratoma, choriocarcinoma, and other trophoblastic tumors.

The incidence of germ cell tumors of the testes is rising. It is estimated that 8090 new cases of testis cancer will be reported in the United States in 2008, but that there will be only 380 cancer-related deaths.[1] Germ cell tumors are seen predominantly in whites and rarely in African Americans. The incidence ratio of whites to African Americans is approximately 5:1. New advances in treatment options for germ cell tumors and the chemo- and radiosensitivity of these tumors give them an excellent prognosis.[2] The 5-year survival rate for all patients who have germ cell tumor is approximately 95%.

These tumors are morphologically diverse and thus can present diagnostic challenges.

[a] Department of Pathology, University of Maryland Medical Center, NBW47, 22 S. Greene Street, Baltimore, MD 21201, USA

[b] Pathology Informatics, Shadyside Hospital, University of Pittsburg Medical Center, 5230 Centre Avenue, Suite WG02.10, Pittsburgh, PA 15232, USA

* Corresponding author.

E-mail address: tali@umm.edu (T.Z. Ali).

Surgical Pathology 2 (2009) 61–159

doi:10.1016/j.path.2008.08.007

Box 1
Classification of testicular neoplasms

Precursor lesions
Intratubular germ cell neoplasia, unclassified

Tumors of one histologic type
Seminoma
    Seminoma with syncytiotrophoblastic cells

Spermatocytic seminoma
    Spermatocytic seminoma with sarcoma

Embryonal carcinoma
Yolk sac tumor
Trophoblastic tumors
    Choriocarcinoma
    Others

Teratoma
    Dermoid cyst
    Monodermal teratoma
    Teratoma with somatic-type malignancy

Tumors of more than one histologic type
Mixed germ cell tumors (combinations of any and various types, specify types and percentage of each component)

Germ cell–sex cord–stromal tumors
Gonadoblastoma
Germ cell–sex cord/gonadal–stromal tumors, unclassified

Sex cord–stromal tumors
Leydig cell tumor
Malignant Leydig cell tumor
Sertoli cell tumor
    Sclerosing Sertoli cell tumor
    Large cell calcifying Sertoli cell tumor
    Sertoli cell tumor, lipid rich variant

Malignant Sertoli cell tumor
Granulosa cell tumors
    Adult-type granulosa cell tumor
    Juvenile-type granulosa cell tumor

Fibroma-thecoma group
Mixed

Tumors of collecting ducts and rete
Adenoma
Carcinoma

Paratesticular tumors
Adenomatoid tumor
Malignant mesothelioma
Benign mesothelioma
    Well-differentiated papillary mesothelioma
    Cystic mesothelioma

Adenocarcinoma of the epididymis
Papillary cystadenoma of epididymis
Melanotic neuroectodermal tumor
Desmoplastic small round cell tumor
Hematopoietic tumors
Mesenchymal tumors of spermatic cord and testicular adnexa
Secondary tumors

Data from WHO Histologic classification of testis tumors. In: World Health Organization classification of tumors, pathology and genetics. Tumors of the urinary system and male genital organs. (Eble JN, Sauder G, Epstein JI, et al, editors. Lyon (France): ARC Press, 1004.)

Pathologists need to become acquainted with the cytomorphologic features of these tumors, because the clinical features and treatments differ among the entities.

Testicular cancers are most common in postpubertal men. These tumors are characterized genetically by the presence of one or more copies of an isochromosome of the short arm of chromosome 12 [i(12p)] or by other forms of 12p amplification and by aneuploidy. The consistent gain of genetic material from chromosome 12 seen in these tumors suggests that it has a crucial role in their development.[3]

Risk factors for testicular cancer include cryptorchidism, which is the most common congenital anomaly, dysgenetic gonads, and a family history of germ cell tumors. In a cohort study of 16,983 men, the risk of testicular cancer among men who were treated surgically for cryptorchidism at age 13 years or older was approximately twice that of men who underwent orchiopexy before the age of 13.[4] An increased incidence of contralateral disease is seen in patients who have a history of germ cell tumors.

A feature unique to testicular germ cell tumors is spontaneous regression. Typically the patient presents with a metastasis and an occult primary tumor. Upon examination of the involved testis, a scar with calcifications but little or no residual tumor is identified. In addition to morphologic overlap, the rarity of the non–germ cell tumors of the testes can pose diagnostic dilemmas. Metastasis to testis is rare.

Table 1 presents the American Joint Commission on Cancer tumor/node/metastasis (TNM) staging system for testicular cancer.

INTRATUBULAR GERM CELL NEOPLASIA, UNCLASSIFIED

OVERVIEW

Intratubular germ cell neoplasia, unclassified (IGCNU) is considered a precursor of all invasive germ cell tumors with the exception of spermatocytic seminoma and prepubertal germ cell tumors. This lesion was described first by Skakkebaek[5] in 1972, who noticed them in infertile men, and was called "carcinoma in situ." Because IGCNU is not an epithelial lesion, the term "carcinoma in situ" currently is not used. IGCNU is seen in association with all the various types of germ cell tumors except spermatocytic seminoma, pediatric yolk sac tumors, and teratomas. IGCNU is the malignant transformation of primordial germ cells and their proliferation within the seminiferous tubules.[6,7]

Table 1
TNM staging of testicular tumors

Classification	Criteria for Classification
Primary tumor (pT)	
pTX	Primary tumor cannot be assessed (if no radical orchiectomy has been performed, TX is used)
pT0	No evidence of primary tumor (eg, histologic scar in testis)
pTis	Intratubular germ cell neoplasia (carcinoma in situ)
pT1	Tumor limited to the testis and epididymis without vascular or lymphatic invasion; tumor may invade into the tunica albuginea, but not the tunica vaginalis
pT2	Tumor limited to the testis and epididymis with vascular or lymphatic invasion or tumor extending through the tunica albuginea with involvement of the tunica vaginalis
pT3	Tumor invades the spermatic cord with or without vascular or lymphatic invasion
pT4	Tumor invades the scrotum with or without vascular or lymphatic invasion
Regional lymph nodes (pN)	
pNX	Unknown nodal status
pN0	No regional node involvement
pN1	Node mass or single nodes $\leq$ 2cm; $\leq$ nodes involved (no node > 2cm)
pN2	Node mass > 2 but < 5cm: or > 5 nodes involved, none > 5cm; or evidence of extranodal tumor
pN3	Node mass > 5cm
Distant metastasis (M)	
MX	Distance metastasis cannot be assessed
M0	No distant metastasis
M1	Distant metastasis
M1a	Nonregional nodal or pulmonary metastasis
M1b	Distant metastasis other than to nonregional lymph nodes and lungs
Serum tumor markers (S)	
SX	No marker studies available
S0	All marker levels normal
S1	LDH < 1.5 $\times$ N1, plus hCG < 5,000 mIU/mL, plus AFP < ng/mL
S2	LDH 1.5–10 $\times$ N1, or hCG 5,000–50,000 mIU/mL, or AFP < 1,000–10,000 ng/mL
S3	LDH > 10 $\times$ N1, or hCG > 50,000 mIU/mL, or AFP >10,000ng/mL

Data from American Joint Committee on Cancer. AJCC cancer staging manual, 6th edition, New York: Springer; 2002;303–8.

Key Features
INTRATUBULAR GERM CELL NEOPLASIA

1. IGCNU cells, like seminoma cells, are oriented along the basement membrane

2. IGCNU cells are large polygonal cells with clear cytoplasm and a large, hyperchromatic, round nucleus with a central nucleolus

3. IGCNU cells are similar to seminoma cells in immunoprofile and ultrastructural appearance

4. The incidence of IGCNU is higher in patients who have cryptorchid testes

5. The contralateral testis to invasive germ cell tumor can harbor IGCNU

6. Untreated IGCNU progresses to germ cell tumors in approximately 50% of cases over a period of 5 years

Differential Diagnosis
INTRATUBULAR GERM CELL NEOPLASIA

- Testicular atrophy with Sertoli cells only can mimic IGCNU

- Prepubertal seminiferous tubules can show large germ cells that can be mistaken for IGCNU

Similarities between the morphology of IGCNU cells and that of primordial germ cells suggest that IGCNU originates from primordial germ cells or gonocytes. It has been suggested that dysgenesis may be caused by aberrant signalling between nurse cells and germ cells that allows embryonic germ cells to survive in the prepubertal and adult testis. Accumulated genetic changes lead to the development of IGCNU, resulting in invasive testicular cancer.[8,9]

Untreated IGCNUs progress to germ cell tumors over a period of 5 years in approximately 50% of cases. IGCNU is identified at a higher rate in 2% to 4% of patients who have cryptorchid testes, a condition with an incidence of 1% to 2%, which is known to carry an increased risk for developing germ cell tumors. Biopsy of cryptorchid testes at the time of orchiopexy showed IGCNU in 0.4% of cases. The lifetime risk for malignancy in the affected testis is 3% to 5%; 80% of the germ cell tumors that occur in these testes are seminomas. Contralateral testis to invasive germ cell tumor also can harbor IGCNU in up to 5% of cases, as can dysgenetic gonads.[6,8–10]

GROSS FEATURES

IGCNU does not form a mass lesion. The cryptorchid testis harboring IGCNU can be atrophic.

MICROSCOPIC FEATURES

IGCNU occurs in atrophic seminiferous tubules with thickened tunica propria and germ cell aplasia. Adjacent tubules may show active spermatogenesis. The cells are similar in appearance to seminoma cells and are oriented along the basement membrane. IGCNU cells are large, polygonal cells with clear cytoplasm and a large, hyperchromatic, round nucleus with a central nucleolus (**Fig. 1**). Mitotic figures, sometimes atypical, are seen. Spermatogenesis almost always is absent in the tubules with IGCNU, and Sertoli cells may be pushed towards the lumen. When IGCNU cells completely replace the Sertoli cells and fill and distend the seminiferous tubules, the condition is called "intratubular seminoma."[10] Intratubular microlithiasis sometimes is associated with IGCNU (**Fig. 2**). IGCNU cells frequently show pagetoid spread along rete testis epithelium (**Fig. 3**).

DIFFERENTIAL DIAGNOSIS

DIAGNOSIS

Immunohistochemistry with placental alkaline phosphatase (PLAP), cKit (CD117), and, recently, OCT3/4 (POU5f1) is used to identify IGCNU. These markers are highly sensitive and specific in identifying IGCNU; with these markers, staining of the non-neoplastic germ cells, as sometimes occurs with periodic acid-Schiff (PAS) stain, is minimal or rare (with PLAP). OCT3/4 is a nuclear stain, whereas PLAP and CD117 show membranous positivity (**Fig. 4**). The immunoprofile and ultrastructural appearance of the IGCNU are similar to that of seminoma cells. PAS stain also can identify most cases of IGCNU but sometimes also

Pitfall
INTRATUBULAR GERM CELL NEOPLASIA

! In patients younger than 1 year, the primordial germ cells and spermatogonia are identical to IGCNU cells in appearance and immunohistochemical profile.

Fig. 1. Atrophic seminiferous tubules with intratubular germ cell neoplasia, unclassified (original magnification ×200). Large neoplastic germ cells are oriented basally, with ample clear cytoplasm and enlarged round nucleus with prominent nucleoli. The tubules show germ cell aplasia with Sertoli cells. Notice the peritubular fibrosis.

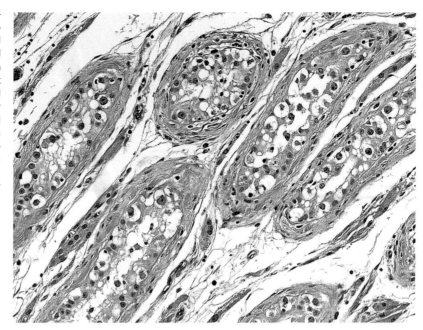

stains non-neoplastic spermatogonia and Sertoli cells.[11] One of the major diagnostic pitfalls is in the diagnosis of IGCNU in patients younger than 1 year old, because the appearance and immunohistochemical profile of the primordial germ cells and spermatogonia in this age group can be identical to the cells of IGCNU. **Box 2** summarizes the markers for IGCNU.

PROGNOSIS

Studies have shown that, if left untreated, up to 90% of testes with IGCNU progress to malignant germ cell tumors within 7 years. The therapy for IGCNU is surgery, irradiation, or watchful waiting.[10,12]

SEMINOMA

OVERVIEW

Classic seminoma is the most common testicular neoplasm. It accounts for up to 50% of the all

---

Box 2
Markers for intratubular germ cell neoplasia

IGCNU is positive for

PLAP: membranous positivity

cKit (CD117): membranous positivity

OCT3/4 (POU5f1): nuclear stain

PAS

Key Features
SEMINOMA

1. Classic seminoma accounts for up to one half of the all germ cell tumors

2. It most often presents as painless testicular enlargement in the fourth decade

3. Grossly seminoma is a demarcated, lobulated, creamy, homogeneous mass, most often without hemorrhages and necrosis

4. Microscopically, large, pale to clear cells with a central nucleus and prominent nucleoli are arranged most commonly in sheets that are divided into lobules by fibrous septa containing lymphocytic infiltrate

5. Approximately 20% of seminomas contain syncytiotrophoblastic giant cells, and 50% show a granulomatous response.

6. Seminomas occasionally can show intertubular, microcystic, or tubular growth patterns and signet-ring cell features

7. Most patients are treated by orchiectomy followed by radiation and chemotherapy

8. The survival rate for patients who have seminoma is greater than 95%, regardless of stage

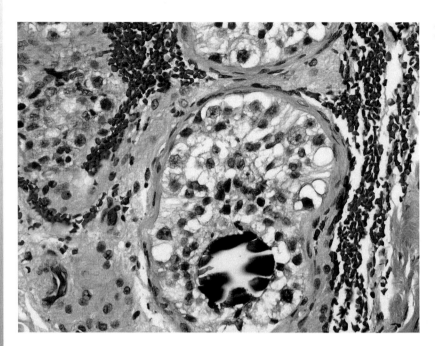

Fig. 2. IGCNU associated with a microlith (original magnification ×400).

germ cell tumors.[13–16] The peak incidence for seminoma occurs in the fourth decade of life, approximately 10 years later than that of NSGCTs. Seminoma most often presents as painless testicular enlargement, occasionally associated with a hydrocele. The characteristic sonographic appearance of seminoma is well-demarcated, somewhat lobulated, and uniformly hypoechoic. Large tumors can give a heterogeneous signal.[17]

GROSS FEATURES

The affected testis is enlarged, and the seminoma forms a bulky, lobulated, pale grey to creamy, soft, homogeneous mass (**Fig. 5**). Hemorrhage, necrosis, and cyst formation are rare. Occasionally, seminoma arises in an atrophic testis. Sometimes nodules separate from the main mass are present, and a multinodular gross appearance occasionally is observed. Large tumors may show areas of necrosis.

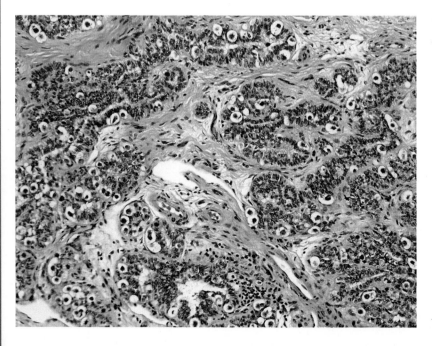

Fig. 3. Pagetoid spread of IGCNU along rete testis epithelium (original magnification ×200).

Fig. 4. Placental alkaline phosphatase immunostain highlighting the malignant cells of IGCNU (original magnification ×200).

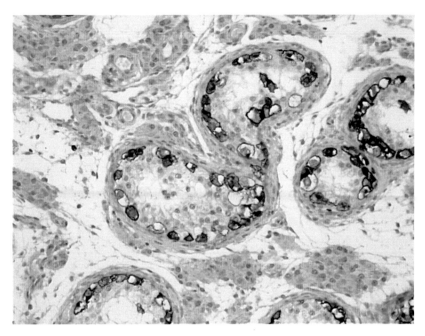

MICROSCOPIC FEATURES

In its most common presentation, seminoma shows a sheetlike growth pattern of large, monomorphic, polygonal cells with ample clear to lightly eosinophilic cytoplasm. The large central nucleus has one or more prominent nucleoli, and the cells show defined cytoplasmic borders. The clear appearance of seminoma cell cytoplasm results from the presence of glycogen. Almost all seminomas have a lymphocytic infiltrate in the fibrovascular septa that divide the tumor cells into lobules, columns, or nests (**Fig. 6**). Occasionally, in classic seminoma a granulomatous response and fibrosis can obliterate the tumor cells almost completely (**Fig. 7**). Mitoses can be brisk. Large tumors show necrosis.

Fig. 5. Gross bivalved testis with seminoma almost replacing the parenchyma, which is present at the superior pole. The typical gross appearance of pure seminoma is a soft, cream-colored lobulated tumor without hemorrhages or necrosis.

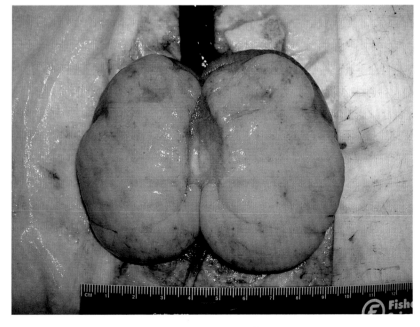

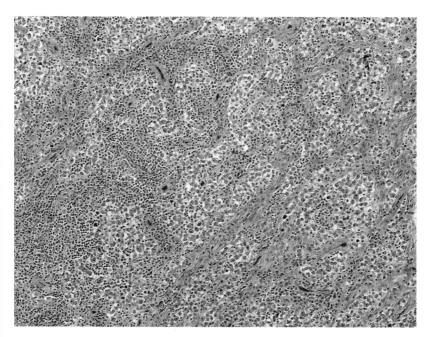

Fig. 6. Low-power view: typical microscopic appearance showing branching fibrous septa dividing sheets of seminoma cells with clear cytoplasm. The septa contain inflammatory infiltrates composed predominantly of lymphocytes (original magnification ×100).

Small seminomas may show an intertubular growth pattern (also known as "interstitial invasion" or "microinvasion"). This arrangement may cause mild enlargement of the testis without an obvious mass and also is seen at the edge of a large tumor (**Fig. 8**). Intratubular growth of seminoma is illustrated by seminiferous tubular lumens filled with seminoma cells. Pagetoid spread of seminoma cells along the rete testis can be seen.

Some seminomas show a microcystic, pseudoglandular, or cribriform pattern, in which the tumor cells form small spaces lined by seminoma cells (**Fig. 9**);[16,18,19] however, this change sometimes may be attributed to edema.[20] The other occasionally seen pattern of seminomas is a solid tubular pattern in which the cells are arranged in elongated nests and tubules that have a palisaded arrangement at the periphery.[19,21]

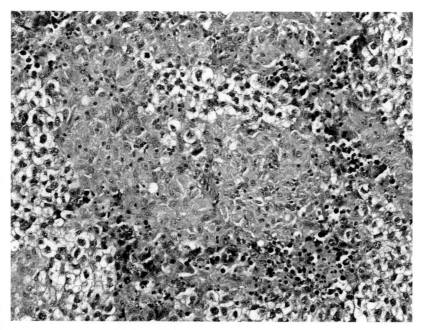

Fig. 7. Granulomatous response in a seminoma (original magnification ×200).

Fig. 8. Seminiferous tubules with IGCNU and intertubular seminoma cells without destruction of the tubules (original magnification ×200). Seminoma cells sometimes are found with a predominant interstitial growth without forming a mass. This pattern is seen commonly at the edge of a seminoma.

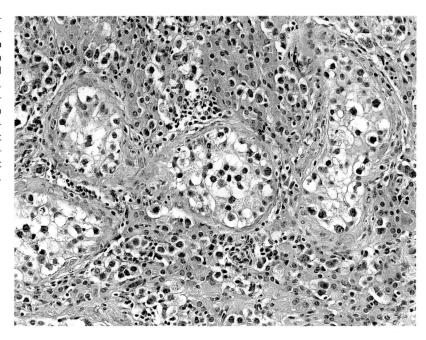

Up to 50% of seminomas show a granulomatous response ranging from scattered or collected epithelioid histiocytes to organized granuloma formation (see **Fig. 7**). The granulomatous reaction can be intense, making identification of tumor cells difficult.[11]

Approximately 20% of seminomas have a scattered population of syncytiotrophoblastic giant cells.[22,23] Usually these cells are dispersed widely and therefore do not cause diagnostic problems (**Fig. 10**), but when they cluster they can be mistaken for choriocarcinoma. The absence of

Fig. 9. Seminoma with microcystic pattern (original magnification ×200).

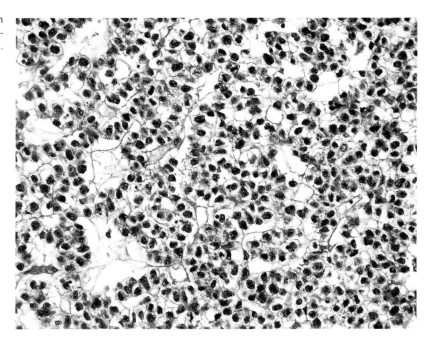

an admixture of syncytiotrophoblastic giant cells with cytotrophoblasts is helpful in ruling out the presence of choriocarcinoma, which shows more nuclear pleomorphism and eosinophilic cytoplasm than seen in seminoma cells.

Recently, two cases of seminomas with conspicuous signet-ring cells, with cytoplasmic contents pushing the nucleus in to an eccentric location, have been described. In one case the cells contained glycogen. In the other case the cells contained empty vacuoles. One was a pure seminoma. The second was part of a mixed germ cell tumor.[12]

DIFFERENTIAL DIAGNOSIS

Occasionally, seminoma can show pleomorphism and a high mitotic rate ("anaplastic seminoma," a term no longer in common use). These tumors may be mistaken for embryonal carcinoma. Embryonal carcinoma, however, has overlapping pleomorphic nuclei with indistinct cell borders, usually forms cords or papillary or glandular structures, and tends to have more necrosis than seminoma. The presence of an inflammatory infiltrate also is helpful in ruling out embryonal carcinoma. PLAP (positive in seminoma) and CD30 (positive in embryonal carcinoma) immunostains can help differentiate between the two entities when cytomorphology is inconclusive.

It may be difficult to differentiate the microcystic pattern of seminoma from that of yolk sac tumor. In seminoma, large polygonal seminoma cells

△△ **Differential Diagnosis**
SEMINOMA

- Embryonal carcinoma: does not have distinct cell borders; nuclei overlap; shows much more pleomorphism and necrosis than seminoma

- Yolk sac tumor has a solid pattern can be confused with seminoma; other areas show regular yolk sac patterns

- Spermatocytic seminoma does not have the regular fibrous septa with lymphocytic infiltrates

- Sertoli cell tumor has no associated IGCNU and is inhibin positive

- Leydig cell tumor has no associated IGCNU and is inhibin positive

- Testicular lymphoma shows interstitial growth and is positive for lymphoid markers

line the cystic spaces; in yolk sac tumor, flattened epithelium lines the microcystic spaces.[20] OCT3/4 and PLAP are positive, and cytokeratin immunostains are negative in seminomas. Rarely, some seminomas may show cytokeratin positivity but not as diffusely as does yolk sac tumor. Other germ cell tumors lack the lymphocytic infiltrate, which is a common helpful diagnostic feature of

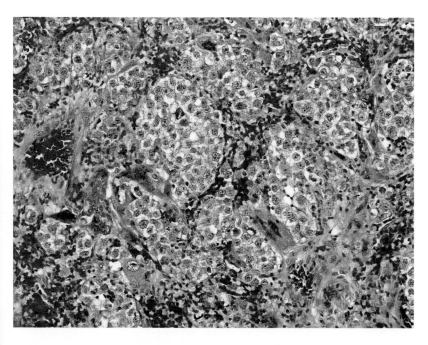

Fig. 10. Syncytiotrophoblastic giant cells are seen in this seminoma (original magnification ×200).

the classic seminoma. Rarely, seminomas may show very focal and scant lymphocytic infiltrates.

The tubular pattern of classic seminoma can cause confusion with a Sertoli cell tumor because of the palisaded arrangement of the tumor cells. Malignant Sertoli cells tumors can show predominant sheetlike growth, clear cells, and prominent nucleoli mimicking seminoma.[24] Adjacent IGCNU can help rule out a Sertoli cell tumor. PLAP and OCT3/4 are positive in seminoma, whereas inhibin is positive in Sertoli cell tumor.[25,26]

The other entity to be considered in the differential diagnosis for seminoma is spermatocytic seminoma. Spermatocytic seminoma usually occurs in an older age group; the cytology is more polymorphous than that classic seminoma, and it lacks a lymphocytic infiltrate. IGCNU is not associated with spermatocytic seminoma. Spermatocytic seminoma is not positive for the immunostains that stain seminoma, except for CD117.[27]

Seminoma with intense granulomatous response may mimic inflammatory granulomatous reactions. In testes idiopathic granulomatous orchitis can show granulomas centered in and on the seminiferous tubules. IGCNU are found in the residual tubules, and immunostains (eg, PLAP) highlight the residual seminoma cells not obliterated by the granulomatous response (**Fig. 11**).

Leydig cell tumors may show clear or vacuolated cytoplasm, thus raising a suspicion for seminoma. This appearance can be problematic during the evaluation of a frozen section. Leydig cell tumors stain with inhibin, whereas seminoma cells are negative.

Rarely, metastatic clear cell renal cell carcinoma to the testis mimics seminoma. In such cases the absence of IGCNU, clinical history, and immunohistochemistry are helpful in ruling out metastatic renal cell carcinoma.

Testicular lymphoma enters the differential diagnosis of seminoma as either a primary testicular lymphoma or as a secondary manifestation. Malignant lymphoma occurs at an older age and may involve bilateral testes. Lymphoma also may show an interstitial growth pattern, unlike most seminomas, and have irregular nuclei with indistinct cell borders and eosinophilic cytoplasm. Immunohistochemistry for CD45 (leukocyte common antigen) and other seminoma markers can be used.

Seminoma with conspicuous signet-ring cells shows positivity with CD117 and PLAP. At a metastatic site these cells can be confused with poorly differentiated adenocarcinoma. These cells are negative for mucicarmine.[12]

DIAGNOSIS

The typical cytomorphologic appearance of the seminoma is the most characteristic and helpful diagnostic feature. Seminoma occurs as testicular enlargement, and approximately 10% of cases

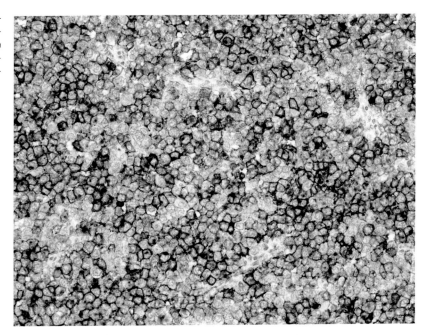

Fig. 11. Placental alkaline phosphatase immunostain in a seminoma with membranous staining (original magnification ×200).

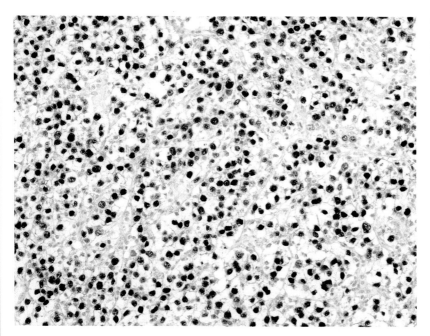

Fig. 12. OCT3/4 (POU5F1) immunostain showing nuclear positivity in seminoma (original magnification ×200).

present with testicular pain. Fewer than 3% of cases present with symptoms related to metastatic disease (eg., back pain secondary to a large retroperitoneal metastasis).[2]

When syncytiotrophoblastic giant cells are present as part of the classic seminoma, they synthesize and secrete human chorionic gonadotropin (hCG). The serum β subunit of hCG is increased, but the value is in 100s, whereas in the presence of choriocarcinoma serum hCG levels are in 1000s (mIU/mL).

Immunohistochemical stains helpful in confirming seminoma include PLAP (see **Fig. 11**), CD117 (cKit), and OCT3/4 (POU5F1) (**Fig. 12**), a recently described nuclear transcription factor that stains seminoma and embryonal carcinoma as well as IGCNU. Recent literature indicates that the monoclonal antibody podoplanin (D2-40) diffusely stains 100% of seminomas, whereas it focally stains only 29% of embryonal carcinomas.[28,29] Rarely, seminomas may show focal positivity with cytokeratins (eg, CAM 5.2); more often, the positivity is in a paranuclear dotlike pattern.[30–32] **Box 3** summarizes the markers for seminoma.

PROGNOSIS

Seminomas are extremely radiation- and chemosensitive, and most patients are treated with both radiation and chemotherapy after orchiectomy. Seminomas rarely invade the spermatic cord and epididymis, and it is unusual for seminomas to involve the vaginal sac.[17] Seminomas

Pitfall
SEMINOMA

! Some seminomas can stain patchily with cytokeratin.

spread to the para-aortic lymph nodes via lymphatics and then to the mediastinal and supraclavicular lymph nodes. Later in the course of the disease, seminoma can spread

Box 3
Markers for seminoma

Seminoma is positive for

PLAP

OCT3/4 (POU5F1)

CD117 (cKit)

The monoclonal antibody D2-40 stains 100% of seminomas diffusely but stains only 29% of embryonal carcinomas focally

Seminoma is negative for

CD30

Inhibin

Epithelial membrane antigen (EMA)

Cytokeratins (rarely, positive; when positive, staining is not as diffuse as in yolk sac tumors)

Mucicarmine

hematogenously to liver, lung, bones, and other organs. Disease is limited to the testis in approximately 75% of cases at the time of initial presentation, 25% of cases show retroperitoneal metastasis, and about 5% have other subdiaphragmatic involvement.[2]

Orchiectomy is followed by ipsilateral retroperitoneal, inguinal, and iliac irradiation of the lymph nodes for stage I, IIA, and IIB seminoma. Large retroperitoneal and supradiaphragmatic metastases are treated with platinum-based chemotherapy. The survival rate for all stages of seminomas is greater than 95%, and approximately 99% of patients who have stage I, IIA, or IIB seminoma are ultimately cured.[33] Overall, the size of the primary tumor, necrosis, vascular space, and tunical invasion have been related to clinical stage at presentation.[30,34]

SPERMATOCYTIC SEMINOMA

OVERVIEW

Spermatocytic seminoma is a rare, distinct testicular tumor composed of cells of three different sizes and is more common in older men. This tumor, initially described by Masson (1946), has a peak incidence at age 55 years[35,36] and is extremely rare in men under 30 years of age.[37] Spermatocytic seminoma comprises 1% to 2% of testicular germ cell tumors.[15,20,36] It occurs only in testis and has no counterparts in the ovary or outside the gonads. There is no elevation of any serum tumor marker. Other clinicopathologic differences from the classic seminoma include:[16,37,38]

- No association with IGCNU
- PLAP negativity (for the most part)
- No association with cryptorchidism or i(12p)
- Rarity of metastasis

Bilateral involvement can occur, metachronously, in up to 9% of cases.[37,39] A case of synchronous bilateral spermatocytic seminomas has been reported recently.[40] The presence of tumor cells that appear polyploid in cases of spermatocytic seminoma has led to the suggestion that this tumor may arise from the "self-fertilization" of germ cells. This hypothesis is in keeping with the location of spermatocytic seminoma in the testis only.[27]

GROSS FEATURES

Spermatocytic seminoma is a slow-growing tumor that presents with painless testicular enlargement. The average size is 7 cm, but tumors as large as 20 cm have been reported.[37] These tumors are

Key Features
SPERMATOCYTIC SEMINOMA

1. Spermatocytic seminoma is a rare tumor, seen usually in men more than 55 years old

2. The gross appearance if bulky, lobulated, bulging, and mucoid

3. It is a distinct testicular tumor composed of cells of three different sizes ranging from 6 to 100 μm

4. Intermediate-sized cells, 15–20 μm in diameter, predominate

5. The nucleus is round with finely granular to lacelike or filamentous "spireme" chromatin

6. Polymorphous cells are arranged in a sheet-like pattern, as in classic seminoma, but fibrous septa with lymphocytic infiltrates are absent

7. The sheets of noncohesive cells often are interrupted by prominent edema

8. Edema can result in a pseudoglandular, nested, or trabecular pattern

9. IGCNU is absent

10. The prognosis is excellent

well demarcated, bulky, and lobulated with a bulging mucoid to gray, solid, fleshy cut surface. Cystic, hemorrhagic, and necrotic areas can be seen with rare extratesticular extension.[41]

MICROSCOPIC FEATURES

The polymorphous cells of spermatocytic seminoma are arranged in a sheetlike pattern resembling classic seminoma, but the regular fibrous septa, lymphocytic infiltrates, and granulomas of classic seminoma are noticeably absent, and there is only scant, inconspicuous stroma (**Fig. 13**). The sheets of noncohesive cells often are interrupted by edema, which can be quite prominent, explaining the gelatinous/mucoid gross appearance. Edema can cause the cells to arrange in a pseudoglandular, nested, or trabecular pattern (**Fig. 14**).[11] Occasionally vascular, tunical, or epididymal invasion can be identified.[37,42,43]

The tripartite cell population is composed of cells that contain uniform round nuclei and are of three different sizes, ranging from 6 to 100 μm:[11,20] small lymphocyte-like cells, intermediate-sized cells, which predominate and average 15 to 20 μm in diameter, and large or giant cells (**Fig. 15**). The

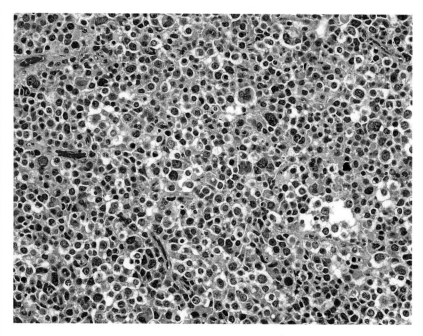

Fig. 13. Spermatocytic seminoma showing sheetlike growth pattern uninterrupted by fibrous septa or inflammatory cells (original magnification ×200). The cytoplasm is eosinophilic. The nuclei are variably sized and appear pleomorphic.

small cells have a pyknotic nucleus with scant eosinophilic cytoplasm. The intermediate-sized cells are round and have variable amounts of eosinophilic cytoplasm. The nucleus is round and has finely granular to lacelike or filamentous "spireme" chromatin, which resembles the chromatin of the primary spermatocytes in meiotic prophase. The large cells have average diameter of 50 to 100 μm. These cells can be multinucleated and may show the spireme chromatin. The cytoplasm can be eosinophilic to amphophilic and does not contain glycogen. Mitotic activity frequently is brisk; atypical mitoses are present. Often, intratubular growth is seen in the seminiferous tubules adjacent to spermatocytic seminoma (Fig. 16). A rare morphologic variant known as

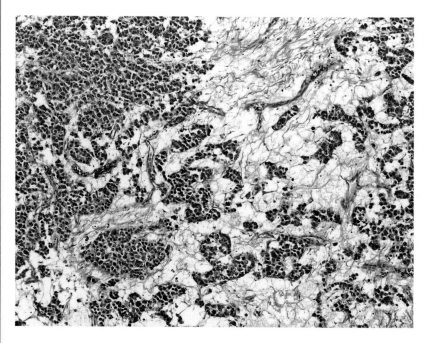

Fig. 14. Edematous stroma gives this area a somewhat trabecular and nested appearance (original magnification ×100).

Fig. 15. Spermatocytic seminoma with three different cell types (original magnification ×400). Small cells with pyknotic nuclei and medium cells with uniform round nucleus predominate. Large cells sometimes can be multinucleated and have the appearance of giant cells. Note the intermediate and large cells with a spireme chromatin pattern similar to that of primary spermatocytes.

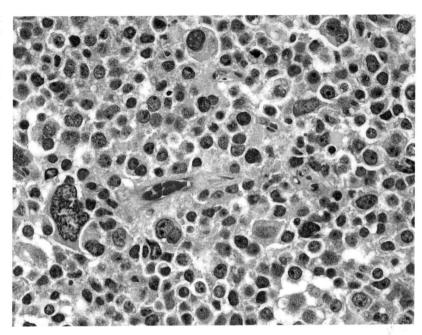

"anaplastic" spermatocytic seminoma shows a monomorphic cell population of intermediate-sized cells with prominent nucleoli. Areas of typical morphology usually can be identified within these tumors and are not thought to portend a worse prognosis,[44] although long-term follow-up and a larger series may be needed to confirm this finding.

DIFFERENTIAL DIAGNOSIS

The differential diagnosis for spermatocytic seminoma includes classic seminoma, testicular lymphoma, and solid variants of embryonal carcinoma and yolk sac tumor.

Embryonal carcinoma, yolk sac tumor, and seminoma all have adjacent IGCNU; spermatocytic seminoma does not.[45] The typical

Fig. 16. Spermatocytic seminoma with inter- and intratubular growth that can mimic IGCNU (original magnification ×200).

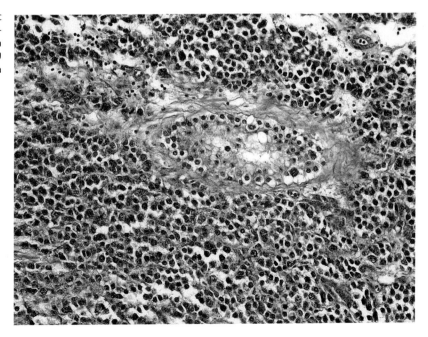

immunohistochemical markers PLAP, D2-40 (for seminoma), alpha-fetoprotein (AFP) (for yolk sac tumor) OCT3/4 (for seminoma and embryonal carcinoma), and cytokeratins and CD30 (for embryonal carcinoma) are negative in spermatocytic seminoma. Focal cytoplasmic staining with CAM5.2 has been reported in some cases.[46] CD117, however, does not discriminate between seminoma, embryonal carcinoma, and spermatocytic seminoma, because it highlights all of them.

Testicular lymphoma, which is the most common testicular neoplasm in older men, shows an interstitial growth pattern, and the chromatin pattern is fine to clumped, whereas the chromatin of spermatocytic seminoma is filamentous. The cellular size is more uniform in lymphoma, and typical lymphoma immunohistochemical markers can help confirm the diagnosis.

DIAGNOSIS

Familiarity with the typical histologic features of spermatocytic seminoma is important. The cells do not stain for glycogen (PAS), nor for OCT3/4 and PLAP [27]; some cases have shown focal positivity with PLAP.[46,47] Only focal cytoplasmic staining with CAM5.2 was noted in some cases, but these tumors are negative for cytokeratins. Positivity for CD117 (cKit)[48] and for the germ cell marker VASA has been reported uniformly.[49]

Ultrastructural examination of these tumors shows that they exhibit structures that make them capable of meiotic division, have specialized junctions, true intercellular bridges and Golgi apparatus.[50] Others found that spermatocytic seminoma represents a better-differentiated variant of seminoma than the classic type, but they oppose the view that spermatocytic seminoma is composed of spermatocytes capable of meiotic division. Spermatocytic seminoma is thought to be composed of cells differentiating in the direction of spermatocytes but that have not yet reached this stage of differentiation.[51] Markers for spermatocytic seminoma are listed in **Box 4**.

PROGNOSIS

Spermatocytic seminoma usually has an indolent course, with extremely rare metastatic potential;[52,53] however, when sarcomatous change occurs, as seen in approximate 6% of cases, the behavior changes dramatically to that of a high-grade sarcoma.[37,54–56] The history then typically is a rapid enlargement of a previously slow-growing mass, and metastases are composed exclusively of the sarcomatous component.[55] Bishop and colleagues[57] noted increased apoptosis in spermatocytic seminoma, possibly mediated by FAS-independent activation of the death receptor pathway. This observation may provide some insight into the excellent prognosis

---

Box 4
Markers for spermatocytic seminoma

Spermatocytic seminoma is positive for

CD117 (cKit)

Germ cell marker VASA

Focal cytoplasmic staining with CAM5.2

Spermatocytic seminoma is negative for

PLAP (may show occasional focal staining)

D2-40 (for seminoma)

AFP (yolk sac tumor)

OCT3/4 (seminoma and embryonal carcinoma)

Cytokeratins (embryonal carcinoma)

CD30 (embryonal carcinoma)

Glycogen (PAS)

for spermatocytic seminoma. The treatment of choice is orchiectomy followed by surveillance. In cases of sarcomatous transformation, the prognosis remains grim even after aggressive chemotherapy.[55,58]

EMBRYONAL CARCINOMA

OVERVIEW

Embryonal carcinoma is a malignant germ cell tumor with primitive cells that show minimal or no differentiation. Pure embryonal carcinoma is relatively rare and accounts for 2% to 3% of all germ cell tumors. After seminoma embryonal carcinoma is the second most common single-cell type of germ cell tumor. Embryonal carcinoma is present as a component in more than 80% of mixed germ cell tumors. Elevated serum AFP and hCG can be detected in most cases. Survival depends largely on the stage of the tumor.[10,59,60]

Pure embryonal carcinoma occurs most frequently in the third and fourth decades, primarily in men between the ages 25 and 35 years; the median patient age at presentation is 32 years. The incidence of embryonal carcinoma peaks at age 30, 10 years earlier than for seminomas. Embryonal carcinoma is rare in patients more than 50 years old. More than 60% of the patients present with distant metastases, including metastasis to retroperitoneal lymph nodes, at the time of diagnosis. Pain is a common presentation in patients who have embryonal carcinoma.[10,11,20]

Key Features
EMBRYONAL CARCINOMA

The typical embryonal carcinoma cell

1. Is polygonal, with an epithelial appearance with large vesicular nuclei and a distinct nuclear membrane
2. Has hyperchromatic pleomorphic nuclei with prominent nucleoli
3. Has voluminous cytoplasm
4. Has an indistinct cell border

GROSS FEATURES

On gross examination, embryonal carcinoma often has a poorly demarcated and variegated mass. These tumors usually are small, as compared with seminomas. The tumor is soft and has a soft gray-tan cut surface with red and brown areas caused by the presence of large foci of hemorrhage and necrosis (**Fig. 17**). When embryonal carcinoma is admixed with other tumors such as a teratoma, grossly cystic areas may be prominent. The tumor may be confined to the testis or may extend to paratesticular tissue.[11]

MICROSCOPIC FEATURES

Histologic examination of embryonal carcinoma reveals a variety of growth patterns including solid, glandular, acinar, tubular, and papillary structures (**Figs. 18 and 19**). There often are large

Fig. 17. Gross image showing bivalved testis with embryonal carcinoma. Note area of hemorrhage. (*Courtesy of* S.G. Silverberg, MD, Baltimore, MD.)

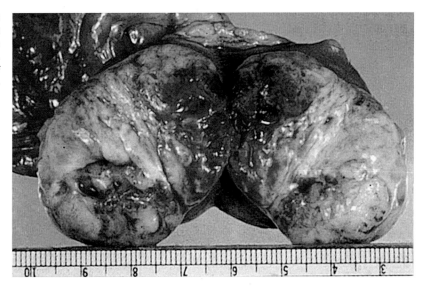

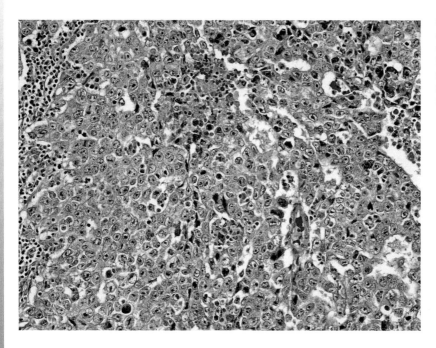

Fig. 18. Solid growth of embryonal carcinoma, with pleomorphic overlapping cells and necrosis. This appearance can mimic seminoma (original magnification ×200).

areas of necrosis and hemorrhage. Embryonal carcinoma often is highly cellular and shows anaplasia, increased mitoses, and pleomorphic, undifferentiated cells. The typical carcinoma cell is polygonal with an epithelial appearance, with large vesicular nuclei and a distinct nuclear membrane.[20,59] The cells have hyperchromatic pleomorphic nuclei with prominent nucleoli. The cytoplasm is voluminous, and the typical cell border is not very distinct (**Fig. 20**). Intratubular germ cell neoplasia or, less commonly, intratubular embryonal carcinoma may be seen in the adjacent testicular parenchyma (**Fig. 21**). Embryonal carcinoma often is admixed with teratoma, yolk sac tumor, or other types of germ cell tumor.[11,20,59] Lymphatic and vascular invasion are more common with embryonal carcinoma than with other germ cell tumors (**Fig. 22**).

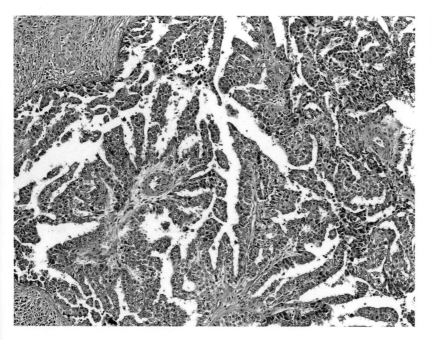

Fig. 19. Papillary growth pattern of embryonal carcinoma with fibrovascular cores (original magnification ×100).

Fig. 20. High-power view of embryonal carcinoma with pleomorphic vesicular overlapping nuclei with prominent nucleoli, amphophilic cytoplasm with indistinguishable cell borders, increased mitoses, and apoptosis (original magnification ×400).

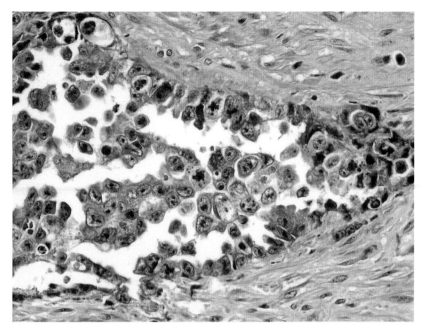

DIFFERENTIAL DIAGNOSIS

Solid embryonal carcinoma can mimic a seminoma in both gross and histologic appearance with some overlapping features. Occasionally, embryonal carcinoma cells may have a clear cytoplasm or a seminomatous component, resulting in a misdiagnosis of seminoma. An important distinguishing feature is that cells are arranged more irregularly in embryonal carcinoma than in a seminoma. Syncytiotrophoblastic cells occasionally are admixed in embryonal carcinoma and should not be confused with a choriocarcinoma component.[11,20,59,61]

Additionally, the solid component of embryonal carcinoma sometimes may have light central cells and dark peripheral cells, mimicking the appearance of a choriocarcinoma. Another pitfall occurs with the tubular form of a seminoma, a rare subtype that may mimic an embryonal carcinoma.[21] For extratesticular masses, the differential diagnosis often includes a somatic carcinoma. Embryonal carcinomas frequently are positive for cytokeratins but are negative for epithelial membrane antigen (EMA), which can help distinguish a metastatic embryonal carcinoma from a somatic carcinoma.[62] The entire specimen always should be sampled carefully and, when appropriate, immunohistochemistry markers should be used to arrive at a correct diagnosis.[10,59,61]

 Differential Diagnosis
EMBRYONAL CARCINOMA

- The gross and histologic appearances of seminoma have some overlapping features with embryonal carcinoma. Embryonal carcinoma cells are more irregularly arranged than cells in a seminoma

- Syncytiotrophoblastic cells occasionally are admixed in embryonal carcinoma and can be confused with a choriocarcinoma component

- The solid component of embryonal carcinoma can have the central light cells and peripheral dark cells seen in choriocarcinoma

- Unlike somatic carcinoma, embryonal carcinoma is negative for epithelial membrane antigen (EMA) even when positive for cytokeratins

DIAGNOSIS

Immunohistochemistry is useful in the diagnosis of embryonal carcinoma and can help distinguish it from other germ cell tumors. Embryonal carcinomas are positive for OCT3/4, CD30, and cytokeratins such as CK7, CAM5.2, and AE1/AE3 and sometimes are positive focally for PLAP. Embryonal carcinomas usually are negative for high

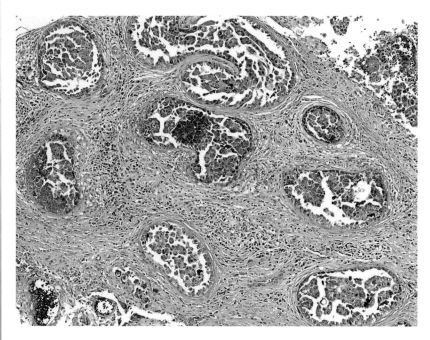

Fig.   21. Intratubular growth of embryonal carcinoma (original magnification ×100).

molecular weight cytokeratins and EMA. PLAP and OCT 3/4 do not distinguish embryonal carcinoma from seminoma. CD30 stains only embryonal carcinoma; it does not stain seminoma, yolk sac tumor, or any other germ cell tumors (**Fig. 23**); frequently, however, metastatic embryonal carcinoma is negative for CD30 after chemotherapy.[28,59,61–63] Markers for embryonal carcinoma are presented in **Box 5**.

PROGNOSIS

Embryonal carcinoma is best treated with orchiectomy followed by combination chemotherapy. Studies have shown that with treatment the overall 5-year survival rate is as high as 88%, and the survival rate is even higher (98%) for patients who have localized disease.[64,65]

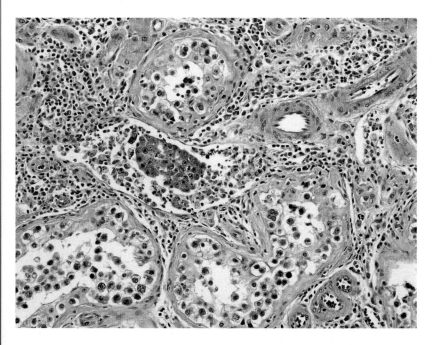

Fig. 22. Lymphovascular invasion by embryonal carcinoma (original magnification ×200). Note adjacent seminiferous tubules with IGCNU.

Fig. 23. A CD30 immu-
nostain with membra-
nous staining of
embryonal carcinoma
(original magnification
×200).

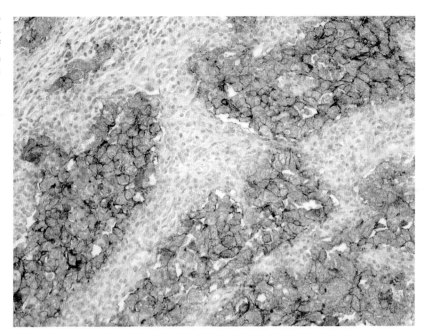

Pitfalls
EMBRYONAL CARCINOMA

! Clear cytoplasm in embryonal carcinoma cells often leads to a misdiagnosis of seminoma.

! The tubular form of a seminoma is a rare subtype that may mimic embryonal carcinoma.

! Incorrect diagnosis can result from sampling less than the entire specimen.

! Use immunohistochemistry markers to arrive at a correct diagnosis.

! After chemotherapy, metastatic embryonal carcinoma frequently is negative for CD30.

Box 5
Markers for embryonal carcinoma

Embryonal carcinoma is positive for

PLAP

OCT3/4

CD-30

Cytokeratins such as CK7, CAM5.2, AE1/AE3

Embryonal carcinoma is negative for

High molecular weight cytokeratins

EMA

After chemotherapy, metastatic embryonal carcinoma can be negative for CD30.

YOLK SAC TUMORS

OVERVIEW

Yolk sac tumor can involve the embryonic yolk sac, allantois, and extra-embryonic mesenchyme.[66] Pure yolk sac tumor is seen predominantly in infants and children younger than 4 years; the mean patient age at presentation is between 16 and 18 months. Pediatric yolk sac tumor is not associated with cryptorchidism or intratubular germ cell neoplasia. Yolk sac tumor is the most common childhood testicular tumor, comprising up to 80% of prepubertal germ cell tumors.[16] Pure yolk sac tumor is extremely rare in adults, but up to 40% of mixed germ cell tumors in adults have a yolk sac component.[59,67–69] In adults, the age range for developing a mixed germ cell tumor with a yolk sac component is 17 to 40 years.[16] Most commonly, patients present with a rapidly growing, painless testicular mass.[59,67,70]

GROSS FEATURES

Yolk sac tumors have a solid, lobulated, tan-yellow to gray-white appearance. The mass often is ill defined with a glistening cut surface. Occasional cases may have hemorrhage, necrosis, and cystic change, most likely caused by the presence of other germ cell elements such as teratoma.[59,71]

MICROSCOPIC FEATURES

Yolk sac tumor presents with a large spectrum of histologic and growth patterns; the architecture

Key Features
YOLK SAC TUMORS

1. Pure yolk sac tumor is seen predominantly in infants and children younger than age 4 years

2. In adults, typical yolk sac tumor is a component of 40% of mixed germ cell tumors

3. Yolk sac tumors commonly contain a mixture of patterns. The most common pattern is the reticular/microcystic pattern with many small, thin-walled cysts lined with flattened cells

4. A characteristic histologic feature is the presence of Schiller-Duval bodies, whose presence is indicative of yolk sac tumor

5. A characteristic histologic hallmark is the presence of round, homogeneous, PAS-positive hyaline globules or droplets most frequently seen in the hepatoid and microvascular areas

6. The presence of yolk sac component in the testicular primary imparts a better prognosis, whereas its presence in the metastasis indicates chemoresistant tumor and portends a poor prognosis

7. More than 90% of pediatric yolk sac tumors present in stage I and therefore have a good prognosis

8. Serum AFP levels can be used to check for recurrence and metastasis

---

Box 6
Classification of yolk sac tumor patterns

1. Reticular (microcystic, honeycomb)
2. Endodermal sinus (perivesicular or festoon)
3. Macrocystic
4. Papillary
5. Solid
6. Glandular-alveolar
7. Myxomatous
8. Sarcomatoid
9. Polyvesicular vitelline
10. Hepatoid
11. Parietal

The solid pattern of yolk sac tumor is characterized by sheets of polygonal epithelial cells with uniform nuclei. The solid areas are interspersed with occasional blood vessels (**Fig. 27**). The alveolar/glandular pattern shows the formation of glandular and papillary structures that are lined by cuboidal or columnar cells which sometimes are pseudostratified. The presence of basal vacuoles can give the glandular pattern an appearance resembling early secretory endometrium (**Fig. 28**). The myxoid pattern is characterized by a loose myxoid stroma with dispersed, scattered, spindle-shaped "fibroblast-like" cells (**Fig. 29**). The hepatoid pattern consists of cellular aggregates of eosinophilic cells reminiscent of liver cells (**Fig. 30**).[59,71]

Another histologic hallmark is the presence of round, homogeneous hyaline globules or droplets that are PAS-positive. These hyaline globules contain AFP or alpha-1 antitrypsin. These hyaline droplets are seen most frequently in the hepatoid and microvascular areas (**Fig. 31**).[71]

DIFFERENTIAL DIAGNOSIS

In adults, a pure yolk sac tumor is rare, but mixed germ cell tumors with a yolk sac tumor component are seen often. It is rare for yolk sac tumors to consist of a single histologic pattern; more usually, two, three, or more histologic patterns are present and can present diagnostic challenges, particularly in a mixed germ cell tumor that has teratoma, embryonal carcinoma, or seminoma.[59,68] The glandular and alveolar patterns of yolk sac tumor lack the muscle layers surrounding the glands and can be mistaken for teratomatous glands. In yolk sac tumors the glands are much more

---

and cellular appearance of the tumor are variable but almost occur in specific patterns that are listed in **Box 6**.[11] The pattern most commonly seen in yolk sac tumors is the reticular/microcystic pattern with many small, thin-walled cysts lined with flattened cells (**Fig. 24**). The macrocystic pattern results from coalesced microcysts (**Fig. 25**). Some other patterns include solid, endodermal sinus, papillary, glandular/alveolar, spindle-shaped, myxoid, parietal, polyvesicular vitelline, and hepatoid patterns.[11] One of these patterns may predominate, but more commonly a mixture of patterns is seen.[59]

A characteristic histologic feature of the endodermal sinus pattern is the presence of Schiller-Duval bodies. In this pattern, there is a papillary formation with a central fibrovascular core that is surrounded by an edematous cystic cavity lined by cuboidal to columnar cells, giving rise to the characteristic Schiller-Duval body (**Fig. 26**). Schiller-Duval bodies are not always present in yolk sac tumors, but their presence is indicative of the endodermal sinus pattern.[59,72]

Fig. 24. Microcystic/reticular pattern of yolk sac tumor (original magnification ×200). Variably sized small cystic spaces are lined by flattened cells. Some cells can resemble lipoblasts.

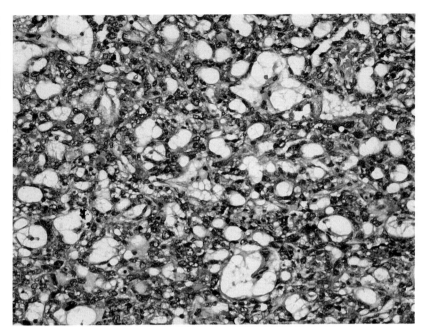

branching than in teratoma, which has simple glands. Teratomatous glands can show AFP positivity but not as diffusely and strongly as in yolk sac tumor. Some yolk sac areas may show pleomorphism and solid growth resembling embryonal carcinoma, leading to misdiagnosis. Immunohistochemistry is useful in this instance, because embryonal carcinoma is positive for CD30 and negative for AFP, whereas yolk sac tumor is negative for CD30 and positive for AFP. Similarly, the solid patterns of a yolk sac tumor can resemble seminoma, leading to a false diagnosis. Solid-pattern yolk sac tumors, however, lack a lymphocytic infiltrate as well as the granulomatous inflammation commonly seen in seminomas.[59,61,68] Rete testis sometimes shows a hyperplastic proliferative response to invasion by germ cell tumors. The hyperplastic

Fig. 25. Macrocystic pattern of yolk sac tumor (original magnification ×100). Small cysts coalesce to form larger cystic spaces (*lower right*) and an endodermal sinus pattern (*upper left*). Festoons of cells line fibrovascular cores.

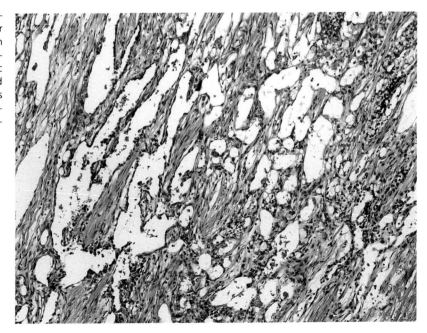

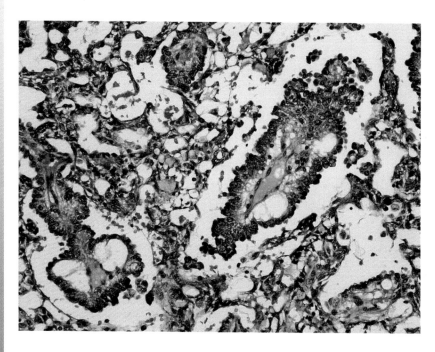

Fig. 26. Endodermal sinus pattern with Schiller Duval bodies, a pathognomonic feature of yolk sac tumor (original magnification ×200).

epithelium has intracytoplasmic hyaline globules mimicking a yolk sac cell component. The cytology usually is bland, and the branching pattern of rete is helpful.[73]

In the pediatric population, the most problematic lesion that can create a diagnostic challenge when dealing with a pure yolk sac tumor is juvenile granulosa cell tumor (JGCT). Both entities occur in the first 6 months of life. Like yolk sac tumor, JGCT has both solid and cystic growth patterns.

Immunohistochemistry is helpful in discriminating the two entities: yolk sac tumor is positive for AFP and negative for inhibin, whereas JGCT is negative for AFP and positive for inhibin.[61,71]

DIAGNOSIS

Yolk sac tumors are positive for AFP (**Fig. 32**), but the staining pattern often is patchy. The hyaline droplets may not stain for AFP but usually stain for

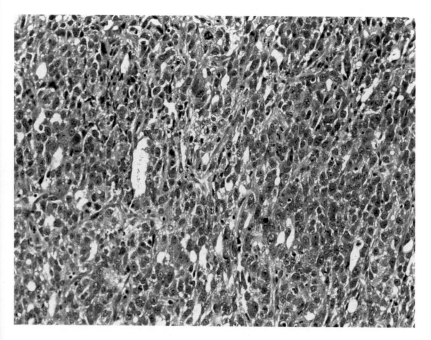

Fig. 27. Solid pattern of yolk sac tumor with pleomorphism (original magnification ×200). This pattern can resemble seminoma.

Fig. 28. Glandular pattern of yolk sac tumor with subnuclear vacuoles resembling secretory endometrium (original magnification ×200).

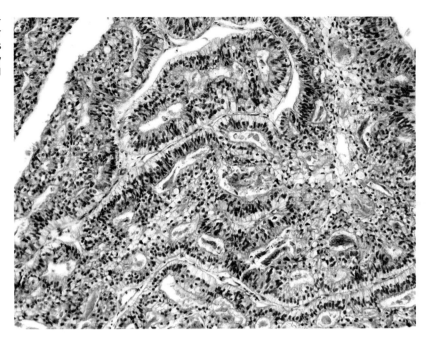

alpha-1 antitrypsin.[74] Low molecular weight cytokeratins usually are positive. Yolk sac tumors have variable positivity for PLAP and alpha-1 antitrypsin. The tumors are negative for CD30, EMA, hCG, and OCT3/4.[75] Glypican 3, a membrane-bound heparin sulfate proteoglycan, is a very sensitive and relatively specific marker for yolk sac tumor.[28,59,71,76,77] **Box 7** summarizes the markers for yolk sac tumors.

PROGNOSIS

The choice of therapy depends on the stage of the disease. Pure yolk sac tumors or mixed tumors with yolk sac elements usually have elevated serum AFP. AFP is a useful serum marker for monitoring response to therapy and for early detection of metastatic and recurrent disease.[59,78] In adult patients who have yolk sac tumors as a component of mixed

Fig. 29. Myxomatous pattern of yolk sac tumor with spindled cells and cords of cells in myxoid stroma (original magnification ×100).

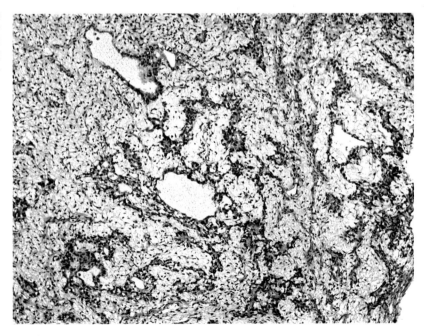

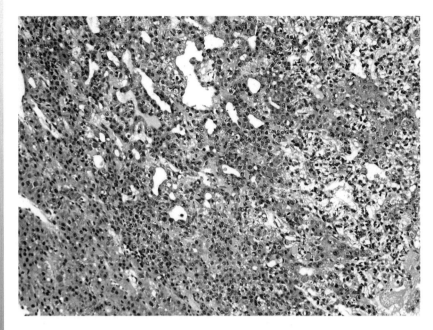

Fig. 30. Hepatoid pattern of yolk sac tumor with eosinophilic cells arranged in hepatocyte-like fashion (original magnification ×200). These cells can be positive for HepPar-1 immunostain.

△△ **Differential Diagnosis**
YOLK SAC TUMORS

Adults

- Embryonal carcinoma: use immunohistochemical studies for CD30 and AFP markers

- Seminoma: solid pattern contains lymphocytic infiltrate and granulomatous inflammation

- Teratoma: yolk sac tumor glandular pattern has complex branching and is more diffusely positive for AFP

- Rete hyperplasia with intracytoplasmic hyaline globules: absence of mitoses and bland cytology, located within the confines of rete

Children

- Juvenile granulosa cell tumor: like yolk sac tumor, has both solid and cystic growth patterns, negative for AFP

 Pitfall
YOLK SAC TUMOR

! Yolk sac tumor may be misdiagnosed as embryonal carcinoma because of the strong similarity in the solid patterns of the two entities.

Box 7
Markers for yolk sac tumors

Yolk sac tumors are positive for

AFP (staining not always uniform and most often patchy)

Low molecular weight cytokeratins

Yolk sac tumors have variable positivity for

PLAP

Alpha-1 antitrypsin (hyaline droplets usually stain for alpha-1-antitrypsin and AFP)

Yolk sac tumors are negative for

CD30

EMA

hCG

OCT3/4

Inhibin

---

germ cell tumor, the treatment and prognosis are the same as for mixed germ cell tumors without a yolk sac component.[79,80]

In children, serum AFP may be normally elevated, and therefore an "elevated" AFP level must be interpreted with clinical and radiologic correlation.[67] For pediatric patients who have clinical stage 1 disease, treatment is orchiectomy

Fig. 31. Scattered eosinophilic round hyaline globules are seen in this high-power image (original magnification ×400). These globules stain for AFP and alpha-1 antitrypsin.

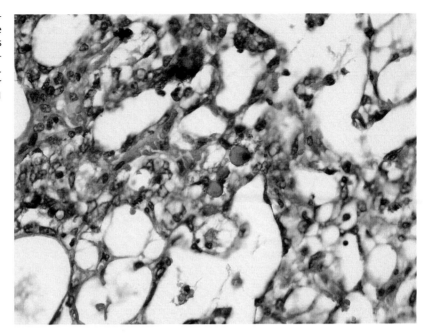

followed by close surveillance.[79,81] Pure yolk sac tumors metastasize to retroperitoneal lymph nodes and lungs.[82] Metastatic yolk sac tumor or recurrent cases are treated with chemotherapy.[80] Overall, the survival of children who have yolk sac tumor is very good.[67,79,80,83]

TERATOMAS

Testicular teratomas include germ cell tumors with somatic differentiation, namely teratomas, epidermoid and dermoid cysts, and monodermal teratomas.

Fig. 32. AFP immunostain in glandular pattern of yolk sac tumor (original magnification ×200). In addition to background staining, AFP immunostain can stain yolk sac tumor very patchily.

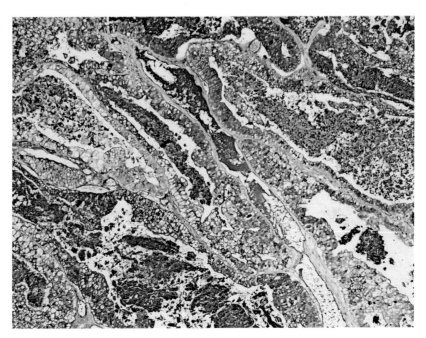

TESTICULAR TERATOMA

OVERVIEW

Testicular teratoma is a testicular germ cell tumor with somatic differentiation and is composed of tissues representing one or more of the germ layers (ie, endoderm, mesoderm, and ectoderm). Testicular teratoma is the second most common tumor in the prepubertal testis,[84] representing approximately 30% of the germ cell tumors in this age group.[85] In young children, it always is benign, even when immature elements are present. In children, it is not associated with IGCNU. The mean patient age at presentation is 20 months; it is rare after 4 years.[38,42,86] In children, teratomas are diploid, and amplification of the short arm of chromosome 12 [i(12p)] is not present.[87] In pure form testicular teratoma comprises about 7% of testicular tumors in adults, and it occurs as a component in 50% of mixed germ cell tumors.[13,42] In postpubertal men, testicular teratomas occur between ages 20 and 40 years[88,89] and are aneuploid. Pure teratoma, even when mature, carries metastatic/malignant potential. A pure teratoma can metastasize as teratomatous elements,[16] or the metastases may contain non-teratomatous elements. Non-teratomatous-type metastases occur in 20% to 40% of teratomas.[88,89] Primary embryonal carcinoma has metastasized as a teratoma.[90] It is postulated that embryonal carcinoma can mature into a teratoma at the metastatic site.[16] Serum tumor markers usually are not elevated in pure teratomas, unless a non-teratomatous element is present at the metastatic site.[38]

GROSS FEATURES

The most common appearance of a teratoma is multinodular, solid, and cystic. Grossly, keratinaceous debris may fill the cysts; mucoid and/or serous fluid may be present also. Bone and gray, translucent nodules of cartilage may be present. Immature elements, when present, appear soft, gray-tan, and solid.

MICROSCOPIC FEATURES

Usually, derivative tissue from all three germ layers that resembles normal mature tissues is present (**Fig. 33**). These tissues can be well organized and resemble normal organ structures (eg, bowel mucosa surrounded by submucosa and smooth muscle layers or recapitulating the bronchial wall) (**Fig. 34**). The stroma of teratoma usually is edematous to fibrous with spindle cells. From the ectoderm, epidermis with adnexa may be seen. Neural

Key Features
TESTICULAR TERATOMA

1. Derivatives of all three germ layers (endoderm, mesoderm, ectoderm) resembling normal tissues are present

2. The testicular mass is firm irregular, nodular, and nontender

3. Significant cytologic atypia and disorganized appearance are seen in the elements of postpubertal teratomas

4. Teratoma with immature elements most commonly has fetal-type neuroepithelium with frequent mitoses

5. Immaturity in postpubertal teratoma has no established significance. These tumors are malignant in the absence of overgrowth of immature neuroepithelium

6. Non-teratomatous-type metastases occur in 20% to 40% of pure teratomas

7. In teratoma with malignant transformation

   - The most common type of somatic malignancy that arises is sarcoma

   - Primitive neuroectodermal tumors (PNET) are identified frequently

   - PNETs show sheets of small, undifferentiated cells with primitive neural-type tubules lined by stratified epithelium or neuroblastic cells in a fibrillary neuropil

   - Various histologic patterns of epithelial malignancies can occur: squamous cell carcinoma, adenocarcinoma, and neuroendocrine carcinoma

8. Pure prepubertal teratomas behave in benign fashion; hence, orchiectomy is curative

9. In adults teratoma is always considered malignant

10. Teratomas with somatic malignancies, when metastatic, have bad prognosis

tissue, sometimes with ependymal differentiation, may be present. The mesoderm is represented by bone, cartilage, skeletal, smooth muscle, and other tissues. The endodermal layer gives rise to various glandular and respiratory-type epithelium. Rarely, pancreatic tissue, salivary gland tissue, liver, or pigmented retinal-type epithelium may be identified.[16,38] The elements of postpubertal teratomas show significant cytologic atypia and

Fig. 33. Mature teratoma with squamous and respiratory type epithelium (original magnification ×100).

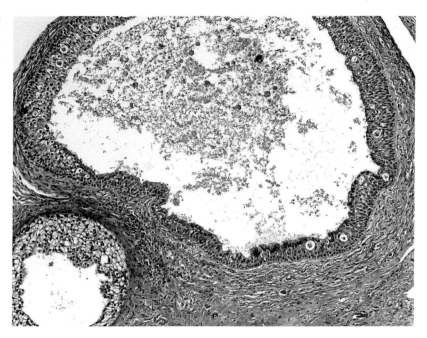

have a disorganized appearance, befitting the aneuploid nature of these tumors.[59]

Teratoma with immature elements most commonly has fetal-type neuroepithelium that shows frequent mitoses (**Fig. 35**). Cellular spindle mesenchymal elements, embryonic skeletal muscle, and immature epithelial elements also are seen intermixed with other mature elements.[59] Immaturity in postpubertal teratomas has no established significance; these tumors are malignant even in the absence of overgrowth of immature neuroepithelium.[20]

Non–germ cell or somatic-type malignancies can develop in a teratoma, a phenomenon known as "malignant transformation of teratoma" or "teratoma with a secondary malignant component." The most common type of somatic

Fig. 34. Mature teratoma recapitulating bronchial wall with cartilage, submucosal glands, and respiratory epithelium (original magnification ×100).

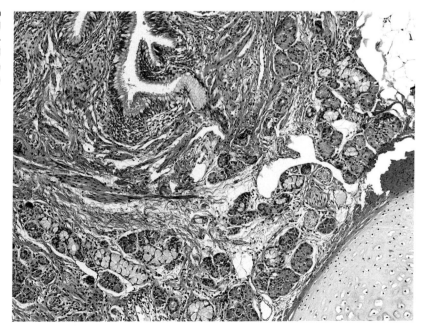

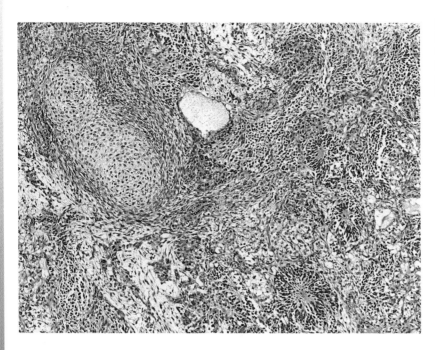

Fig. 35. Teratoma with immature fetal-type neuroepithelium forming rosettes and immature cartilage (original magnification ×100).

malignancy that arises is sarcoma.[91] Sarcomas derived from striated and smooth muscle (rhabdomyosarcoma and leiomyosarcoma, respectively) are common, although 50% of sarcomas are undifferentiated. Rare forms include chondro-, fibro- and osteosarcomas.[42] Primitive neuroectodermal tumors (PNET) are being recognized increasingly.[91–95] These tumors show sheets of small, undifferentiated cells with primitive neural-type tubules lined by stratified epithelium or neuroblastic cells in a fibrillary neuropil (**Fig. 36**). The various histologic patterns of PNETs occurring in the testis include neuroblastoma, medulloepithelioma, peripheral neuroepithelioma, and ependymoblastoma. These tumors stain with neuroendocrine markers (synaptophysin, chromogranin, CD57) and can be cytokeratin and S-100 positive.[42] Nephroblastoma-like tumors are rare in the testes but are common at the metastatic site. They more commonly arise after chemotherapy in patients who have metastatic germ cell tumors.[96] Nephroblastoma-like tumors have primitive tubular structures, blastema, and stroma. These tumors are not positive for neuroendocrine markers. Epithelial malignancies also arise, albeit less commonly, in teratomas with malignant transformation. These tumors stain with EMA, cytokeratins, and occasionally CEA.[42] Various histologic patterns, including squamous cell carcinoma, adenocarcinoma, and neuroendocrine carcinoma, have been reported.[97–102]

DIFFERENTIAL DIAGNOSIS

Pure mature teratoma in adults must be distinguished from dermoid and epidermoid cysts, which are benign cystic lesions not associated with IGCNU. Epidermoid cyst is a simple squamous epithelium-lined cyst filled with keratinaceous debris.

 Differential Diagnosis
TESTICULAR TERATOMA

Dermoid and epidermoid cysts
- Unlike teratoma, there is no association with IGCNU
- Pilosebaceous units are organized around the squamous epithelium in a skinlike fashion. The cytologic atypia present in adult teratomas are lacking
- Frequent lipogranulomatous reaction is also present

Metastatic malignancies
- Residual teratomatous elements may be identified
- In metastatic lesions to testis, adjacent seminiferous tubules lack IGCNU

Yolk sac tumor (children)
- Check AFP levels

Fig. 36. Teratoma with PNET showing sheets of small undifferentiated cells with primitive neural-type tubules lined by stratified epithelium or neuroblastic cells in a fibrillary neuropil (original magnification ×100).

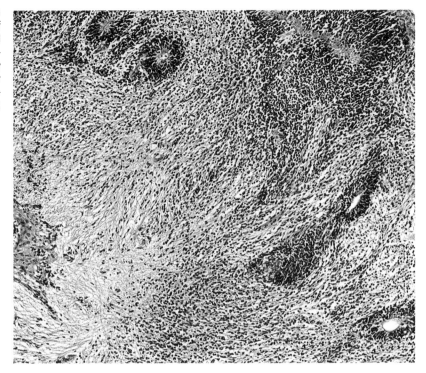

Dermoid cyst contains keratinaceous debris in addition to hair. The pilosebaceous units are organized around the squamous epithelium in a skinlike fashion. There is no cytologic atypia, which is noted in adult teratomas, and frequently a lipogranulomatous reaction is present.[16,61,103–106]

Other differential diagnostic considerations include metastatic malignancies versus teratoma with malignant transformation showing sarcomas, carcinomas, PNETs, and other entities. Residual teratomatous elements may be identified. In metastatic lesions to testis, the adjacent seminiferous tubules lack IGCNU.

DIAGNOSIS

Teratomas present with testicular swelling. A testicular mass sometimes may present with symptoms associated with metastases.[59] The testicular mass is firm, irregular, nodular, and nontender. Serum AFP levels are helpful in distinguishing teratoma from yolk sac tumor in children.[85,107] Teratomas have distinctive histologic features that usually can be recognized easily, and most of the epithelia seen are positive for cytokeratins and EMA. Vimentin and desmin highlight the stromal and muscle tissue, respectively. AFP immunohistochemistry may be positive in the intestinal- or respiratory-type epithelium.[108]

To arrive at the diagnosis of malignant transformation of teratoma, the non–germ cell malignancy should show an expansile or infiltrative growth and occupy at least one low-power (4×) microscopic field.[11,42] These tumors can arise at the primary testicular or metastatic site. In teratomas with malignant transformation, CD99 stains the PNET component, actin and desmin highlight the muscle derivative sarcomas, and stains for PLAP, AFP and hCG are negative.

Teratomas in children are diploid and lack amplification of chromosome 12p, whereas teratomas in postpubertal males are aneuploid and have the typical i(12p) amplification.[87] Non–germ cell malignancies arising in teratoma retain the characteristic cytogenetic change seen in germ cell tumors of i(12p).[97,109] **Box 8** summarizes markers for teratoma.

Pitfall
TESTICULAR TERATOMA

! Malignant transformation of teratoma: a non–germ cell malignancy should show an expansile growth that occupies at least one low-power (4×) microscopic field.

Testicular teratomas are positive for

Cytokeratins

AFP may be positive in the intestinal- or respiratory-type epithelium

EMA

Non–germ cell malignancies arising in teratomas:

PNETs stain with CD99, neuroendocrine markers (synaptophysin, chromogranin, CD57) and can be cytokeratin and S-100 positive

Nephroblastoma-like tumors lack positivity for neuroendocrine markers

Epithelial malignancies in teratomas stain with EMA and cytokeratins and occasionally with CEA

AFP levels distinguish teratoma from yolk sac tumor in children

Actin and desmin highlight muscle-derivative sarcomas

Stains for PLAP, AFP, and HCG are negative.

PROGNOSIS

Pure prepubertal teratomas behave in benign fashion; therefore orchiectomy is curative. Leibovitch and colleagues[88] found that 37% of adult patients who have pure teratoma present with advanced disease. In adults who have teratoma, there is a 25% risk of metastasis after orchiectomy. Pure teratomas and teratomas in mixed germ cell tumors are treated as NSGCTs.[110] The prognostic differences in prepubertal and postpubertal teratomas are explained by the pathogenetic model: prepubertal testicular teratoma and epidermoid and dermoid cysts have a benign germ cell as the precursor cell, but the postpubertal teratoma is derived from a malignant germ cell (ie, IGCNU), which gives rise to a non-teratomatous germ cell tumor that, in turn, differentiates into teratomatous elements.[20] This pathogenetic model is supported by the similar patterns of allelic loss in postpubertal teratomas and the other germ cell tumors that co-exist with them.[111] This model explains the presence of IGCNU in postpubertal teratomas, metastases of non-teratomatous type, and the rarity of pure postpubertal teratoma.[20]

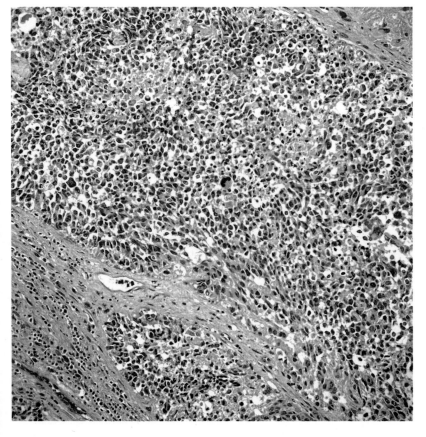

Fig. 37. Primitive neuro-ectodermal tumor arising in teratoma (original magnification ×200). Note increased mitoses and necrosis.

Teratoma with malignant transformation becomes significantly resistant to chemotherapeutic agents, and surgical resection is the treatment of choice.[112] Nephroblastoma-like secondary malignancy in teratoma has a much better prognosis than do PNETs (**Fig. 37**). When these secondary malignancies are limited to the testis, the overall prognosis remains the same as for testicular teratoma.[102] When these malignancies develop at the metastatic site, however, the prognosis is affected gravely.[91,93,97,102] PNETs, when identified in postchemotherapy resections of testicular germ cell tumors, portend a bad prognosis.[93]

EPIDERMOID AND DERMOID CYSTS

OVERVIEW

Epidermoid cysts are benign testicular tumors that, as the name indicates, are composed of squamous epithelial-lined cysts. Epidermoid cysts account for 3% of pediatric and 1% of adult testicular tumors.[106,113] The tumor presents as a nontender, palpable testicular mass between the second and fourth decades of life.[106] Serum levels of tumor markers are negative.[114] Ultrasound study reveals a well-demarcated intratesticular lesion with mixed echogenicity. A fibrous cyst wall sharply separates the lesion from the adjacent testis parenchyma and appears hyperechoic.[114] Although most epidermoid cysts are intraparenchymal, they also can involve the tunica and the epididymis.[115]

On the cut surface, epidermoid cysts are well-circumscribed, pearly white to yellowish lesions with a capsule of variable thickness and with laminated contents. They range in size from 0.5 to 10.5 cm, with a mean size of 2.0 cm.[106]

Microscopically they have fibrous wall lined by simple keratinizing squamous epithelium with granular cell layer. There are no skin appendages or any cytologic atypia (**Fig. 38**). Granulomatous reaction to keratin debris can be identified next to an area of rupture. There is no associated IGCNU.[116,117]

In the differential diagnosis, it is important to note the absence of other teratomatous elements and IGCNU to distinguish epidermoid cyst from teratoma. Epidermoid cysts lack the typical chromosome 12p abnormalities seen in other germ cell tumors; therefore, interphase fluorescence in situ hybridization analysis for i(12p) can be used in difficult cases.[113]

Epidermoid cysts have a benign course. Conservative local excision and testis-sparing surgery can be attempted when feasible.[114]

Testicular dermoid cysts are rare tumors classified separately from mature testicular teratoma which, in postpubertal males, has a metastatic potential.[88,118] Testicular dermoid cysts are composed of cyst lined by mature, keratinizing, squamous epithelium with skin appendages, including hair and sebaceous glands.

Fig. 38. Epidermoid cyst showing simple keratinizing squamous epithelium with granular cell layer and no adnexal structures (original magnification ×40). Keratinaceous debris fills the cyst.

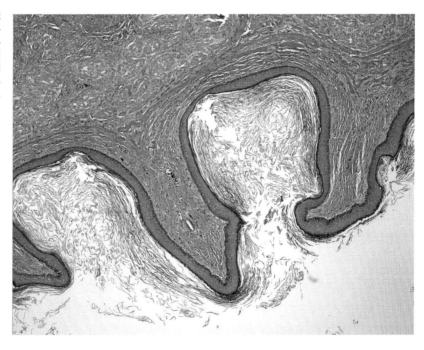

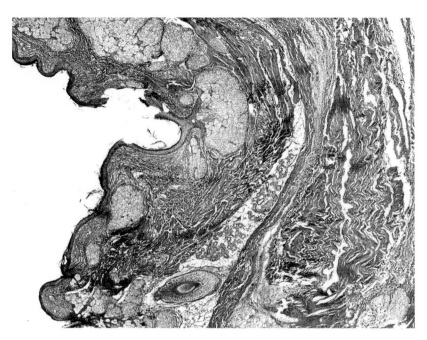

Fig. 39. Dermoid cyst wall is lined by organized skinlike epithelium with associated cutaneous appendages, with well-formed hair follicles, sebaceous glands, and sweat glands (original magnification ×40).

On gross examination these tumors have the friable keratinaceous/cheesy debris, sometimes mixed with hair, filling a cyst with a thick, fibrous wall.

Microscopically, the cyst wall is lined by organized skin-like epithelium with associated cutaneous appendages, with well-formed hair follicles, sebaceous glands, and sweat glands (**Fig. 39**).[61] Additionally, limited amounts of glands lined by intestinal or ciliated epithelium, as well as islands of cartilage, may be seen. These teratomatous elements always are well organized. The cellular elements lack any cytologic atypia, and lipogranulomatous reaction is seen frequently.[61]

Thus dermoid cysts may have noncutaneous teratomatous elements, and an important key to their diagnosis is the lack of IGCNU. Therefore, unlike teratoma, these tumors are believed to arise from a nonmalignant germ cell rather than from a malignant germ cell.[104] Orchiectomy is curative.

MONODERMAL TERATOMAS

OVERVIEW

Monodermal teratomas are germ cell tumors that are composed of derivatives of only one of the three germ layers. Primary pure carcinoid tumor of the testis is considered a form of monodermal teratoma. The entity is discussed in detail in the section on testicular carcinoid.

PNET of the testis also is considered a monodermal teratoma. These tumors most often develop as secondary malignant components, overgrowths of the immature neural elements of teratoma, but rarely they may represent a primary pure testicular PNET.[92,93,119]

Grossly, they are gray-white and are partially necrotic.

Microscopically, monodermal teratomas are composed of sheets of primitive, poorly differentiated tumor cells with scant cytoplasm and foci of fetal neural-type tubules lined by stratified epithelium and forming the ependymal-type rosettes. In a neuroblastoma-like tumor, the rosettes can have neuroblastic cells in a fibrillary neuropil background. Synaptophysin, chromogranin, and CD99 are variably positive.[119] Only PNET occurring in the metastasis are associated with a bad prognosis.[93]

CHORIOCARCINOMA

OVERVIEW

Choriocarcinoma is a rare malignant germ cell tumor that is composed of a mixture of cytotrophoblastic and syncytiotrophoblastic cells. This neoplasm recapitulates placental tissue development (trophoblastic differentiation). Choriocarcinoma usually occurs in patients between the ages of 20 and 30 years.[120] Choriocarcinoma is an aggressive neoplasm and usually presents with an early hematogenous spread to the lungs,[20,121,122] liver, gastrointestinal tract, and brain.[120,123–126] As a consequence, choriocarcinomas are more likely to present with symptoms caused by metastatic disease. Some of the clinical presentations include hemoptysis, gastrointestinal bleeding, and neurologic symptoms. The testicular primary usually is small and may be regressed. Choriocarcinoma occurs in the descended and undescended testis as well as in extratesticular sites.[20] Pure choriocarcinomas are seen in fewer than 1% of patients who have testicular tumors. More commonly, choriocarcinoma occurs as a component in up to 15% of mixed germ cell tumors.[20,61,127]

GROSS FEATURES

Grossly, in the testis, choriocarcinoma has the appearance of a small, hemorrhagic nodule, most often surrounded by a grayish white rim of tissue at the periphery. Occasionally, the tumor has a "burnt out" appearance with only a fibrous scar.

MICROSCOPIC FEATURES

Histologic evaluation shows that choriocarcinoma has a mixture of two cell types, syncytiotrophoblasts and cytotrophoblasts, in juxtaposition (**Fig. 40**).[20] Syncytiotrophoblasts are large, multinucleated cells with abundant vacuolated eosinophilic cytoplasm and with many large, hyperchromatic nuclei; syncytiotrophoblasts have a smudgy appearance.[20,61] Cytotrophoblasts are polygonal cells with a uniform appearance and distinct cell borders. They have abundant clear to pale cytoplasm and single, irregular nuclei with one or two nucleoli. The cytotrophoblasts are arranged in clusters within a background of hemorrhagic necrosis and are surrounded by the multinucleated

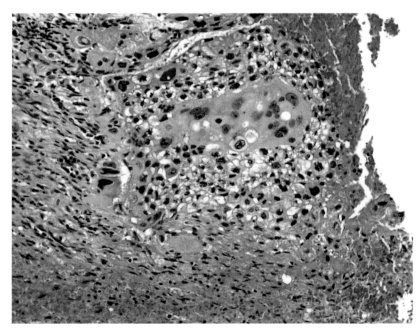

Fig. 40. High-power view of choriocarcinoma with syncytiotrophoblasts, large multinucleated cells that have abundant vacuolated eosinophilic cytoplasm and many large and hyperchromatic nuclei, with a smudgy appearance, next to cytotrophoblasts with vacuolated cytoplasm (original magnification ×400).

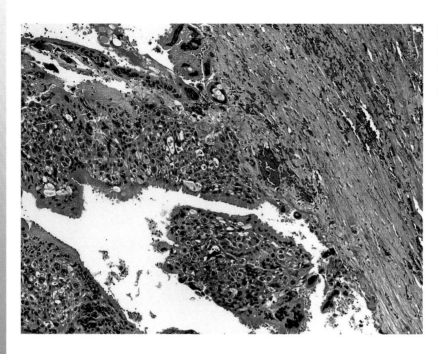

Fig. 41. Cytotrophoblasts with capping of syncytiotrophoblasts in a hemorrhagic background typical for choriocarcinoma (original magnification ×200)

syncytiotrophoblasts (**Fig. 41**).[10,121] The syncytiotrophoblasts drape over the smaller clusters of cytotrophoblasts to form a border. In addition, the tumor has intermediate trophoblasts that are larger than cytotrophoblasts and have eosinophilic cytoplasm with irregular hyperchromatic nuclei (**Fig. 42**).[10,61,128]

DIFFERENTIAL DIAGNOSIS

Seminomas with scattered syncytiotrophoblasts are seen frequently and should not be called "choriocarcinoma admixed with seminomas." Rare cases of seminoma with choriocarcinoma do occur. Cytotrophoblasts may resemble the solid

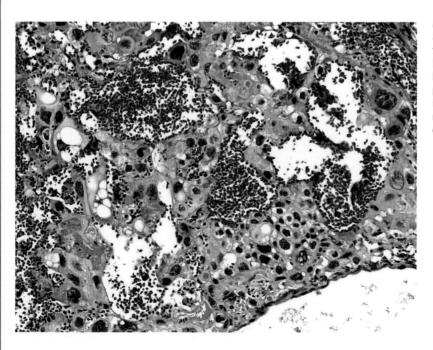

Fig. 42. Choriocarcinoma also has intermediate trophoblasts that are larger than cytotrophoblasts and have eosinophilic cytoplasm with irregular hyperchromatic nuclei (original magnification ×400).

Differential Diagnosis
CHORIOCARCINOMA

- Seminoma with scattered syncytiotrophoblasts
- Seminoma with choriocarcinoma (rare)
- Solid variant of yolk sac tumor can resemble cytotrophoblasts
- Monophasic choriocarcinoma resembles seminoma, embryonal carcinoma, or solid variant of yolk sac tumor (rare)

Pitfalls
CHORIOCARCINOMA

! Choriocarcinoma can be difficult to distinguish from embryonal carcinoma, particularly the cytotrophoblasts. Immunohistochemistry using CD30 may be helpful.

! Pure choriocarcinomas are extremely rare in patients who have testicular tumors. More commonly, choriocarcinoma occurs as a component in mixed germ cell tumors.

variant of yolk sac tumor.[61] Immunohistochemistry with AFP may be useful. Embryonal carcinoma can be difficult to distinguish from choriocarcinoma, particularly the cytotrophoblasts. Immunohistochemistry using CD30 may be helpful.[10,121]

Monophasic choriocarcinoma consists mainly of monomorphic cytotrophoblasts with single nuclei. The syncytiotrophoblastic cells are rare and inconspicuous. These monophasic choriocarcinomas, although rare, may present diagnostic difficulties because of their resemblance to seminoma, embryonal carcinoma, or the solid variant of yolk sac tumor. Immunohistochemistry and careful correlation with serum markers are necessary.[10,61,127]

DIAGNOSIS

β-hCG is a glycoprotein with the same alpha subunit as thyroid-stimulating hormone, follicle-stimulating hormone, and luteinizing hormone. hCG serum levels are markedly elevated in choriocarcinoma (>100,000 mIU/mL). As a result of the elevated hCG and because of the presence of the alpha subunit that is present in other hormones, some patients may present with endocrine abnormalities such as gynecomastia and hyperthyroidism. An ultrasound scan may show mixed echogenicity with hemorrhage, necrosis, and calcifications.

Syncytiotrophoblasts are positive for hCG, EMA, inhibin, pregnancy-specific beta-1 glycoprotein (SP1), and human placental lactogen (HPL). Intermediate trophoblasts are positive for inhibin, hCG, HPL, and SP1. Cytotrophoblasts usually are negative or weakly positive for hCG and negative for SP1 and HPL. Cytokeratins and PLAP immunostaining is positive in about 50% of choriocarcinomas (all cell types).[28,129] Glypican 3 also is positive in choriocarcinomas..[20,28,130] Markers for choriocarcinoma are summarized in **Box 9**.

PROGNOSIS

Pure choriocarcinomas have a worse prognosis than other testicular germ cell neoplasms and than mixed germ cell tumor with choriocarcinomatous component. In general, the greater the amount of choriocarcinoma admixed with other germ cell tumors, the worst is the effect on

Box 9
Markers for choriocarcinoma
Syncytiotrophoblasts are positive for
hCG
EMA
Inhibin
SP1
HPL
Intermediate trophoblasts are positive for
Inhibin
hCG
HPL
SP1
Cytotrophoblasts usually are negative or weakly positive for hCG
Cytotrophoblasts are negative for
SP1
HPL
Choriocarcinomas are positive for
Cytokeratins (50% cases)
PLAP (50% cases)
Glypican 3

survival.[131–133] Choriocarcinomas and mixed germ cell tumors are treated as NSGCTs. The management of choriocarcinomas is similar to that of the other histologic types of NSGCT.[10,134–136] The prognosis of choriocarcinoma as part of a mixed germ cell tumor depends on the tumor stage, which includes the serum hCG levels. A high serum level of hCG (> 50,000 mIU/mL) correlates with poor prognosis. Pure choriocarcinoma is not as sensitive to chemotherapy as mixed NSGCT.[131,133–137]

MIXED GERM CELL TUMORS

OVERVIEW

Mixed germ cell tumors are also called NSGCTs. These tumors show two or more components in any combination and distribution of the various germ cell tumor types described thus far, except spermatocytic seminoma and seminoma with syncytiotrophoblastic giant cells. Mixed germ cell tumors are composed of embryonal carcinoma, immature or mature teratoma, yolk sac tumor, seminoma, choriocarcinoma, and other rare trophoblastic tumors, in decreasing order of frequency.[127] Mixed germ cell tumors rarely, if ever, occur in the prepubertal testis but comprise 30% to 50% of germ cell tumors in adults and are the second most common testicular tumor in adult men.[15,42,59,138] They are seen from puberty through the fifth decade of life; the mean patient age at presentation is 30 years.[16] Mixed germ cell tumors that contain seminoma as a component occur at a later age than those that do not contain seminoma. Serum elevation of AFP and hCG is common.[139] Polyembryoma and diffuse embryoma are rare types of mixed germ cell tumors with polyembryoma that have a distinctive arrangement of yolk sac tumor and embryonal carcinoma, recapitulating the very early embryonic development. Diffuse embryoma and polyembryoma patterns are seen more commonly as a portion of mixed germ cell tumor than as pure forms.[20]

GROSS FEATURES

Mixed germ cell tumors present as painless or painful testicular swelling. The appearance of the cut surface is variegated because of the various types of components. These tumors can be soft or firm, with solid and cystic areas; hemorrhage and necrosis also are seen commonly (**Fig. 43**).

MICROSCOPIC FEATURES

The various types of germ cell tumors are arranged haphazardly, with the combination of embryonal carcinoma, yolk sac tumor, seminoma, and embryonal carcinoma with teratoma (teratocarcinoma) being the more common mixtures (**Fig. 44**).[15] Embryonal carcinoma is the most

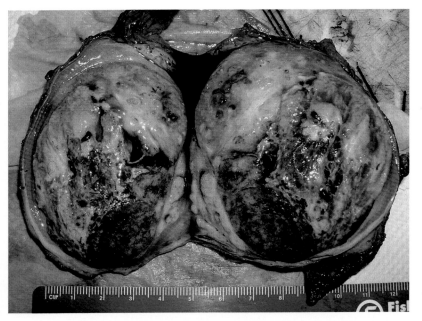

Fig. 43. Gross bivalved testis showing mixed germ cell tumor with nearly complete replacement of the testicular parenchyma. The cut surface is heterogeneous with hemorrhage and necrosis and solid and cystic areas.

Fig. 44. Mixed germ cell tumor with cartilage and stroma representing teratoma and adjacent pleomorphic embryonal carcinoma with necrosis (original magnification ×100).

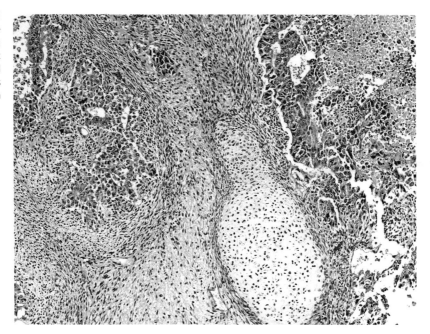

commonly present component in mixed germ cell tumors; yolk sac tumor is the most frequently overlooked component.[138] The histologic appearance of each of the components in a germ cell tumor is similar to that of the component's pure form. Syncytiotrophoblastic giant cells are present in 40% of mixed germ cell tumors (**Fig. 45**).[42]

Polyembryoma has a mixture of embryonal carcinoma, yolk sac tumor, and teratomatous elements forming embryoid bodies with an associated amnionlike cavity in myxoid stroma of extra-embryonic mesenchyme (**Fig. 46**). Diffuse embryoma has an organized ribbonlike arrangement with a layer of embryonal carcinoma surrounded by a single, flattened layer of yolk

Fig. 45. Mixed germ cell tumor with syncytiotrophoblastic giant cells (original magnification ×200).

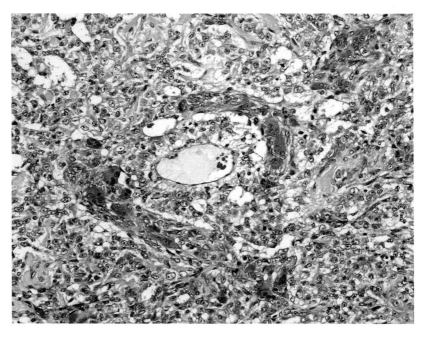

Key Features
MIXED GERM CELL TUMOR

1. These NSGCTs show more than one germ cell tumor type

2. Mixed germ cell tumors can have any combination of embryonal carcinoma, immature or mature teratoma, yolk sac tumor, seminoma, and choriocarcinoma

3. Mixed germ cell tumors are the second most common germ cell tumor in the adult testis

4. Serum elevation of AFP and hCG is common

5. These tumors present as painless testicular swelling

6. The cut surface can be variegated, soft, firm, or cystic; hemorrhage and necrosis are common

7. Teratocarcinoma (teratoma with embryonal carcinoma) is most common combination; embryonal carcinoma is the most common single entity

8. Tumors containing embryonal carcinoma alone behave more aggressively than tumors that have teratoma as a component

9. Lymphovascular invasion in the primary tumor is predictive of relapse and nodal metastasis

10. Favorable findings in metastasis of retroperitoneal lymph node dissection specimens are the presence of necrosis, fibrosis, and mature teratoma

Differential Diagnosis
MIXED GERM CELL TUMOR

The differential diagnosis of mixed germ cell tumor includes

- Embryonal carcinoma
- Yolk sac tumor
- Teratoma

carcinoma, and OCT3/4 also stains seminoma; and HCG stains the trophoblasts. **Box 10** lists currently identified markers for germ cell tumors.

PROGNOSIS

Tumors consisting of embryonal carcinoma alone behave more aggressively than those composed of embryonal carcinoma and teratoma.[141] A yolk sac tumor component also alters the prognosis of a mixed germ cell tumor favorably.[142] The presence of vascular/lymphatic invasion in the primary tumor is predictive of relapse and nodal metastasis.[140,142–144]

sac tumor, with equal proportions of both elements.[11]

DIFFERENTIAL DIAGNOSIS
DIAGNOSIS

Each of the components present in the mixed germ cell tumor should be mentioned in the pathology report, along with their estimated amount. These tumors also may present with signs and symptoms of metastatic disease. The histology of metastases is similar to that of the primary tumor in 88% of cases.[140]

Immunohistochemistry can be used to identify the various elements. AFP stains the yolk sac and some glandular teratomatous elements; CD30 and OCT3/4 stain embryonal

Pitfalls
MIXED GERM CELL TUMOR

! Yolk sac tumor is the most frequently overlooked component in mixed germ cell tumor.

! A yolk sac tumor component favorably alters the prognosis of a mixed germ cell tumor.

! Unfavorable findings in a retroperitoneal lymph node dissection include the presence of embryonal carcinoma, viable seminoma, yolk sac tumor, and choriocarcinoma.

! Watch for the presence of vascular/ lymphatic invasion in the primary tumor, because it is predictive of relapse and nodal metastasis.

! The pathology report must include each of the components present in the mixed germ cell tumors and the estimated percentage of each component.

Fig. 46. Embryoid body of polyembryoma. The outer cavity is amnion like with a layer of embryonal carcinoma and a layer of yolk sac tumor (original magnification ×200).

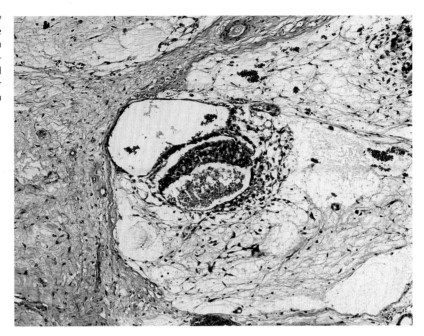

In retroperitoneal lymph node dissections (RPLND) specimens, favorable findings are the presence of necrosis, fibrosis, and mature teratoma in metastasis (**Fig. 47**). Unfavorable findings include the presence of embryonal carcinoma, viable seminoma, yolk sac tumor, and choriocarcinoma.[110] These tumors are treated as NSGCT, and the treatment depends on tumor stage, percentage of embryonal carcinoma, and finding of angiolymphatic invasion.[110]

REGRESSED GERM CELL TUMOR

Occasionally, germ cell tumors of the testis show the phenomenon of spontaneous

---

Box 10
Markers for mixed germ cell tumor

AFP staining (yolk sac tumor and some glandular teratomatous elements)

CD30 (embryonal carcinoma)

OCT3/4 (embryonal carcinoma and seminoma)

CD117 and PLAP (seminoma)

hCG (trophoblasts)

---

regression. The classic scenario and the most common presentation of regressed germ cell tumor is a patient presenting with a retroperitoneal germ cell tumor who is found, upon investigation, to have metastasis from a regressed testicular primary.[10,20,145] One study noted that 10% of patients who died of metastatic germ cell tumors had such a scar in their testicular primaries at autopsy.[146]

Gross examination of the testis most often shows a distinct scarred or fibrous area, which can be nodular, multinodular, or stellate (**Fig. 48**).[145] Calcification may be obvious. On microscopic examination of the testis, there are findings of atrophy, hyalinized "scar" with lymphoplasmacytic infiltrates, hemosiderin-laden macrophages, prominent vascularity, and coarse calcifications (**Fig. 49**). Adjacent to the scar, IGCNU, intratubular calcification, and prominent Leydig cells are identified frequently. These patients are believed to have regression of most of or of the entire primary testicular tumor.

A minor component of viable tumor, such as seminoma, teratoma, or IGCNU, may be seen in association with the scar (**Fig. 50**). Ghost remains of the tubules can be identified that are believed to be regression of neoplastic area (eg, in the intertubular growth of germ cell tumor, which is seen

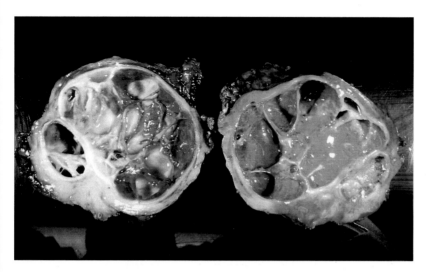

Fig. 47. Gross bisected retroperitoneal lymph node with metastatic mature teratoma after chemotherapy for a mixed germ cell tumor. (*Courtesy of* A. Brown, MD, Baltimore, MD.)

quite frequently in seminoma).[20] Choriocarcinoma probably is the tumor most prone to regression, and seminoma accounts for the most cases.[145] When regression occurs in embryonal carcinoma, coarse intratubular calcification representing the remains of the comedonecrosis that occurs in intratubular embryonal carcinoma may provide evidence of previous viable tumor.[20] These findings are helpful in differentiating a non-neoplastic scar resulting from trauma or vascular disease from the scar of regressed/regressing germ cell tumor.[61]

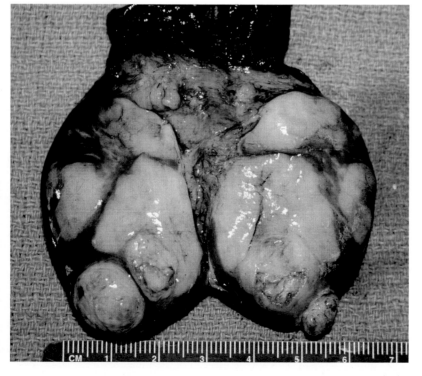

Fig. 48. Gross bivalved testis showing scar, leiomyomatous nodules, and calcification from a regressed testicular germ cell tumor that presented with a large retroperitoneal metastasis.

Fig. 49. Calcification and scarring in a regressed germ cell tumor (original magnification ×40).

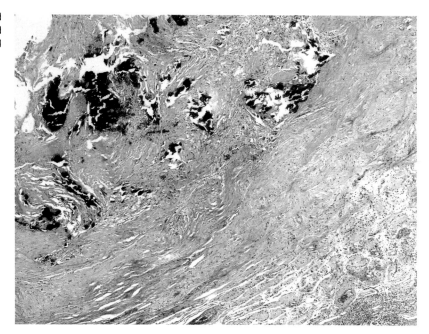

TESTICULAR CARCINOID TUMOR

OVERVIEW

Primary testicular carcinoid tumors are rare, representing less than 1% of testicular tumors.[42] Although these tumors more commonly occur as pure neoplasms, up to 20% occur as part of a teratoma.[147–149] These tumors have not been seen in association with non-teratomatous germ cell tumors. When these tumors occur as pure testicular carcinoid tumors, there is no associated IGCNU in the adjacent testis.[16,150] Fluorescence in situ hybridization and immunohistochemistry showed that the carcinoids associated with teratomas have i(12p) and overexpression of 12p.[151] The pure primary carcinoids, however, do not show these cytogenetic abnormalities seen in germ cell tumors.[152]

Fig. 50. Focal residual teratomatous elements seen in a nearly completely regressed germ cell tumor (original magnification ×100).

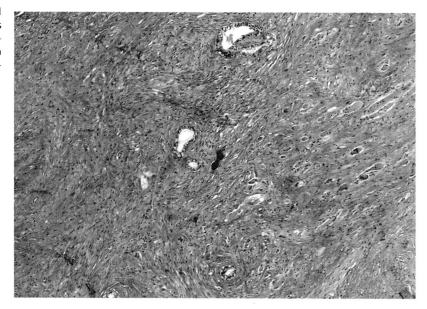

Key Features
TESTICULAR CARCINOID TUMOR

1. Testicular carcinoid tumor is rare (less than 1% of testicular tumors)

2. Nearly one quarter occur as part of teratoma

3. Trabecular and nesting patterns with frequent rosettes are separated by thin fibroconnective tissue

4. The tumor is well demarcated but unencapsulated

5. Cells have eosinophilic cytoplasm, uniform round to oval nuclei with granular chromatin, some showing nucleoli

6. Mitotic activity is rare; hemorrhage and necrosis may be seen

7. Primary testicular carcinoid tumors are rare

8. In pure testicular carcinoid tumor there is no associated IGCNU in the adjacent testis

9. Mean patient age at presentation is 46 years (range, 10–83 years)

Differential Diagnosis
TESTICULAR CARCINOID TUMOR

- Pure primary carcinoid tumor: does not show cytogenetic abnormalities seen in germ cell tumors

- Component of testicular teratoma: might have adjacent IGCNU, unlike primary carcinoids

- Carcinoids associated with teratomas show i(12p) and overexpression of 12p

- The presence of other teratomatous elements confirms testis as the primary location for carcinoid arising in a teratoma

- Metastatic involvement of the testis by carcinoid tumor: frequently bilateral, lymphovascular invasion; extratesticular carcinoid sometimes is present

- Sertoli cell tumors: may show carcinoid like appearance

- Granulosa cell tumors: Call-Exner bodies may be mistaken for rosettes

- Inhibin and calretinin would be positive in these sex cord–stromal tumors

Traditionally, testicular carcinoids are divided into three categories:

1. Pure primary carcinoid tumor

2. Carcinoid occurring as part of a testicular teratoma

3. Metastatic involvement of the testis by carcinoid tumor

The mean patient age at presentation is 46 years,[147] but ranges from 10 to 83 years.[16,42] Approximately 10% of cases are associated with carcinoid syndrome.[153,154]

GROSS FEATURES

These tumors present with unilateral, usually painless testicular swelling, sometimes of prolonged duration spanning years. The size ranges from 1 cm to 9.5 cm with a mean size of 4.6 cm. The tumors are well demarcated but unencapsulated, solid, pale tan to dark tan, with occasional calcifications.[42,150]

MICROSCOPIC FEATURES

In testes, carcinoid tumors most commonly show the trabecular and nesting patterns with frequent rosettes separated by thin fibroconnective tissue, similar to the pattern seen in midgut carcinoids (**Fig. 51**). These tumors are unencapsulated,[150] and the cells have eosinophilic cytoplasm and uniform round to oval nuclei with granular chromatin; some show nucleoli (**Fig. 52**). Mitotic activity is rare; hemorrhage and necrosis may be seen.[148,155] Intracytoplasmic membrane-bound

Pitfalls
TESTICULAR CARCINOID TUMOR

! Some Sertoli cell tumors stain with neuroendocrine markers.

! Metastatic carcinoids have poor prognosis and therefore should be ruled out carefully.

! Larger tumors and tumors presenting with carcinoid syndrome are more likely to metastasize.

Fig. 51. Low-power view of a pure testicular carcinoid tumor (original magnification ×20). Note unencapsulated tumor with nests and islands of cells separated by thin fibroconnective tissue. Upper left corner shows adjacent testicular parenchyma.

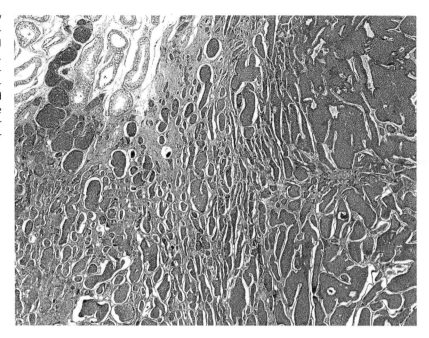

granules have been identified on electron microscopic examination.[148,156]

DIFFERENTIAL DIAGNOSIS

Metastatic carcinoids frequently are bilateral[157] and show lymphovascular invasion; sometimes the presence of extratesticular carcinoid is known.[158] The presence of other teratomatous elements confirms testis as the primary location. Primary carcinoids do not have adjacent IGCNU, but carcinoids associated with teratoma might.

Additional differential diagnostic considerations are Sertoli cell tumors, which may show carcinoid-like appearance, as do some granulosa cell

Fig. 52. Testicular carcinoid tumor with nested appearance showing small acini and rosettes (original magnification ×100).

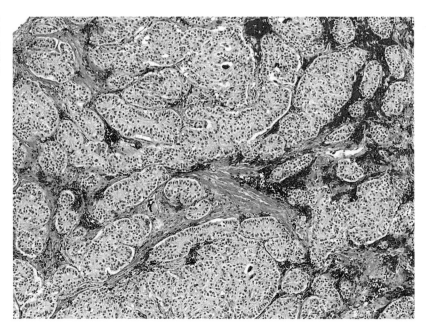

tumors, in which the Call-Exner bodies may be mistaken for rosettes. In these sex cord–stromal tumors, neuroendocrine stains are negative, and inhibin and calretinin are positive. Rare Sertoli cell tumors have shown positivity with the usual neuroendocrine markers.[159]

DIAGNOSIS

Testicular carcinoids, like carcinoid tumors elsewhere in the body, are positive for synaptophysin, chromogranin, and cytokeratin[150] in addition to neuron-specific enolase and serotonin. They are negative for OCT3/4, ckit (CD117), CD30, CDX2, TTF1,[151] p53, EGFR, and PLAP.[150] **Box 11** presents the markers for carcinoid tumor.

PROGNOSIS

Testicular carcinoids, even those that occur in association with teratoma, have excellent prognosis. Orchiectomy with close follow-up is the treatment of choice.[156] Rare cases of malignant metastasizing testicular carcinoids have been reported.[157,159–162] The metastatic sites included regional lymph nodes, liver, skin, and the skeletal system.[163] Larger tumors and tumors presenting with carcinoid syndrome are more likely to metastasize.[148]

GONADOBLASTOMA

OVERVIEW

Gonadoblastoma is a rare neoplasm that has the potential for malignant transformation.[164]

Box 11
Markers for carcinoid tumors

Carcinoid tumors are positive for
Synaptophysin
Cytokeratin
Neuron-specific enolase
Serotonin

Carcinoid tumors are negative for
OCT3/4
cKit (CD117)
CD30
CDX2
TTF1
p53
EGFR
PLAP

Gonadoblastoma was first described in 1953 by Scully,[165] who noted that this neoplasm resembles a normally developing gonad and is composed of germ cells and sex cord derivatives resembling immature granulosa and Sertoli cells.[165,166] Subsequent studies have shown that gonadoblastoma is a mixed germ cell–sex cord–stromal tumor.[165–169] Most of these tumors are identified within the first 2 decades of life.[164,169–174]

Gonadoblastoma is the most common testicular neoplasm in patients who have dysgenetic gonads and who have Y-chromosomal material such as 45,X, 46,XY in their genome.[173,175] Therefore, it occurs mostly in patients who have pure or mixed gonadal dysgenesis or in male pseudohermaphrodism. Phenotypically, 80% of patients who have gonadoblastoma are females, and 20% are males.[170,171] Gonadoblastoma is present in approximately 7% to 10% of patients who have Turner syndrome.[172,176] Recent studies have shown that testis-specific protein Y-encoded gene (*TSPY*) is a tandem-repeat gene located at the gonadoblastoma locus on Y chromosome, which is closely associated with initiation and various stages of gonadoblastoma development.[167,177]

GROSS FEATURES

Grossly, pure gonadoblastomas are very small, slightly lobulated, and soft to firm, gray-tan to brown, tumors. They have a "gritty" cut surface because of the presence of diffuse or focal calcification.[164]

HISTOLOGIC FEATURES

Histologically, the tumor is composed of tumor nests with an organoid growth pattern that is surrounded by stromal elements.[166] The surrounding stroma may be loose or hyalinized. There are two main cell types. The first is similar to the large germ cells found in seminomas with clear cytoplasm and large, round vesicular nuclei. The second cell type resembles small, immature Sertoli cells with small nuclei (**Fig. 53**). A third type of cell similar to the Leydig cells may be seen in the stroma. Brisk mitotic activity may be observed.[164,166,178]

The tumor cells form nests or aggregates with calcifications. If the germ cell components outgrow these discrete aggregates, the lesion is a seminoma arising in a gonadoblastoma (**Fig. 54**). As the seminomatous component grows, it may obscure the architecture of gonadoblastoma. Other causes of obliteration of the

Fig. 53. High-power image detailing a tumor nest of gonadoblastoma with two main cell types (original magnification ×400). One cell type is similar to the large germ cells found in seminomas with clear cytoplasm and large, round vesicular nuclei. The second cell type resembles small, immature Sertoli cells with small nuclei oriented around hyalinized eosinophilic basement membrane material.

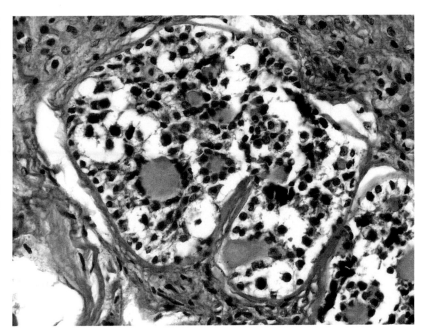

gonadoblastoma may be diffuse hyalinization and calcification.[164,166]

DIFFERENTIAL DIAGNOSIS

The pathologic diagnosis of gonadoblastoma can be challenging. The differential diagnosis of a gonadoblastoma includes a pure seminoma, a sex cord tumor with annular tubules, and or an unclassified germ cell–sex cord–stromal tumor. These tumors may elevate serum levels of β-HCG. Gonadoblastoma often is misdiagnosed as a NSGCT. Only a few cases of NSGCTs, such as yolk sac tumors and teratomas, have been reported in patients who have gonadoblastoma.[164,172,179,180]

Fig. 54. Low-power view of gonadoblastoma forming organoid nests/aggregates with calcifications (original magnification ×100). The germ cell elements appear to be overgrowing. If the germ cell components outgrow these discrete aggregates, the lesion is a seminoma arising in a gonadoblastoma.

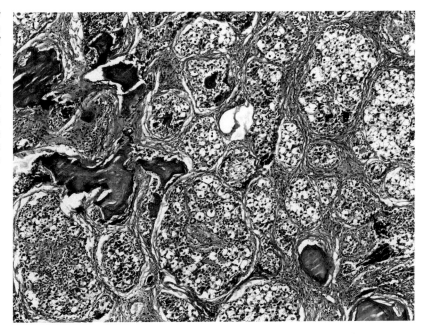

DIAGNOSIS

Chromosome analysis is important for the diagnosis of gonadoblastoma. At birth, the karyotype is used as a screening test in neonates who have abnormal genitalia. Many studies have confirmed that the presence of a mosaic karyotype with a Y chromosome is a risk factor for developing gonadoblastoma in the intersex population.[173,174,176] Tumors usually are discovered when a young patient who has intersex features is evaluated.[181] Histologic features that are important for diagnosis are the nests containing seminoma-like germ cells and stromal cells of granulosa-Sertoli–type. The germ cells are positive for cKit or PLAP, and the stromal cells are positive for inhibin.[63,182] The diagnosis of seminoma in a patient who has dysgenic gonads and a Y chromosome is an indication of a concurrent gonadoblastoma.[170,172,183]

PROGNOSIS

Early gonadectomy is recommended in patients at risk for gonadoblastoma. The current recommendation for patients who have an intersex disorder or Turner syndrome is to proceed with prophylactic removal of the dysgenic gonad before gonadoblastoma develops.[172] Overall, the prognosis of patients who have gonadoblastoma is excellent if the tumor is removed before transformation to a malignant germinoma or seminoma occurs. Gonadoblastoma by itself is benign, but about 50% of the tumors may have local overgrowth by the germ cell tumor component, and about 10% of these seminomas may have metastases.[164,172]

SEX CORD GONADAL–STROMAL TUMORS

OVERVIEW

Sex cord gonadal–stromal tumors comprise approximately 4% to 6% of adult testicular tumors and more than 30% of testicular tumors in the pediatric population. This group of tumors, although a minority, can pose diagnostic difficulties.[11] Approximately 10% of these tumors show malignant potential with metastases; however, there are no definite morphologic criteria to predict such behavior. Malignant potential is almost always seen in adults only.

Tumors included in this group are Leydig cell tumors, Sertoli cell tumors, granulosa cell tumors, and tumors of the fibroma/thecoma group.[42]

LEYDIG CELL TUMOR

OVERVIEW

Leydig cell tumors are the most common tumors classified in the sex cord gonadal–stromal tumor group. Also known as "interstitial cell tumor," they account for 2% to 3% of testicular tumors in adults.[11,16,184] Three percent of testicular tumors in infants and children are Leydig cell tumors, and they comprise 14% of the stromal tumors in this population.[185] Five percent to 10% of Leydig cell tumors are associated with cryptorchidism.[184] Patients who have Klinefelter syndrome occasionally develop these tumors.[16] Although these tumors occur in all age groups, they are most common in patients between the ages of 20 and 50 years,[10]

Key Features
LEYDIG CELL TUMORS

1. Leydig cell tumors are the most common tumors of the sex cord–stromal tumor group

2. Most occur in patients aged 20 to 50 years with a smaller peak in patients aged 5 to 10 years

3. Gynecomastia is the presenting feature in about one third of cases; these tumors behave benign

4. Children who have Leydig cell tumors almost always present with isosexual pseudoprecocity

5. In adults, approximately 10% of Leydig cell tumors become metastatic; there are no reports of malignant Leydig cell tumors in children

6. The tumors nodules are 2 to 5 cm in size, solid, well circumscribed, and often encapsulated

7. Histologically, polyhedral cells have ample pink cytoplasm, ovoid nuclei with prominent nucleoli, grow in sheets, nests, cords, or ribbonlike patterns, and have fibrous to edematous stroma

8. In one third intra- or extracytoplasmic Reinke crystalloids may be seen; fifteen percent contain lipofuscin pigment

9. Orchiectomy is curable for benign Leydig cell tumors; malignant cases are treated with orchiectomy with RPLND

10. Malignant Leydig cell tumors are insensitive to radiation and chemotherapy

with a smaller peak at the age of 5 to 10 years.[186] Gynecomastia is present in one third of cases and can be the presenting symptom.[16,184] Children who have Leydig cell tumors almost always present with isosexual pseudoprecocity because of the androgenic hormone (ie, testosterone, androstenedione and dihydroepiandrosterone) elaboration by the tumor.[10,11] Levels of other hormones (eg, estrogen and progesterone) also may be elevated.[42] Estrogen-producing tumors may cause loss of libido and infertility.[187,188] These tumors usually present as painless testicular swelling. Small tumors can be detected on ultrasound examination. Only 3% of Leydig cell tumors are bilateral.[184] Approximately 10% of Leydig cell tumors behave aggressively. There are no reports of malignant Leydig cell tumors in children.

On imaging, Leydig cell tumors appear as hypoechoic, well-demarcated nodules that may show cystic areas. Sonographically they may be indistinguishable from germ cell tumors.[42]

GROSS FEATURES

Leydig cell tumors are solid, well-demarcated, often encapsulated, ovoid, sometimes lobulated masses and occasionally have fibrous bands. The cut surface is homogeneous yellow to tan to dark brown. These tumors range in size from 0.5 to 10 cm, more commonly being 2 to 5 cm.[184] In children Leydig cell tumors present as small tumors.[11] There may be occasional foci of hemorrhage and necrosis. Extratesticular extension may be seen in 10% to 15% of cases.[184]

MICROSCOPIC FEATURES

The most common histologic appearance is a diffuse, sheetlike growth of large, polygonal cells with ample eosinophilic cytoplasm and a central round to ovoid nucleus showing a prominent central nucleolus (**Fig. 55**). Nuclear size may vary slightly, and binucleation or multinucleation sometimes is observed. Mitoses are rare.[42] Other frequently seen patterns are nesting, ribbons, and cords with prominent fibrous stroma; the stroma, however, may be edematous.[11] The cytoplasm occasionally contains lipid, giving it a bubbly to vacuolated appearance, depending on the amount. In one third of cases, Reinke crystalloids, rod-shaped, bright eosinophilic crystals, are seen in the intracytoplasm or interstitium.[11] More commonly seen are rounded intracytoplasmic eosinophilic bodies that are considered precursors to Reinke crystalloids.[11] Lipofuscin pigment is seen in up to 15% of Leydig cell tumors.[11,42]

Two unique patterns described in Leydig cell tumors are tumors with prominent microcystic areas[189] and tumor cells that are spindled and arranged in fascicles. Calcification and foci of adipose metaplasia can be seen occasionally.[190]

DIFFERENTIAL DIAGNOSIS

The major differential is from benign entities, Leydig cell hyperplasia, and multinodular tumors of the adrenogenital and Nelson syndromes. Leydig cell hyperplasia has an interstitial growth with preserved intervening seminiferous tubules rather

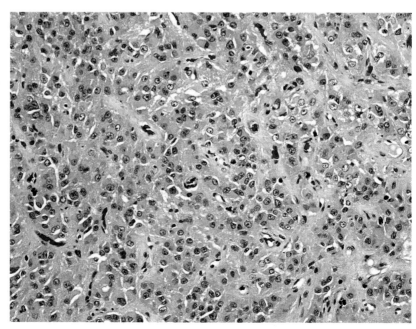

Fig. 55. Large polygonal cells with eosinophilic cytoplasm and round nuclei with central nucleoli in a diffuse growth pattern are seen most commonly in Leydig cell tumors (original magnification ×200). Occasional cells with brown lipofuscin pigment are seen in the lower half of the image.

△△ Differential Diagnosis
LEYDIG CELL TUMORS

- Leydig cell hyperplasia
- Multinodular tumors of the adrenogenital and Nelson syndromes (may be synaptophysin positive)
- Classic seminoma
- Malakoplakia
- Large cell calcifying Sertoli cell tumor
- Microcystic pattern may resemble yolk sac tumor
- Metastatic prostatic carcinoma

⊘ Pitfall
LEYDIG CELL TUMORS

! Leydig cell tumors can be patchily cytokeratin positive.

The lipid contents of Leydig cell cytoplasm may give them a somewhat clear-cell appearance resembling seminoma. The lack of IGCNU, fibrous septa with inflammatory infiltrates, and the use of immunostaining confirm the diagnosis of Leydig cell tumor.[11] Malakoplakia can mimic Leydig cell tumor; Michaelis-Gutmann bodies, the presence of other inflammatory cells, prominent intratubular growth, and positive staining with CD68 are discriminating features of malakoplakia. Large cell calcifying Sertoli cell tumor (LCCSCT) is a consideration in the differential diagnosis, but these tumors frequently occur as part of clinical syndromes, namely Carney's and Peutz-Jeghers syndromes, and can be multifocal and bilateral. LCCSCT can show an intratubular growth and have calcifications, whereas Leydig cell tumors do not have intratubular growth and rarely have calcifications.[11,110]

The microcystic growth pattern can resemble yolk sac tumor, which is positive for AFP. The presence of other areas typical for Leydig cell

than the expansile growth of Leydig cell tumors. Tumors of adrenogenital and Nelson syndromes usually are bilateral, multifocal, and dark brown (containing ample lipofuscin) and show cellular pleomorphism and hyalinized stroma. Clinical history is important in these cases.[11,42] Recently, synaptophysin positivity has been documented in tumors of adrenogenital syndrome and may help differentiate these tumors from Leydig cell tumors.[191]

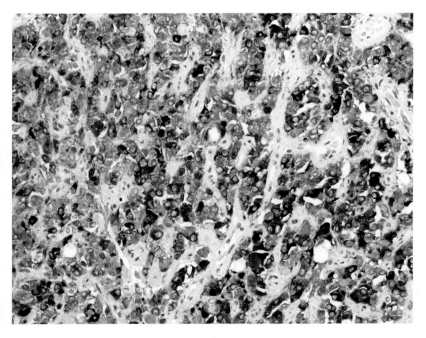

Fig. 56. Inhibin immunostain highlighting the cytoplasm of Leydig cell tumor (original magnification ×200).

Fig. 57. Malignant Leydig cell tumor with hyperchromatic and pleomorphic nuclei with coarse chromatin and obvious mitoses (original magnification ×200).

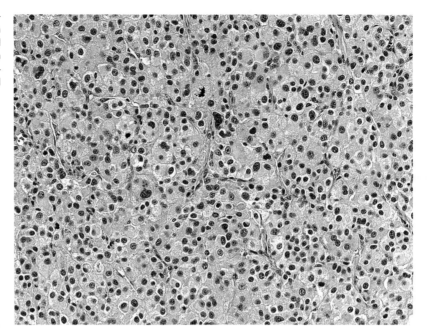

tumors is helpful, as is adequate sampling of sex cord–stromal tumors.

Rarely, metastatic prostatic carcinoma may be considered in the differential diagnosis of a Leydig cell tumor. Stains for cytokeratin and prostate-specific antigen and lack of inhibin staining provide clarification.

DIAGNOSIS

More than 90% of Leydig cell tumors stain with inhibin (**Fig. 56**), melan-A, and calretinin. S-100 might be positive also.[192] Vimentin always is positive. Steroid hormones can be demonstrated by immunohistochemistry.[11] Leydig cell tumors occasionally may have patchy cytokeratin

Fig. 58. Malignant Leydig cell tumor with necrosis (original magnification ×200).

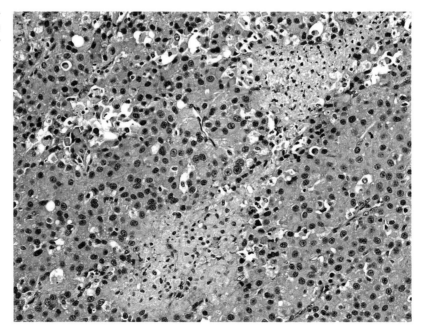

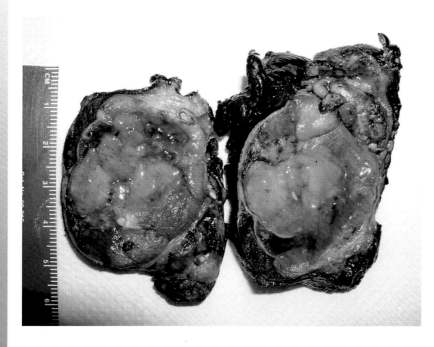

Fig. 59. Gross retroperitoneal lymph node with metastatic malignant Leydig cell tumor. Note the variegated appearance with hemorrhage and necrosis.

staining.[11,41] The microcystic areas and the spindle cells of Leydig cell tumors retain the usual immunomarkers for these tumors.

Electron microscopic examination reveals ample smooth endoplasmic reticulum, mitochondria with tubular cristae, and intracytoplasmic lipid droplets, features of steroid hormone–producing cells. Reinke crystalloids and membranous whorls sometimes can be seen on ultrastructural examination. Reinke crystals can have variable appearance and can appear as parallel lines, a prismatic or hexagonal lattice, or a dotlike pattern.[193–195]

PROGNOSIS

Most Leydig cell tumors follow a benign course with remission following orchiectomy. Recently testis-sparing surgery with clear margins documented by intraoperative frozen section is being considered for Leydig cell tumors, especially in children and young men.[196,197] Tumors presenting with gynecomastia almost always have a benign course.[184] Ten percent of Leydig cell tumors show malignant behavior, have large size (> 5 cm), occur in older individuals, and show nuclear pleomorphism (**Fig. 57**), necrosis, vascular invasion, and an increased mitotic rate (3–5 mitoses/ 10 high-power-fields) with abnormal mitoses (**Fig. 58**), increased ki-67 (> 5%), and DNA aneuploidy.[184,198] Malignant Leydig cell tumor is treated with orchiectomy and RPLND, because these tumors are insensitive to radiation and chemotherapy (**Fig. 59**). The tumors can recur after many years.[199] There are three documented

reports of sarcomatoid differentiation in Leydig cell tumors.[190,200,201] One showed sarcomatoid differentiation positive for muscle specific actin in metastases that occurred 17 years after orchiectomy.[200] The sarcomatoid differentiation seems to lose the usual staining pattern for Leydig cell tumors in the testis.[190]

SERTOLI CELL TUMOR

OVERVIEW

Sertoli cell tumor is a sex cord neoplasm with Sertoli cell differentiation.

Key Features
SERTOLI CELL TUMORS

1. Malignant tumors may present as lymph node metastasis

2. Most tumors are benign

3. Sertoli cell tumor patterns are cords, sheets, and tubular or retiform structures

4. Neoplastic cells may be eosinophilic to pale or have a vacuolated cytoplasm

5. A common pattern is tubule formation with or without a lumen, lined by radially arranged cells cytologically resembling normal testicular Sertoli cells

CLINICAL FEATURES

Sertoli cell tumors are rare, constituting less than 1% of testicular tumors. They occur at all ages.[202] Approximately 15% occur in children.[203] On rare occasions, these tumors may develop in patients who have androgen insensitivity syndrome and Peutz-Jeghers syndrome. Most Sertoli cell tumors are benign,[204] but malignant tumors represent approximately 10% of all Sertoli cell tumors.[10,24,71,169,204–206] In one report, only 6 of 66 cases of Sertoli cell tumors were associated with metastasis.[207]

Most Sertoli cell tumors are painless testicular masses; however, malignant tumors may present as lymph node metastases. In some cases, the tumor is an incidental ultrasound finding. Sertoli cell tumors are less likely than Leydig cell tumors to be hormonally active, but gynecomastia can occur. Virilization may be seen in children.[205,206,208,209]

Three common subtypes have been described: the classic Sertoli cell tumor, LCCSCT with characteristic calcifications,[210] and the rarer sclerosing form.[211] Other rarer subtypes include Sertoli cell adenoma and the Sertoli-Leydig cell tumor.[204] These rarer subtypes are not discussed further.

LCCSCT is a subtype with large areas of calcification that are seen readily with ultrasound. This subtype has been associated with Peutz-Jeghers syndrome and Carney syndrome (See the section on Larger Cell Calcifying Sertoli Cell Tumor).[71,210,212]

Serum markers, including AFP, hCG, lactate dehydrogenase (LDH), and PLAP, are always negative in Sertoli cell tumors. Sertoli cell tumors generally are hypoechoic on ultrasound. Genetic studies using comparative genomic hybridization performed in 11 cases of Sertoli cell tumors showed that the most frequently detected aberrations were gain of chromosome X (in 5 of 11 cases) followed by loss of all or part of chromosomes 2 and 19 (in three cases).[213]

ΔΔ **Differential Diagnosis**
SERTOLI CELL TUMORS

- Tubular seminoma
- Leydig cell tumors, particularly with cytoplasmic vacuolation
- Rete testis carcinoma, particularly when the Sertoli cell tumor has a retiform growth pattern
- Well-differentiated adenocarcinoma, particularly at metastatic sites

---

GROSS FEATURES

Sertoli tumors usually are well-circumscribed, unilateral, firm, round to lobulated masses. Most tumors are unifocal. Cystic and/or hemorrhagic areas may be seen, rarely, particularly in larger tumors.[71] The tumors have a yellow-tan or white appearance with an average diameter of 3.5 cm. Sertoli cell tumors of the sclerosing subtype tend to be smaller, with a mean diameter of 1.5 cm.[71,204]

MICROSCOPIC FEATURES

Sertoli cell tumors exhibit a variety of growth patterns including cords, sheets, and tubular or retiform structures. The neoplastic cells may be eosinophilic to pale or have a vacuolated cytoplasm. The nuclei are round to oval, with a regular appearance; some may have grooves, and on rare occasions inclusions may be seen.[61] Nucleoli may be seen also. Tumors with a retiform growth pattern show a network of irregularly branching, elongated, narrow tubules and cysts in which the papillary structures may project (**Fig. 60**).[204] A common pattern is tubule formation with or without a lumen, lined by radially arranged cells, cytologically resembling normal testicular Sertoli cells (**Fig. 61**).[61,214] The sclerosing subtype has anastomosing tubules and cords of epithelial cells within a dense, fibrous matrix.[61,71] Ultrastructural examination may show Charcot-Böttcher filaments.

DIFFERENTIAL DIAGNOSIS

The differential diagnosis includes seminoma (eg, a tubular seminoma), but other features of seminoma, such as lymphoid reaction, granulomas, and intratubular germ cell neoplasia, are absent. Immunohistochemistry is helpful in distinguishing the two. Sertoli cell tumors should be negative for cKit and PLAP and positive for inhibin. Leydig cell tumors, particularly those with a cytoplasmic vacuolation, may mimic the appearance of Sertoli cell tumors. Inhibin stain tends to be more diffuse and intense in Leydig cell tumors than in Sertoli cell tumors.[61,204]

Pitfall
SERTOLI CELL TUMORS

! Sertoli cell neoplasm may be mistaken for carcinoma. Immunohistochemistry, particularly using inhibin, often is helpful in discriminating carcinoma from Sertoli cell tumors.

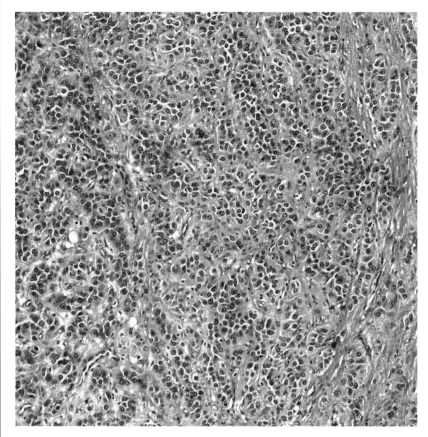

Fig. 60. Sertoli cell tumors with retiform growth pattern, a network of irregularly branching, elongated, narrow tubules and cysts in which the papillary structures may project (original magnification ×100).

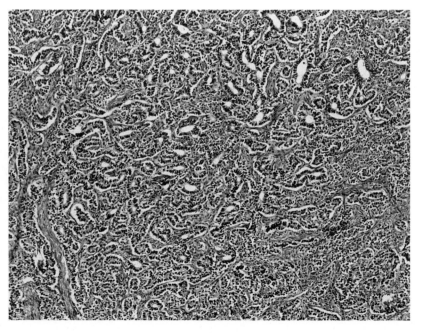

Fig. 61. A common pattern of Sertoli cell tumor with tubule formation, with or without a lumen, lined by radially arranged cells (original magnification ×100).

Rete testis carcinoma mimics the appearance of Sertoli cell tumor, particularly Sertoli cell tumor with a retiform growth pattern. Rete testis carcinoma is negative for inhibin and positive for EMA.[61]

Another entity in the differential diagnosis, particularly at metastatic sites, is well-differentiated adenocarcinoma. Immunohistochemistry, particularly using inhibin, often is helpful in distinguishing carcinoma from Sertoli cell tumors.[61,204]

IMMUNOHISTOCHEMISTRY

Neoplastic cells express vimentin, cytokeratins, inhibin (40% of the cases), and S-100 (30%, focally). The neoplastic cells are negative for EMA, PLAP, AFP, and hCG.[214–216] **Box 12** lists the markers for Sertoli cell tumors.

PROGNOSIS

Malignant tumors may metastasize. Treatment for benign Sertoli cell tumor is orchiectomy. Malignant Sertoli cell tumors may be treated additionally with RPLND.[206,209,217]

LARGE CELL CALCIFYING SERTOLI CELL TUMOR

OVERVIEW

LCCSCT, a rare tumor, usually occurs in young males.[218] Approximately 30% of these tumors occur as part of Carney's syndrome and less

---

Box 12
Markers for Sertoli cell tumors

Neoplasms express vimentin, cytokeratins, inhibin, and S-100 (30%, focally)

Neoplastic cells are negative for

EMA

PLAP

AFP

hCG

CKIT

PLAP

Neoplastic cells are positive for inhibin. (Inhibin stain tends to be less diffuse and intense in Sertoli cell tumors than in Leydig cell tumors.)

---

commonly in Peutz-Jeghers syndrome; overall, 60% are sporadic.[42] Of the limited number of cases reported in the literature (around 50), about 20% behaved in malignant fashion.[42] The age range for presentation of benign LCCSCT is 2 to 38 years, with a mean age of 17 years; the age range for the presentation of LCCSCT with malignant behavior is 28 to 51 years with a mean age of 39 years.[210] The syndromic tumors commonly are multifocal, bilateral, and behave in a benign fashion. Reported malignant tumors were unilateral and solitary.[210] Various endocrine symptoms, most commonly gynecomastia and precocious

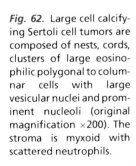

Fig. 62. Large cell calcifying Sertoli cell tumors are composed of nests, cords, clusters of large eosinophilic polygonal to columnar cells with large vesicular nuclei and prominent nucleoli (original magnification ×200). The stroma is myxoid with scattered neutrophils.

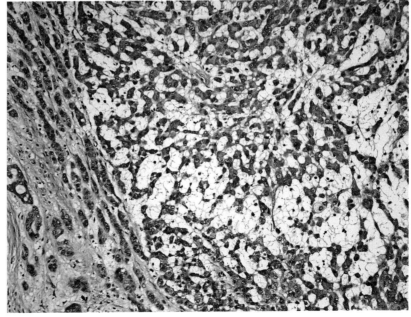

puberty, are manifested with these tumors.[42] In the ovary, the tumor associated with Peutz-Jeghers syndrome is sex cord tumor with annular tubules that lack calcifications. Rarely, in testes, similar tumors can be seen with this syndrome.

GROSS FEATURES

LCCSCT usually are small tumors (most < 2 cm) contained within the testis; up to 25% are bilateral

and may be multifocal.[11] The cut surface is yellow to tan and gritty because of calcifications.[11] Malignant tumors typically are larger than 4 cm and may have areas of hemorrhage and necrosis.

MICROSCOPIC FEATURES

LCCSCT are composed of nests and cord and clusters of large eosinophilic polygonal to columnar cells with large vesicular nuclei and prominent nucleoli (**Fig. 62**). These cells show frequent intratubular growth. The stroma can be myxoid to hyalinized with scattered neutrophils; prominent laminated calcifications are seen in 50% of intratubular as well as in extratubular tumor cells (**Fig. 63**). Mitoses are rare in benign tumors but are seen readily in malignant tumors.

DIFFERENTIAL DIAGNOSIS

LCCSCT can be mistaken for Leydig cell tumors because of the presence of eosinophilic cells; however, these cells frequently show intratubular growth and calcifications, which are lacking in Leydig cell tumors.[11,110]

DIAGNOSIS

Immunohistochemical positivity for inhibin, vimentin, S-100, desmin, and EMA and focal positivity for cytokeratin are seen (**Box 13**).[210,219,220]

Ultrastructural studies and the presence of Charcot-Böttcher filaments support the Sertoli cell derivation of these tumors.[219,221]

PROGNOSIS

Features associated with aggressive behavior include size greater than 4 cm, extratesticular growth, gross or microscopic necrosis, high-grade cytologic atypia, vascular space invasion, and a mitotic rate greater than three mitoses/10 high-power fields.[210]

Box 13
Markers for large cell calcifying Sertoli cell tumors
LCCSCT are positive for
Inhibin
Vimentin
S-100
Desmin
EMA
Cytokeratins (focally)

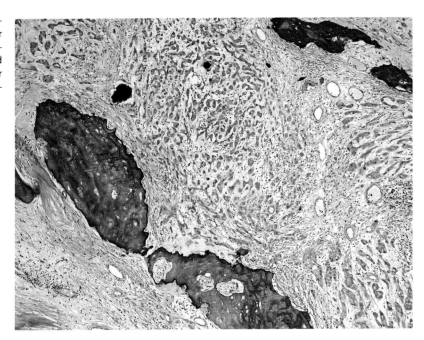

Fig. 63. Large cell calcifying Sertoli cell tumor with prominent calcifications in the stroma and associated with tumor cells (original magnification ×40).

Only one case of this tumor in Carney's syndrome had a malignant course,[210] and none of the tumors associated with Peutz-Jeghers syndrome behaved in a malignant fashion.

The treatment for benign tumors is orchiectomy or testis-sparing therapy. For suspected malignant tumors, orchiectomy with RPLND can be performed.[110]

ADULT GRANULOSA CELL TUMOR

OVERVIEW

Granulosa cell tumors (GCT) in the testis are quite rare; they resemble the more common ovarian granulosa cell tumor.[222–224] These tumors may present with gynecomastia (in 25% of cases). The age range of patients at presentation is 16 to 76 years (mean age, 44 years).[42] Granulosa cell tumors usually have an indolent course, but 20% of the reported cases behaved in a malignant fashion.[225]

GROSS FEATURES

Granulosa cell tumors present with unilateral testicular swelling, sometimes of long duration. Tumors are well demarcated and may show encapsulation. They are firm with a white to yellow cut surface, often are lobulated, and may be cystic. They range in size from 1 to 13 cm.

MICROSCOPIC FEATURES

Granulosa cell tumors are cellular tumors with cells characteristically having scant cytoplasm. The nuclei are round to ovoid, pale, and may show the typical "coffee bean" grooves well known for this entity in the ovary. There may be some focal cytologic atypia. Mitoses are rare. The cells commonly are arranged in a microfollicular pattern with Call-Exner bodies (palisaded cells surrounding central eosinophilic material) or may have a solid arrangement (**Fig. 64**). Macrofollicular, insular, gyriform, trabecular, and pseudosarcomatous patterns also have been observed (**Fig. 65**). Occasionally, the cells at the periphery of the tumor may appear to infiltrate around the seminiferous tubules and may invade tunica albuginea.[42] These tumors sometimes can have smooth muscle and focal osteoid.[222]

DIFFERENTIAL DIAGNOSIS

These tumors might be diagnosed as unclassified sex cord–stromal tumors with granulosa cell features in the testis; however, when the predominant tumor shows granulosa cell features, it should be diagnosed as such.[110] The presence of focal

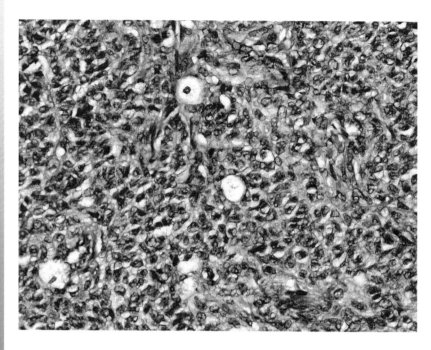

Fig. 64. Adult granulosa cell tumor with diffuse growth pattern, composed of cells with coffee bean–shaped nuclei and Call-Exner bodies (original magnification ×400).

luteinized cells may suggest gonadoblastoma; negative staining with CD117, PLAP, and OCT3/4 should clarify the diagnosis.[110]

DIAGNOSIS

Adult granulosa cell tumor of the testis may be the rarest tumor of the sex cord–stromal group.

Tumors cells label with antibodies to vimentin, smooth muscle actin, and CD99 (O13) and focally with cytokeratin.[11,226,227]

PROGNOSIS

Approximately 20% of testicular adult granulosa tumors have metastasized.[186,225,228,229] Size

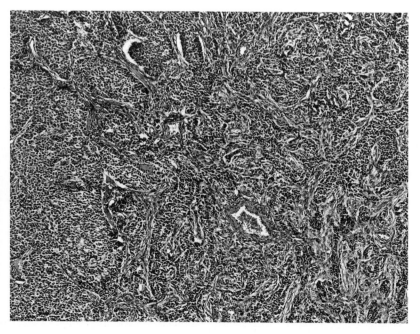

Fig. 65. Gyriform and trabecular growth pattern of adult granulosa cell tumor (original magnification ×100).

greater than 7 cm, lymphovascular invasion, hemorrhage, and necrosis portend aggressive behavior.[228] Orchiectomy is curative; RPLND can be performed when metastasis is suspected.[229] Metastases have been noted several years after orchiectomy.[228] In one case, orchiectomy with chemotherapy and resection of lung metastases provided remission.[225]

JUVENILE GRANULOSA CELL TUMOR

OVERVIEW

JGCTs occur predominantly in the first 6 months of life.[71] Although rare, they are the most common tumor in this age group. JGCT commonly is associated with abnormal sex chromosomes (45XO/46XY, and 45XO/46X isoYq mosaicism), intersex syndromes, and ambiguous genitalia (in 20% of cases), but isosexual precocity or gynecomastia has not been observed.[42,110] The most common associated abnormality is mixed gonadal dysgenesis and, secondly, hypospadias. These tumors most often occur in descended testis, but about 30% occur in abdominal testes. Presentation after the first year of life is exceptional.[42] A single case of JGCT recently was reported in a 27-year-old man.[230] Ultrasonography reveals a complex, multiseptated, and hypoechoic mass.[231]

GROSS FEATURES

This rare gonadal stromal tumor can present as a scrotal or abdominal mass. Bilateral JGCT has been reported as large masses in abdominal testis.[232] The testis is enlarged, and the mass has solid and cystic areas. The tumor may show partial encapsulation. The size ranges from 0.8 to 5 cm.[233] The cut surface shows gray to yellow solid areas with interspersed cysts containing viscid fluid.[11]

MICROSCOPIC FEATURES

These tumors have follicular cystic and solid components.[233] The follicles that give this neoplasm a multicystic appearance have cells arranged in multilayered fashion; solid nests and nodules of cells separated by hyalinized stroma also are present. The contents of the follicles are eosinophilic to basophilic and can stain with mucicarmine (**Fig. 66**).[234] Depending on the cystic dilatation of the follicles, the tumors are lined on the inner aspect by granulosa-like cells, and the outer layers have theca-like cells. The outer layers have columnar cells with scanty cytoplasm. The outermost layers become spindled, apparently corresponding to theca externa. The inner granulosa-like cells are polyhedral and have moderate pale to eosinophilic and sometimes vacuolated cytoplasm with hyperchromatic, rounded nuclei (**Fig. 67**). Frequent mitoses can be seen in the inner layers. Call-Exner bodies may be seen in the cells lining the follicles. Occasional tumor cells can be seen in the adjacent seminiferous tubules.[234,235]

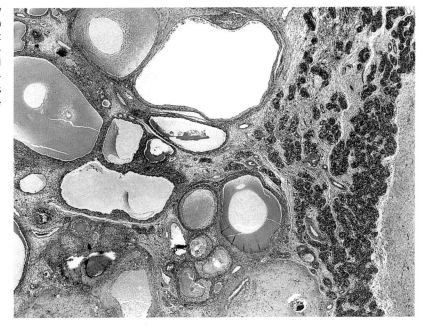

Fig. 66. Low-power view of juvenile granulosa cell tumor, with cystic spaces containing basophilic material (original magnification ×40). Adjacent fetal seminiferous tubules are seen on the right side.

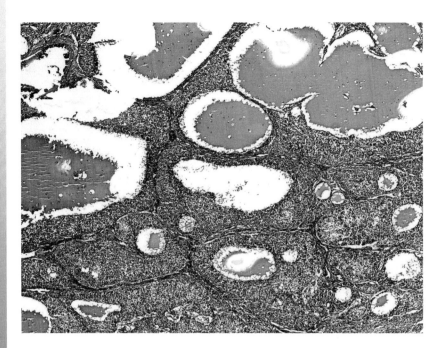

Fig. 67. Solid and cystic area of juvenile granulosa cell tumor, with follicles lined by granulosa cells and variable cysts (original magnification ×100).

DIFFERENTIAL DIAGNOSIS

The major differential diagnostic consideration is with **y**olk sac tumor. Both tumors have solid and cystic areas, cytologic atypia, and a high mitotic rate.[233,236] Yolk sac tumor occurs in older children, and the presence of other yolk sac patterns, along with AFP positivity confirms the diagnosis. Awareness that serum AFP is physiologically elevated in neonates can clarify the issue further.[11]

DIAGNOSIS

The granulosa-like cells in these tumors are uniformly inhibin, vimentin, cytokeratin, CD99, and S-100 positive. The outer thecalike (spindle) cells show diffuse smooth muscle actin and vimentin positivity with focal desmin staining.[11,42,234,237] These tumors are believed to be derived from common specialized gonadal stroma, because they show ultrastructural features of both primitive Sertoli cells and preovulatory granulosa cells, with a dual epithelial and smooth muscle differentiation.[238,239]

PROGNOSIS

JGCTs are considered benign, and the prognosis is excellent. Orchiectomy is curative. Testis-sparing surgery can be considered.[231,240] No metastasis or recurrences have been reported thus far.[236,237,241,242]

FIBROMA/THECOMA

OVERVIEW

Fibroma/thecomas are rare tumors in the testis. Less than 50 cases have been described. The tumors are slow-growing masses usually seen in the third to fourth decades of life. Patients present with unilateral, sometimes painful, testicular masses.[1] These tumors resemble the fibroma/thecoma tumors of the ovary and are not associated with increased hormonal function.[170,243–246]

GROSS FEATURES

These tumors are solid, firm, yellow-gray-white, and well circumscribed. Most are not encapsulated. There is no hemorrhage or necrosis.[244]

HISTOLOGIC FEATURES

Fibromas are composed of acellular collagenized plaques and hypercellular areas of fibroblastic spindle cells growing in a storiform fashion or in fascicles (**Fig. 68**).[1] No definite neoplastic sex cord elements are present, although rare cases with minor sex cord–stromal elements have been described.[247] Occasionally, entrapped seminiferous tubules and germ cells are interspersed with occasional blood vessels. Mitosis is present very infrequently.[244]

Fig. 68. This fibroma is composed of collagenized stroma and hypercellular areas of fibroblastic spindle cells growing in a storiform arrangement (original magnification ×200).

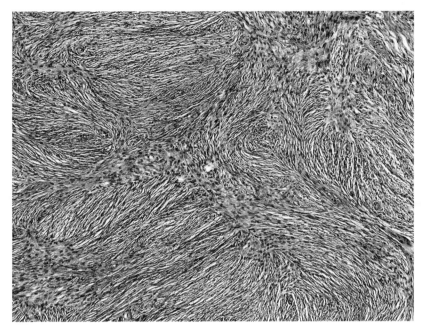

DIFFERENTIAL DIAGNOSIS

Entities in the differential diagnosis include unclassified sex cord–stromal tumors, fibroma arising in the tunica, solitary fibrous tumor, neurofibroma, and smooth muscle tumors. The differential diagnosis also includes stromal tumors and some malignant tumors, such as primary paratesticular or extratesticular sarcoma of the testis.[170,245,246,248–250]

DIAGNOSIS

Ultrasound is useful for identifying the location of the mass (testicular versus paratesticular) but not for distinguishing the type of the lesion.[251] Immunohistochemically, the neoplastic cells are positive for vimentin and smooth muscle actin and less frequently are positive for desmin, cytokeratin, and S-100.[1] The tumor cells are negative for inhibin and CD99. Ultrastructurally, these tumor cells have features of both fibroblasts and myofibroblasts.[244]

PROGNOSIS

Tumors of the fibroma/thecoma group have a good prognosis. No recurrences or metastases have been reported.[170,245,246]

MIXED AND UNCLASSIFIED SEX CORD–STROMAL TUMORS

OVERVIEW

The category of mixed sex cord–stromal tumors includes tumors that have recognizable sex cord gonadal–stromal elements containing more than one type of cell (ie, Leydig cells, Sertoli cells, and granulosa cells) in variable proportions. The unclassified group includes tumors that are recognizable as sex cord– or gonadal-stromal tumors but lack specific differentiation or have abortive differentiation. These tumors occur over a wide age range and present with unilateral testicular swelling. Gynecomastia is present in 15% of these cases.[11,206]

GROSS FEATURES

These tumors vary widely in size, ranging from small nodules to large, lobulated masses replacing the testis. The cut surface is gray-white to yellow.

MICROSCOPIC FEATURES

The mixed tumors have the histologic features of the various types of well-differentiated components. The unclassifiable sex cord gonadal–stromal tumors make up a heterogeneous group of neoplasms. The predominant morphology in many of these tumors is spindle cells.[252,253] The spindle cell tumors have either relatively short spindled cells with prominent nuclear grooves and intermixed epithelioid cells or elongated spindle cells that are reminiscent of smooth muscle.[252] The concurrent presence of some morphologic and immunohistochemical features of both Leydig and granulosa cell lines in these tumors suggests their origin from a stromal stem cell, possibly capable of dual differentiation but with maturation arrested at an early phase of differentiation.[253] The histologic, immunohistochemical, and ultrastructural features of the spindle cell tumors are similar to those of granulosa cell tumors. Reactivity for S-100 protein and smooth muscle actin is characteristic of these tumors.[252] Unlike ovarian granulosa cell tumors, however, these tumors and other testicular granulosa cell tumors are either negative or only patchily positive for cytokeratin.[42]

Sertoli-Leydig cell tumors are common in ovary but extremely rare in testis.[254] Two examples of unclassified sex cord gonadal–stromal tumors are shown in **Figs. 69** and **70**. One of these tumors has some Sertoli cell features forming tubules and cords with clear cells, the stroma being fibrotic. The second has cells with vacuolated cytoplasm reminiscent of some Leydig cell tumors. Both these tumors had focal staining with either inhibin or melan A, but the histology was not typical of any one of the sex cord gonadal–stromal tumors; hence these tumors were designated as unclassified sex cord gonadal–stromal tumors.

DIFFERENTIAL DIAGNOSIS

When these tumors show spindle cell morphology, care should be taken to rule out a testicular or paratesticular sarcoma. Gross examination to ascertain the testicular origin, in addition to immunohistochemistry for identification of epithelial differentiation in a tumor with prominent spindle morphology, can help place these tumors in the sex cord gonadal–stromal category.[110]

DIAGNOSIS

Each of the differentiated elements stains as their pure counterparts do. Undifferentiated components may show positivity for S-100, smooth muscle actin, desmin, and cytokeratins.[252,255,256] Ultrastructural analysis of the spindle cell tumors revealed desmosomes, numerous thin filaments, and focal dense bodies.[252] Reticulin enveloped aggregates of cells of various sizes but not individual cells.[252]

PROGNOSIS

Tumors occurring in children younger than 10 years of age have behaved innocuously; however, lesions in older individuals and of large size have a guarded prognosis. Approximately 20% of these tumors are malignant.[257,258] Large tumor size, cellular atypia, hemorrhage, necrosis, and lymphovascular invasion are predictive of aggressive behavior.[257]

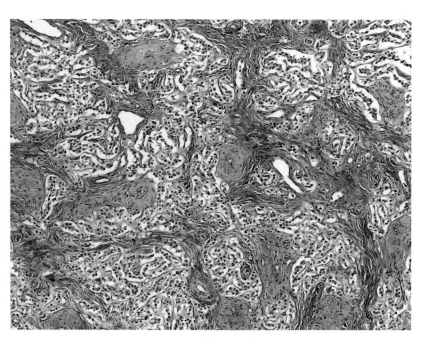

Fig. 69. This sex cord gonadal stromal tumor shows some features of Sertoli cell tumor with trabeculae and cords of clear cells arranged in a hyalinized fibrotic stroma (original magnification ×100). Inhibin immunostaining is positive.

Fig. 70. This sex cord gonadal stromal tumor
(original magnification
×200) has a uniform vac-
uolated appearance
throughout the tumor,
as seen focally in some
Leydig cell tumors. This
tumor has patchy melan
A positivity.

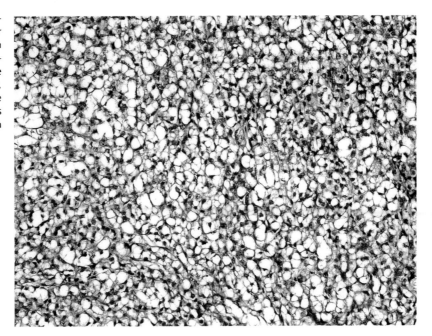

Typically orchiectomy alone is the treatment of choice. When there is metastasis or suspicion for metastatic behavior based on pathologic examination, RPLND may be undertaken.

RETE TESTIS LESIONS

CYSTIC DYSPLASIA

OVERVIEW

Cystic dysplasia is considered a developmental anomaly, because it is seen in infants and children associated with ipsilateral renal agenesis,[259–261] multicystic renal dysplasia,[262] and bilateral rete cystic dysplasia with renal adysplasia (bilateral renal agenesis).[263] Cystically dilated rete testis causes compression atrophy of the testicular parenchyma and forms a scrotal mass, which can be painful.

ADENOMATOUS HYPERPLASIA

OVERVIEW

Adenomatous hyperplasia of rete testis can be an incidental finding in a background of other testicular pathology; in 50% of cases it presents as a solid or cystic mass. This condition is seen commonly with testicular atrophy.[264–266] It is characterized by complex interconnecting proliferation of tubulo-papillary channels lined by cytologically bland, cuboidal to low columnar cells. These channels may show cystic dilatation;[266] contiguity to the

non-hyperplastic rete supports its origin in the rete (**Fig. 71**).[267]

Adenomatous hyperplasia of rete testis can be seen in patients who have germ cell tumors, cryptorchidism and chronic hepatic insufficiency, and bilateral renal dysplasia.[268] In the background of germ cells tumors, rete testis can have proliferation of the epithelium, with cells containing intracytoplasmic eosinophilic hyaline globules, sometimes filling the channels, which in turn may be expanded. This pattern can be mistaken for yolk sac tumor.[73]

ADENOMA

OVERVIEW

Rete testis adenomas, grossly circumscribed benign tumors are centered on rete testis, have a proliferation of cytologically bland cuboidal to low columnar epithelium forming either a solid mass of closely packed tubules or mild papillary proliferations with cellular stratification and budding in cystically dilated spaces. These rare tumors have been reported in patients 21 to 79 years of age. The tumors range in size from 1.5 to 3.6 cm.[268] The various designations of these tumors (adenoma, adenofibroma, cystadenoma, and papillary cystadenoma) is based on their morphologic/architectural appearance.[264,268]

Sertoliform cystadenoma of rete testis is a distinct tumor with areas of solid tubules and proliferations within cystically dilated rete spaces. The

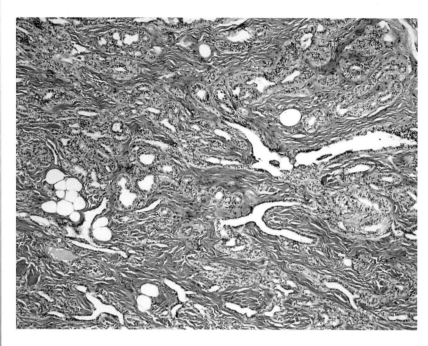

Fig.   71. Adenomatoid hyperplasia of rete testis showing interconnecting proliferation of tubulo-papillary channels lined by cytologically bland, cuboidal to low columnar cells (original magnification   ×100). Contiguity to the non-hyperplastic rete is seen.

cells resemble the cells of Sertoli cell tumors of the testicular parenchyma.[269,270] These tumors have been reported in adults and range in size from microscopic to 3 cm. The proliferation in dilated rete channels consists of tall columnar cells with ample eosinophilic to pale cytoplasm and basally oriented nuclei with prominent central nucleoli (**Fig. 72**). These tumors also can show intratubular

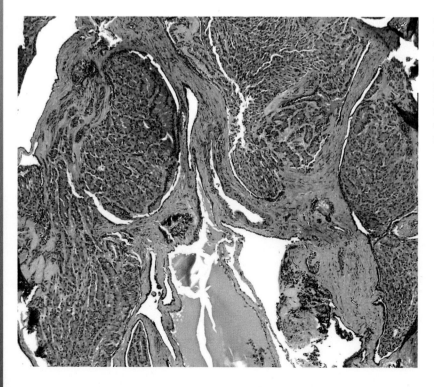

Fig. 72. Sertoliform cystadenoma with proliferation in dilated rete channels of tall columnar cells with ample eosinophilic to pale cytoplasm and basally oriented nuclei with prominent central nucleoli (original magnification ×100).

growth within adjacent tubules (**Fig. 73**). The remarkable resemblance of sertoliform cystadenoma of rete testis to Sertoli cell tumors and its positivity for inhibin supports its putative origin from the rete testis (ie, from both sex cord and mesonephros).[267]

RETE TESTIS ADENOCARCINOMA

OVERVIEW

Rete testis adenocarcinoma is a rare tumor (approximately 35 cases have been reported); hence a diagnosis of exclusion is needed. Strict criteria for a diagnosis of primary rete testis adenocarcinoma have been established:[264,267,271,272]

1. Absence of histologically similar extrascrotal tumor that could prove to be the primary site
2. Tumor centered on the testicular hilum
3. Morphology incompatible with any other type of testicular or paratesticular tumor
4. Immunohistochemical exclusion of other locally arising malignancies, namely malignant mesothelioma and papillary serous carcinoma

Transition from benign to neoplastic rete epithelium, when identified, is also a useful finding, but a large tumor may obliterate the normal structures.[11,267]

Patients may present with testicular pain, swelling, features of epididymitis, hydrocele, hematocele, nodules in scrotal skin, metastasis to suprapubic skin, or signs and symptoms of distant metastatic disease.[11,268,273–277] These tumors occur over a wide age range, 8 to 91 years. Prognosis is dismal, with average survival of 8 months. Rare long-term survival of 4 years has been reported.[11,267,268,271,272,278]

MICROSCOPIC FEATURES

These tumors form a large, solid to cystic or solid, firm to rubbery mass centered at the testicular hilum, with satellite nodules involving spermatic cord in about one third of cases. Tumor may extend to the epididymis, spreading to the para-aortic, iliac, and other lymph nodes, to viscera, and to bone. The size ranges from 1 to 10 cm.

Microscopically, large cellular nodules and small clumps are identified with a range of glandular patterns. The most common pattern is tubuloglandular, with elongated and compressed, slitlike branching tubules. Solid tubular or mildly papillary growth within cystic spaces, solid growth with tiny slitlike channels, and biphasic epithelial and spindle patterns have all been described (**Fig. 74**).[11,271,272,278] The cells are cuboidal to sometimes columnar with eosinophilic cytoplasm. Moderate pleomorphism, nuclear stratification, and scattered mitoses are seen. The stroma may be inflammatory or desmoplastic (**Fig. 75**). Necrosis is variable.[11] Treatment is orchiectomy with RPLND.

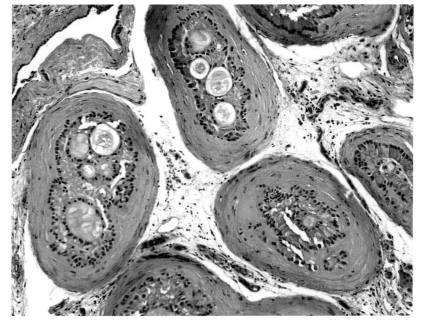

Fig. 73. Cells of sertoliform adenoma with intratubular growth within adjacent tubules (original magnification ×200).

Key Features
RETE TESTIS ADENOCARCINOMA

1. Rete testis adenocarcinoma is a rare tumor. Approximately 35 cases have been reported

2. Criteria for diagnosis are

- Absence of histologically similar extra-scrotal tumor that could prove to be the primary site

- Tumor centered on the testicular hilum

- Morphology incompatible with any other type of testicular or paratesticular tumor

- Immunohistochemical exclusion of other locally arising malignancies, namely malignant mesothelioma and papillary serous carcinoma

3. Rete testis adenocarcinoma may present with unilateral testicular pain, swelling, features of epididymitis, hydrocele, hematocele, nodules in scrotal skin, metastasis to suprapubic skin, and signs and symptoms of distant metastatic disease

4. Growth patterns can be papillary, solid tubular, branching tubular (retiform), spindled, or cystic. Stroma is inflammatory or desmoplastic

5. There are frequent mitoses; pleomorphic cells have with eosinophilic to amphophilic cytoplasm; nuclei have clumped chromatin and may have prominent nucleoli

6. Prognosis is dismal, with average survival of less than 1 year. Only 36% of patients available for follow-up were disease free after treatment

7. Orchiectomy with RPLND is the treatment of choice

Differential Diagnosis
RETE TESTIS ADENOCARCINOMA

- Paratesticular mesotheliomas
- Metastatic adenocarcinomas
- Ovarian-type epithelial tumors
- Epididymal adenocarcinoma
- Malignant Sertoli cell tumors
- Germ cell tumor embryonal carcinoma

DIFFERENTIAL DIAGNOSIS

The differential diagnostic considerations for this entity include malignant mesothelioma, certain ovarian-type tumors, metastatic adenocarcinoma, epididymal adenocarcinoma, and malignant Sertoli cell tumors.[11,265,268,271] Mesotheliomas can be distinguished by combined gross and microscopic features in most cases. Mesotheliomas typically coat the tunica vaginalis surfaces with multifocal nodules, with typical tubulopapillary microscopic architecture lined by bland-appearing cells compared with rete carcinomas. Finally, immunomarkers, including calretinin, WT1, CK5/6 (for mesothelioma) and Leu-M1, Ber EP4, and B72.3 (for adenocarcinoma) can be used.[267]

Müllerian-type tumors, namely serous tumor of low malignant potential and occasionally endometrioid carcinoma, may pose a diagnostic challenge with rete carcinoma. Serous tumors typically are predominantly cystic with bland cytology; psammoma bodies and divergent mucinous or squamous differentiation sometimes are seen in serous carcinomas. These tumors typically are centered in the epididymo-testicular grove. Finally CA-125 and WT1 immunomarkers can be used to confirm the Müllerian origin of these tumors.[267]

Metastatic adenocarcinomas frequently are bilateral and multifocal, show lymphovascular invasion, and may have an interstitial growth around rete channels. A history of carcinoma elsewhere in the body, even though remote, helps clarify the definitive diagnosis.[267]

Epididymal adenocarcinomas are extremely rare tumors that can be solid, widely destructive, and invade the paratesticular tissues. Less often they form a localized cystic mass.[279] These tumors have a predominantly tubular pattern but may have cystically dilated and papillary areas creating a tubulocystic to tubulopapillary appearance. The cells are cuboidal to columnar with ample clear to amphophilic to eosinophilic cytoplasm. Epididymal adenocarcinomas sometimes have much less atypia and mitotic activity than rete carcinomas. The presence of prominent

Pitfall
RETE TESTIS ADENOCARCINOMA

! Large tumors may obliterate normal structures, so identifying origin from the rete testis may be challenging.

Fig. 74. Low-power view of rete testis adenocarcinoma with tubuloglandular, solid tubular, and mildly papillary growth within cystic spaces (original magnification ×40). This lesion is centered on rete testis. The stroma is inflammatory and desmoplastic.

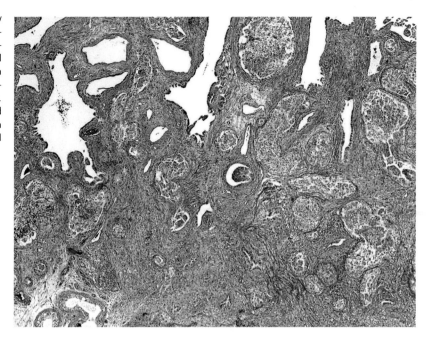

clear cells in a tubular carcinoma of this region favors an epididymal adenocarcinoma over rete testis adeocarcinoma.[267]

Sertoli cell tumors are distinguished from rete carcinoma by their predominant location within the testis parenchyma, so gross evaluation is of crucial importance.[267]

TESTICULAR LYMPHOMA, PLASMACYTOMA, AND LEUKEMIA

OVERVIEW

Malignant lymphoma can arise in the testis or paratesticular tissues, namely the epididymis and spermatic cord. Secondary testicular

Fig. 75. Rete testis carcinoma with contiguity to rete testis channels (original magnification ×100). The cells are cuboidal to columnar with eosinophilic cytoplasm. Moderate pleomorphism and nuclear stratification are seen.

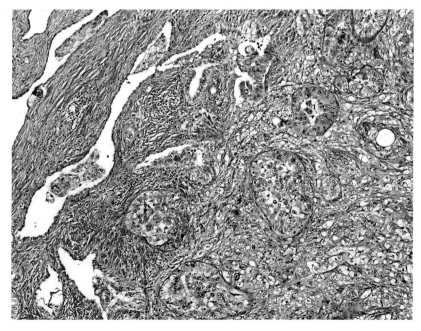

involvement is more common with plasmacytoma and leukemia. Malignant lymphomas account for 5% of testicular tumors; however, they comprise one half of the testicular tumors in men older than 60 years,[280–282] and also are the most common testicular tumor in men 60 to 80 years of age.[282–285] Childhood primary testicular lymphomas are rare. When they do occur, it is usually before puberty, between the ages of 3 and 10 years.[286,287] The rate of secondary testicular involvement by systemic childhood lymphoma is 5%.[288]

Lymphomas are bilateral in 10% to 15% of cases.[10] Bilaterality is most often metachronous.[282,283] Involvement of contralateral testis is more common (10%–40%) at the time of lymphoma recurrence.[284,289,290] Simultaneous bilateral involvement is typical for lymphoblastic lymphoma.[42,281] B-symptoms are rare in primary tumors.[42] Twenty-five percent of adult testicular lymphomas are a manifestation of systemic disease.

Ultrasonography may not be able to distinguish between a lymphoma and a germ cell tumor. Lymphomas also are hypoechoic but often are bilateral and multifocal and involve the extratesticular tissues much more frequently than germ cell tumors.[42,291,292]

Primary plasmacytoma of the testis is rare. The mean patient age at presentation is around 55 years. Testicular involvement usually is a manifestation of systemic disease.[293]

GROSS FEATURES

Testicular lymphomas present with painless unilateral enlargement of the scrotum or the inguinal region. Lymphoma may replace the testicular parenchyma partially or completely and form a poorly demarcated, fleshy or firm, single or multinodular mass that has a pale tan, pale pink or gray, sometimes necrotic and hemorrhagic cut surface. Extratesticular invasion is common. It also may cause diffuse enlargement of the testis or paratesticular tissues.[294]

Plasmacytomas appear tan to gray-white and fleshy with foci of hemorrhage.[11]

MICROSCOPIC FEATURES

Microscopically, lymphoma cells have a primarily intertubular/interstitial growth, with preservation of the seminiferous tubules (Figs. 76 and 77); however, they may efface or invade the tubules. Significant sclerosis may be seen in about 30% of cases of lymphoma but not in plasmacytomas. Vascular invasion is seen in 60% of these lesions. Sheets of noncohesive large cells, often with irregular nuclei, variable size, and sometimes prominent nucleoli, are seen (Fig. 78).

Testicular plasmacytomas have the same morphology as plasmacytomas elsewhere in the body, with sheets of atypical plasma cells that may be binucleate or multinucleate and show an interstitial growth pattern. The seminiferous tubules are effaced towards the center of the lesion; an interstitial growth with preservation of the tubules is more common at the periphery.[295,296]

The histologic picture of leukemic involvement of the testis is similar to that of lymphoma. Granulocytic sarcomas (tumorous myeloid leukemic infiltrates) can have primitive-appearing cells with scant cytoplasm or may have bright, eosinophilic,

Fig. 76. Low-power view of primary testicular lymphoma showing interstitial growth around the seminiferous tubules (original magnification ×40).

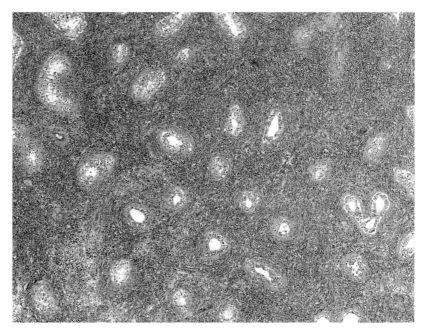

occasionally granular cytoplasm, consistent with a myeloid lineage. The nuclei are round and can be eccentric. Associated sclerosis may be present.[297]

DIFFERENTIAL DIAGNOSIS

The primary consideration in the differential diagnosis is the distinction from germ cell tumors, namely seminoma, spermatocytic seminoma, and embryonal carcinoma,[293,298] and from other types of hematologic malignancies.[297] The use of immunohistochemistry can sort through these lesions. Seminoma is positive for PLAP, CD117, OCT3/4, and D2-40; embryonal carcinoma is positive for CD30, OCT3/4, and cytokeratin; spermatocytic seminoma is positive for CD117 and is

Fig. 77. Lymphoblastic lymphoma involving the testis, sparing the seminiferous tubules (original magnification ×200).

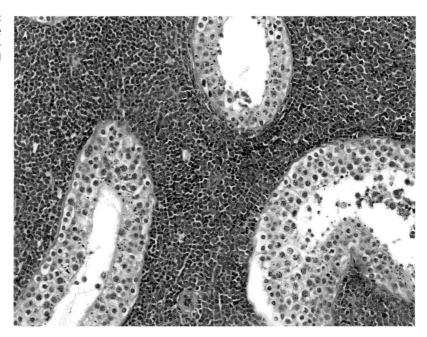

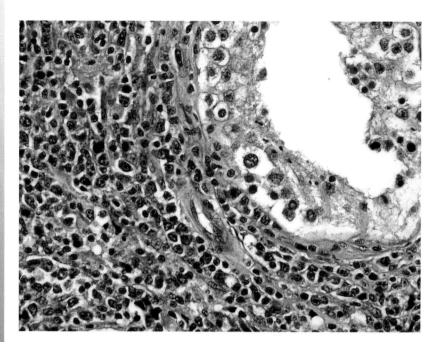

Fig. 78. High-power view of diffuse large B-cell lymphoma with sheets of noncohesive large cells with irregular nuclei, variable size, and prominent nucleoli (original magnification ×400).

negative for hematologic markers. Lymphoma and plasmacytoma are seen rarely in the adjacent seminiferous tubules, whereas seminoma and embryonal carcinoma have adjacent IGCNU and intratubular growth. Spermatocytic seminoma also frequently has intratubular growth.

Certain inflammatory conditions such as nonspecific granulomatous orchitis may resemble a lymphoma. The cell population in this entity is variable and polyclonal, consisting mostly of histiocytes and plasma cells.

DIAGNOSIS

In adults, primary diffuse large B cell lymphoma is the most common entity, comprising 70% to 80% of cases. Rare examples of Burkitt's lymphoma have been reported in adults,[299] and Burkitt's lymphoma remains the most common lymphoma involving the testes in children.[281] Anaplastic large-cell lymphoma,[298] primary T-cell lymphoma,[300] and CD56-positive Epstein-Barr virus associated T/natural killer cell lymphoma of nasal type[301] also have been described as rare testicular lymphomas. Hodgkin's lymphoma involving the testis has been reported only rarely.[302]

Follicular lymphomas can present, rarely, as primary testicular lymphomas in younger adults; however, most of these tumors have been described in children.[303] Some of the notable differences between primary testicular lymphomas and nodal follicular lymphomas are grade at presentation (stage I for most nodal follicular lymphomas, versus stage III for most testicular follicular lymphomas) and the lack of BCL2 expression and *BCL2* gene rearrangement. Primary testicular lymphomas and follicular nodal lymphomas have similar immunophenotypes and share an excellent prognosis.[303]

At autopsy, microscopic involvement of the testis has been found in about 60% patients who

---

△△ *Differential Diagnosis*
TESTICULAR LYMPHOMA, PLASMACYTOMA, AND LEUKEMIA

- Seminoma
- Spermatocytic seminoma
- Embryonal carcinoma, diffuse pattern
- Other hematologic malignancies
- Certain inflammatory conditions such as nonspecific granulomatous orchitis

---

 Pitfall
TESTICULAR LYMPHOMA, PLASMACYTOMA, AND LEUKEMIA

! Spermatocytic seminoma occurs in the same age group as primary testicular lymphoma.

have acute leukemia and in about 20% of patients who have chronic leukemia. Bilateral leukemic testicular involvement is common.

On rare occasions (5%), granulocytic sarcoma of the testis is the initial manifestation of acute myeloid leukemia.[297,304] Granulocytic sarcomas are associated with more widespread regional extratesticular involvement and may have sclerosis. Expression of myeloperoxidase, lysozyme, leukocyte common antigen, and CD43, but not of B-cell-specific or T-cell-specific antigens, is seen.

PROGNOSIS

Approximately 25% of testicular lymphomas present with stage II disease; the remaining cases either are confined to the testis or involve only adjacent structures (ie, stage I). Testicular lymphomas with best prognosis are the ones that present at stage I and at a younger age and have sclerosis.[280,281] Overall, primary lymphomas of testis and spermatic cord have the worst prognosis of all extranodal lymphomas, with a 5-year overall survival rate of 70% to 79%.[284,290] Relapses are common, occurring in more than 50% of cases. Extranodal sites are involved in 71% to 91% of cases, with the contralateral testis involved in 10% to 40% of cases and central nervous system parenchymal involvement in 20% to 27% of cases.[284,289,290]

Multiple myeloma with testicular involvement usually is present at a more widespread, advanced stage of the disease.[293] Primary plasmacytoma of the testis has a better prognosis.[293,296]

OVARIAN-TYPE EPITHELIAL TUMORS

OVERVIEW

Ovarian-type epithelial tumors are rare paratesticular and sometimes testicular tumors resembling surface epithelial tumors of the ovary. Most commonly found in this region are the serous borderline tumors. Other variants, including serous carcinomas, mucinous tumors and carcinomas, endometrioid carcinomas, clear cell adenocarcinomas, and benign and malignant Brenner tumors, have been described in this location.[267,305–307] Histology identical to that of ovarian tumors permits the various criteria and nomenclature used for the ovarian tumors to be applied to their male counterparts.[267] These tumors are believed to arise from Müllerian metaplasia of the tunica vaginalis, Müllerian rests in the paratesticular tissues, or the appendix testis. Intratesticular tumors are believed to arise from metaplasia of the mesothelial inclusions. Brenner tumor may arise from the Walthard rests of the tunica.[267,305,307]

Key Features
OVARIAN-TYPE EPITHELIAL TUMORS

1. These rare tumors are commonly paratesticular, sometimes testicular, and resemble surface epithelial tumors of the ovary

2. The tumors most commonly described in this location are serous borderline tumors

3. The various criteria and nomenclature used for ovarian tumors are applied to these tumors

4. These tumors arise either from Müllerian metaplasia of tunica vaginalis, Müllerian rests in paratesticular tissues, appendix testis, or metaplasia of mesothelial inclusions in the testis

5. The mean patient age at presentation is in the fifties. The mean tumor size at presentation is 3.5 cm

6. The tumor may present as a painless or painful swelling, hydrocele, or palpable mass

7. Serum CA-125 is elevated (recurrence may be predicted by serum CA-125 levels)

8. Grossly, these mostly are cystic cystadenoma and borderline tumors or solid carcinomas and may extend beyond the tunica vaginalis

9. Microscopically, blunt end papillary fibrovascular cores are lined by stratified cuboidal cells with little atypia in serous borderline tumors. Atypia and invasion are seen in carcinomas. Psammoma bodies are common

10. Mucinous cystadenomas have endocervical-type lining. Mucinous borderline tumor and carcinomas have intestinal-type epithelium. Mucin extravasation may be present

11. Cystadenomas and borderline tumors have excellent prognosis. Carcinomas can metastasize and have poor overall prognosis

The mean patient age at presentation of these tumors is in the fifties, with a range from the second to the eighth decade. These tumors may present with hydrocele, painful or painless swelling, or a palpable mass. Their mean size is 3.5 cm.[305,306,308,309] The serum CA-125 level usually is elevated. The gross appearance may be cystic in the presence of a cystadenoma (only mucinous type seen in this location) or borderline tumor with single or multiple small exophytic lesions studding the surface of tunica vaginalis or solid and infiltrative when carcinomas are present. Mucinous tumors may have gelatinous contents. Serous tumors usually are paratesticular, but a subset of mucinous tumors is intratesticular, raising the question of a teratoma. The absence of teratomatous or other germ cell elements, absence of IGCNU, and an older patient age at presentation suggest an ovarian-type epithelial tumor.[305,306,308,309]

MICROSCOPIC FEATURES

Microscopically, serous borderline tumors are cystic and have blunt end papillary cores lined by stratified cuboidal cells with mostly mild atypia and variable mitoses (**Fig. 79**). Psammoma bodies, ciliated and hobnail cells typical of serous differentiation, may be present. Focal areas of invasion can be seen (microinvasion), rarely. Overall, prognosis is excellent for completely excised serous borderline tumors.[308,310] Serous carcinomas have papillary structures with highly atypical lining cells, psammoma bodies, and frank invasion with desmoplasia. These carcinomas can have recurrences and metastases.[264,279] The distinction of serous borderline tumor from mesothelioma and rete testis adenocarcinoma is discussed in the sections describing mesothelioma and rete testis.

Mucinous cystadenomas are lined by bland columnar endocervical-type epithelium, with basally oriented nuclei (**Fig. 80**); mucinous cystic tumors of borderline malignancy and mucinous carcinomas have intestinal-type epithelium. Borderline tumors have intracystic complex papillary and cribriform architecture, rarely with highly atypical cells, as in intraepithelial carcinoma, or microinvasion (< 3 mm). Mucin extravasation, calcification, or ossification may be present in the adjacent tissues.[264,305,306] In a follow-up extending for up to 12 years (median, 2 years), mucinous cystadenoma and borderline tumors had an excellent prognosis and no recurrences.[306] Mucinous carcinomas, on the other hand, can have intraperitoneal spread. Besides teratoma, other differential diagnostic considerations for mucinous tumors are metastatic adenocarcinoma and extension of appendiceal mucinous tumor along hernia sac to scrotum.[306,311] History of a carcinoma elsewhere, bilaterality, and lymphovascular invasion are seen in metastases. CK7 can be used as a discriminatory marker for ovarian-type tumor (positive) and metastasis from lower gastrointestinal tract (negative).[267]

DIFFERENTIAL DIAGNOSIS

DIAGNOSIS

It is important to be aware of the existence of these very rare tumors. They may be underreported because of incorrect diagnosis.

METASTATIC TUMORS TO THE TESTIS

OVERVIEW

Metastatic tumors to the testis and paratestis are rare, with an incidence less than 1% of all testicular tumors. Most of these tumors are seen in

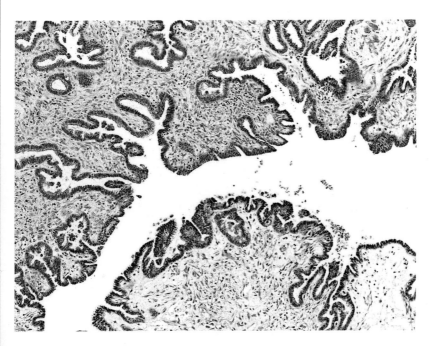

Fig. 79. Serous tumor of borderline malignant potential showing blunt end papillary cores lined by stratified cuboidal cells with mostly mild atypia (original magnification ×100).

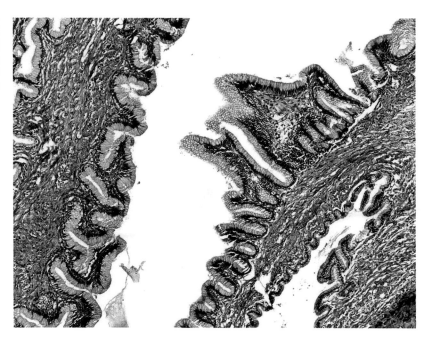

Fig. 80. Mucinous cystadenoma lined by bland columnar endocervical type epithelium, with basally oriented nuclei (original magnification ×100).

patients who are more than 50 years old. Most patients who have metastases to the testis have a known history of prior malignancy.[312–317]

The most common tumor types include renal cell carcinoma clear cell type[318] and prostatic adenocarcinoma.[319,320] Other neoplasms include metastatic melanoma and colon, pancreas, and lung carcinoma. Patients who have metastatic tumors to the testis generally are older than the patients who have testicular germ cell tumors. Another feature common to metastatic tumors to the testis is the absence of IGCNU. Also, bilateral disease is more common in patients who have metastatic tumors and is seen in 15% to 20% of cases.[10,312,314–317,321]

GROSS FEATURES

The size and appearance of metastatic tumors varies, depending on the primary origin of the tumor. In general, metastatic tumors are more nodular and are multifocal and bilateral.

HISTOLOGIC FEATURES

The morphologic appearance and the location of the tumors vary, depending on the origin.

△△ Differential Diagnosis
OVARIAN-TYPE EPITHELIAL TUMORS

- Serous tumors (negative for calretinin): mesothelioma and rete testis adenocarcinoma

- Mucinous tumors (always CK7 positive): teratoma, metastatic adenocarcinomas, and extension of appendiceal mucinous tumor along a hernia sac to the paratesticular area

- Clear cell carcinoma: papillary cystadenoma and adenocarcinoma of the epididymis have predominantly clear cells but little atypia

---

Key Features
METASTATIC TUMORS TO TESTIS

1. Metastatic tumors to the testis are rare, occurring mostly in patients more than 50 years old who have a history of prior malignancy

2. Renal cell carcinoma clear cell type and prostatic adenocarcinoma are the most common types of metastatic tumor to testis

4. Less common metastatic tumors are melanoma, colon, pancreas, and lung cancer

5. A feature common to metastatic tumors to the testis is the absence of IGCNU

6. Metastatic tumors are present in the interstitium but also may involve the tubules, and vascular involvement is usually present

Metastatic prostatic carcinoma may have a solid growth pattern with rounded nuclei and prominent nucleoli, similar to seminoma. Melanoma may have melanin pigment, nuclear and/or cytoplasmic inclusions, or prominent binucleation. In general, metastatic tumors are present in the interstitium but also may involve the tubules. Vascular involvement is usually present. Immunohistochemistry to confirm the origin of the metastatic tumor is useful.[10,314,321]

DIFFERENTIAL DIAGNOSIS

It is critical to obtain a good patient history to avoid the wrong diagnosis of a seminoma or other primary testicular neoplasm. Clear cell renal cell carcinoma and prostatic carcinoma with clear cell areas may mimic seminoma because of the presence of rounded nuclei, prominent nucleoli, and pale to clear cytoplasm. The growth pattern may be tubular or glandular growth, a feature commonly seen in seminomas. S-100 positivity for melanoma should be interpreted with caution, because S-100 also may be positive in some primary sex cord–stromal tumors. Another melanoma marker, melan-A, may stain sex cord–stromal tumors such as Leydig cell tumors.[312,313,321]

DIAGNOSIS

Radiologic evaluation such as an ultrasound scan is useful for tumor localization and for identifying multifocal and bilateral tumors, which are seen more commonly with metastatic tumors.[313] Prostatic carcinoma is a common metastatic carcinoma in the testis. Immunohistochemistry for prostate-specific antigen, prostatic acid phosphatase, or prostein is useful to confirm the diagnosis of metastatic prostate carcinoma in patients who have a known history of prostatic carcinoma or when dealing with a testicular tumor with features of prostatic carcinoma.[320] Similarly, immunohistochemistry may be extremely helpful for correctly diagnosing other metastatic tumors such as melanoma and lung carcinoma. For clear cell renal

Differential Diagnosis
METASTATIC TUMORS

- Seminoma
- Other primary paratesticular neoplasms (malignant mesothelioma, Müllerian-type carcinomas, rete testis carcinoma, and epididymal carcinoma)
- Sex cord gonadal–stromal tumors

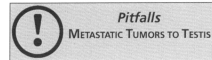

Pitfalls
METASTATIC TUMORS TO TESTIS

! Incorrect diagnosis of seminoma or other primary testicular neoplasm can be avoided by obtaining a good patient history

! Because S-100 and melan-A may be positive in some primary sex cord–stromal tumors, S-100 and melan-A positivity should be interpreted with caution

cell carcinoma, immunostaining for renal cell carcinoma antigen may be helpful. OCT4 immunostain is strongly reactive in seminoma and negative in almost all metastatic tumors. TTF1 immunostain may be useful in the diagnosis of non–small cell carcinomas of the lung.[312] Currently used markers for metastatic tumors to the testis are listed in **Box 14**.

PROGNOSIS

The prognosis for metastatic tumors to the testis usually is poor because the metastatic disease typically is at an advanced stage. An accurate diagnosis of the primary tumor may help in selecting the appropriate chemotherapy and management.[10,312,313]

PARATESTICULAR TUMORS

SOFT TISSUE LOCATIONS

The paratesticular region has many tumors that also can occur in other soft tissue locations of the body with identical clinical and pathologic features. Some of these entities are described here in some detail; others are mentioned here because of

---

Box 14
Markers for metastatic tumors to testis

Prostate-specific antigen: metastatic prostate carcinoma

Prostatic acid phosphatase: metastatic prostate carcinoma

Prostein: metastatic prostate carcinoma

Renal cell carcinoma antigen: clear cell renal cell carcinoma

OCT4 immunostain: strongly reactive in seminoma and embryonal carcinoma and negative in almost all metastatic tumors

TTF1 immunostain: non–small cell carcinomas of the lung

some unique aspect of the morphology or clinical presentation.

ADENOMATOID TUMORS

OVERVIEW

Adenomatoid tumors are rare, benign tumors and account for approximately 30% of all paratesticular masses.[322,323] Occasionally adenomatoid tumor occurs as an intratesticular mass. It now is generally accepted that the adenomatoid tumors are of mesothelial origin.[324] The Wilms tumor 1 (*WT1*) gene also has been implicated in the development of adenomatoid tumor, further supporting the mesothelial origin of this tumor type.[325]

Adenomatoid tumors are the most common paratesticular neoplasms.[322,325] Adenomatoid tumors occur mostly in the third to fifth decades of life; the mean patient age at presentation is 36 years.[323,326] These tumors also can occur in young children or older adults. They occur in the epididymis, spermatic cord, prostate, and ejaculatory duct. Most frequently, adenomatoid tumors arise within or around the lower or upper pole of the epididymis, occurring with equal frequency on either side.[327] Intratesticular adenomatoid tumors originate in the tunica albuginea, resulting in their peripheral location. They also may be found in the tunica vaginalis and rete testis.[323]

Clinically, adenomatoid tumors may present as an incidental finding or as a slow-growing (months to years) scrotal mass. Adenomatoid lesions

Key Features
ADENOMATOID TUMORS

1. Rare benign tumor, of mesothelial origin

2. Most common paratesticular neoplasm

3. Occur mostly in the third to fifth decades of life; mean patient age at presentation is 36 years

4. Present as an incidental finding or as a slow-growing (months to years) intrascrotal mass

5. Ultrasound typical appearance is a hypoechoic and homogeneous mass

usually are painless unless there is an accompanying infarct; enlargement usually is painless, with normal scrotal skin and surrounding adnexa. Very rarely, adenomatoid tumors have presented with testicular pain and inflammation. In 2006 Piccin and colleagues[328] described a case of adenomatoid tumor as an incidental finding in a patient being treated with imatinib for chronic myeloid leukemia. On ultrasonography, an adenomatoid tumor typically appears as a hyperechoic and homogeneous mass.[323]

GROSS FEATURES

Grossly, adenomatoid tumors are usually small, solid, firm, gray to white to tan and poorly to

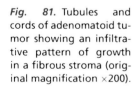

Fig. 81. Tubules and cords of adenomatoid tumor showing an infiltrative pattern of growth in a fibrous stroma (original magnification ×200).

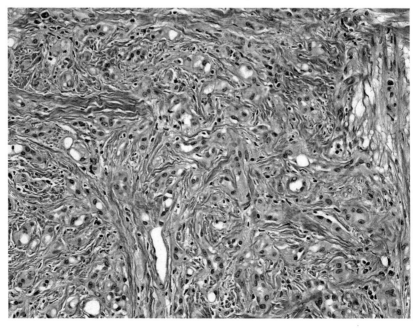

well-circumscribed masses. They usually are smaller than 3 cm and very rarely are larger than 5 cm. They are situated between testicular tissue and tunica albuginea or lamina parietalis tunica vaginalis. They also can appear as flattened and plaquelike masses. On frozen section, atrophic tubules with fibrous stromal proliferation are seen.[329]

MICROSCOPIC FEATURES

Adenomatoid tumors may show a wide spectrum of histologic growth patterns including tubular/ glandular, angiomatoid, solid, or cystic patterns.[325] The tumors have an infiltrating growth pattern within fibrous tissue and smooth muscle (**Fig. 81**). The tumors appear as eosinophilic mesothelial cells in a pattern of solid cords as well as dilated tubules that may look endothelial in origin (**Fig. 82**).

   The characteristic cellular feature is a vacuolated cytoplasm. Some of the cells may have an attenuated appearance. Nuclei usually are small with inconspicuous nucleoli. The stroma usually is fibrous but may consist of smooth muscle,[323,329]

> △△ **Differential Diagnosis**
> **ADENOMATOID TUMORS**
>
> - Adenocarcinoma of testes
> - Hemangioma
> - Malignant mesothelioma
> - Yolk sac tumor
> - Metastatic carcinoma of prostate
> - Lymphoma
> - Other testicular masses and tumors

with occasional smooth muscle proliferation. This tumor generally is unencapsulated; therefore the pattern of growth is uncharacteristic of benign neoplasms and frequently invades the surrounding tissue.[330] The tumor cells stain positively for hyaluronidase-sensitive mucosubstance with Alcian blue stain.[326]

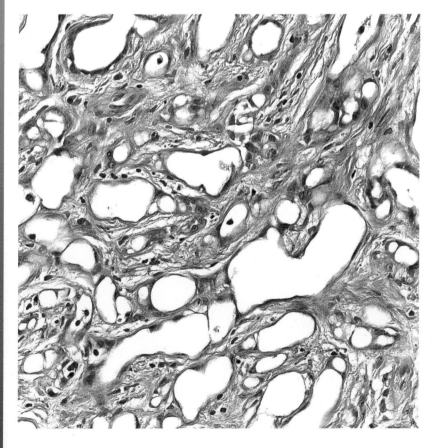

Fig. 82. Adenomatoid tumor with cells lining dilated tubules that look like vascular spaces lined by endothelium (original magnification ×400).

DIFFERENTIAL DIAGNOSIS

The differential diagnoses include adenocarcinoma of testes, hemangioma, malignant mesothelioma, yolk sac tumor, metastatic carcinoma of prostate, lymphoma, and other testicular masses and tumors.

Absence of serum tumor markers such as hCG, AFT, and LDH helps exclude a malignant lesion.

Absence of inhibin expression helps exclude adrenal cortical and sex cord–stromal neoplasms.

Absence of staining for vascular makers such as CD34 excludes vascular tumors and mesenchymal lesions.

DIAGNOSIS

Ultrasonography demonstrates the extratesticular nature of the lesion, which usually is hypoechoic and solid. Absence of serum tumor markers such as hCG, AFP, and LDH help exclude a malignant lesion. Histologic evaluation of the specimen results in definitive diagnosis that also is supported by immunohistochemistry.

Immunohistochemistry shows an expression of WT1, calretinin, and vimentin.[325] Adenomatoid tumors also have been reported to show positivity for high and low molecular weight cytokeratin, EMA, and primary mesothelial monoclonal antibody 1.[326] Adenomatoid tumors are negative for CEA, CD15, Ber-EP4, and CD34. Absence of staining for vascular makers such as CD34 excludes vascular tumors and mesenchymal lesions. Absence of inhibin expression helps exclude adrenal cortical and sex cord–stromal neoplasms.[331] **Box 15** summarizes the currently used markers for adenomatoid tumors.

PROGNOSIS

Adenomatoid tumors never have been known to recur or to show malignant degeneration.[325] The adequate use of tumor marker studies, ultrasonography, and intraoperative frozen sections can

---

Box 15
Markers for adenomatoid tumors
Adenomatoid tumors are positive for
WT1
Calretinin
Vimentin
High and low molecular weight cytokeratin
EMA
Primary mesothelial monoclonal antibody 1
Adenomatoid tumors are negative for
CEA
CD15 (Leu-M1)
Ber-EP4
CD34

---

facilitate organ-sparing surgery. The overall goal is to prevent unnecessary orchiectomy.[329]

MESOTHELIOMA

OVERVIEW

Tunica vaginalis can be involved by benign cystic mesothelioma, by well-differentiated papillary mesothelioma, and by malignant mesothelioma.[265,332–337] These tumors can originate from the tunica vaginalis or tunica albuginea. Although these tumors are rare, they are second in frequency after primary intrascrotal sarcomas. Bilateral tumors have been reported.[338,339]

Benign cystic mesothelioma presents as a scrotal swelling. Well-differentiated papillary mesothelioma most often presents as a recurrent hydrocele. These tumors occur most commonly in younger men in the second and third decades of life. Both these tumors are identical to the same name lesions occurring in the peritoneum of both sexes. The presentation of malignant mesothelioma can vary; hydrocele, either acute or recurrent, is a common accompaniment; there may be local soreness and pain; the tumor may be discovered incidentally in a hernia repair; or it may present as a palpable scrotal mass.

Sonography of well-differentiated papillary mesothelioma shows a hydrocele with a homogeneous, well-encapsulated extratesticular mass with echogenicity similar to that of the normal testis.[340] The ultrasonographic appearance of malignant mesothelioma is typical, demonstrating multinodular masses in a hydrocele with irregular contours.[341] Asbestos exposure is the only known risk factor for tunica vaginalis mesothelioma; the

---

Pitfalls
ADENOMATOID TUMORS

! May be incorrectly diagnosed as a metastatic carcinoma with signet-ring cells.

! Infarction can cause necrosis and reactive fibroblastic proliferation, obscuring the lesion and causing reactive atypia in the remaining tumor.

Key Features
MESOTHELIOMA

1. Three variants can occur in the tunica vaginalis:

- Benign cystic mesothelioma
- Well-differentiated papillary mesothelioma
- Malignant mesothelioma

2. Mesothelioma is the second most common malignant paratesticular tumor

3. Mesothelioma most commonly presents as recurrent hydrocele

4. Diagnosis can be made on cytology of the aspirate

5. Benign cystic mesotheliomas are multicystic lesions, with thin, translucent walls and slightly mucinous clear contents

6. Well-differentiated papillary mesothelioma can be a single nodule or multifocal or can appear as granular deposits on the surface of hydrocele sac

7. Malignant mesothelioma has multiple tan, friable nodules and excrescences; invasion into adjacent testicular structures (epididymis, hilum of testis, or spermatic cord) may be grossly visible as firm, tan masses

8. Microscopically, cuboidal bland cells line the papillary architecture in well-differentiated papillary mesothelioma and epithelioid malignant mesotheliomas. Diffuse sheetlike growth can show atypia

9. The sarcomatoid variant can have a varying amount of spindle cell component with atypia and epithelioid components and usually is cytokeratin positive

10. Ultrastructurally, long, branching microvilli, cytoplasmic microfilaments, and desmosomes are seen

Differential Diagnosis
MESOTHELIOMA

Benign cystic mesothelioma must be differentiated from lymphangioma

Reactive mesothelial hyperplasia is the most common consideration

Other entities to be excluded are

- Metastatic adenocarcinomas
- Rete testis adenocarcinoma (calretinin negative)
- Sarcoma from sarcomatoid variant of mesothelioma
- Ovarian surface-type serous borderline tumor

5 cm in diameter with a thin, translucent wall and slightly mucinous clear contents.[343] Well-differentiated papillary mesothelioma usually is a single nodule but can be multifocal. These tumors also can appear as granular deposits on the surface of hydrocele sac. The tunica vaginalis, when involved by malignant mesothelioma, is thickened with multiple, tan, friable nodules and excrescences, sometimes involving tunica albuginea. The hydrocele fluid is clear to hemorrhagic. Invasion into adjacent testicular structures (epididymis, hilum of testis, or spermatic cord) may be grossly visible as firm, tan masses.[42]

MICROSCOPIC FEATURES

Microscopic examination of benign cystic mesothelioma demonstrates multiple cystic spaces lined by flat to low cuboidal cells with occasional hobnail cell features and no atypia or mitoses. The cysts are separated by fibrous septa with areas of acute and chronic inflammation and slight stromal cell proliferation.[343] Well-differentiated

incidence of tunica mesothelioma following asbestos exposure has been reported to be between 23% and 40%.[336,342]

GROSS FEATURES

Benign cystic mesothelioma are composed of multicystic lesions that impart a somewhat spongelike gross appearance and cysts 0.2 to

Pitfalls
MESOTHELIOMA

! The presence of occasional psammoma bodies causes these tumors to be confused with ovarian-type serous tumors.

! Sarcomatoid variants can appear as sarcomas.

papillary mesotheliomas can form papillae and tubules that have a single row of cuboidal or flattened mesothelium lining papillary fibrovascular cores (**Fig. 83**). These tumors lack stromal invasion but may have rare mitoses.[336,344–346]

Approximately 75% of malignant mesotheliomas are purely epithelial, and about 25% are biphasic with variable amounts of sarcomatoid element.[336,342] The epithelioid mesotheliomas show predominant papillary and tubulopapillary architecture, often with areas of solid sheets of cells. One or more layers of mesothelial cells line the papillary structures (**Fig. 84**). These cells usually appear bland and are round to cuboidal but can be hyperchromatic with mild atypia.[42] Papillary architecture can be arborizing and complex. The sheetlike growth has pleomorphic cells and increased mitoses. These lesions may have highly pleomorphic epithelioid cells with necrosis-forming cords, nests, small tubules, and irregular slitlike spaces with intracystic proliferation (**Fig. 85**). Nuclei have prominent nucleoli, and the cytoplasm is eosinophilic. Occasional psammoma bodies and clusters of foamy macrophages can be seen.[110,264,267,336] The biphasic pattern has sarcomatoid elements composed of spindled cells with nuclear pleomorphism, arranged in fascicles or a storiform pattern (**Fig. 86**).[342] Rarely, a pure spindle or sarcomatoid pattern is present; the desmoplastic variant must be differentiated from sarcomas.[264,336,342] These tumors may show

adjacent in situ lesion with atypia of the surface mesothelial cells.[336] Invasion of paratesticular soft tissue, skin of the penis, scrotum, or the testis with intratubular growth of mesothelioma has been observed rarely.[264]

DIFFERENTIAL DIAGNOSIS

Benign cystic mesothelioma must be distinguished from lymphangioma. Immunohistochemical analysis with endothelial markers (CD34, CD31) versus mesothelial markers (calretinin, WT1, and cytokeratin) clarifies the diagnosis.[332,336]

For the other mesotheliomas, the major entities in the differential are reactive mesothelial hyperplasia, metastatic adenocarcinomas, rete testis adenocarcinoma, sarcoma from sarcomatoid variants, and ovarian surface-type neoplasms, namely serous borderline tumor that can arise in the paratesticular region.[264]

Reactive mesothelial hyperplasia does not form a gross mass or have complex arborizing papillae. It may have an intense inflammatory reaction, with fibrosis and small tubules within the stroma, but it has a layered appearance parallel to the surface rather than the haphazard arrangement seen in malignancy.[264]

The papillae of serous borderline tumor are broad based compared with mesothelioma and have cellular budding and stratification rather than uniform cells lining the papillae. Psammoma bodies are rare in mesotheliomas but can be

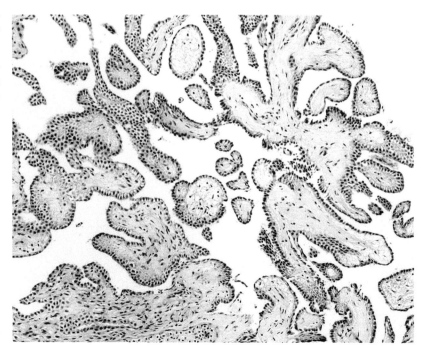

Fig. 83. Well-differentiated papillary mesothelioma showing fibrovascular cores lined by a single cuboidal layer of bland mesothelial cells (original magnification ×100).

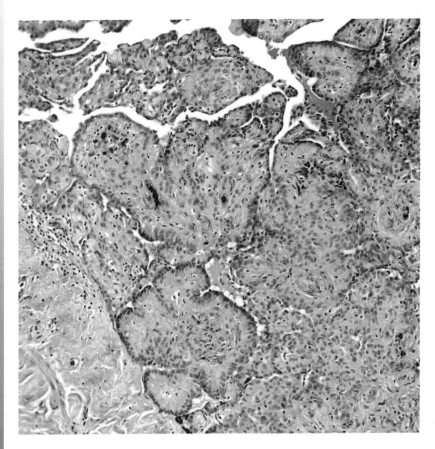

Fig. 84. Papillary malignant mesothelioma with branching fibrovascular cores, lined by single or multiple layers of cells (original magnification ×100).

abundant in serous tumors. Immunomarkers such as calretinin (for mesothelioma), and B72.3 (for serous carcinoma) can be used also.[264,347]

Features that distinguish rete carcinoma from mesotheliomas are their predominant or exclusive location within the rete testis and microscopic continuation with the rete epithelium. Immunostains such as WT1 (for mesothelioma), B72.3 and Leu-M1 (for adenocarcinoma) may prove helpful.[264,267]

Immunohistochemistry is required to distinguish high-grade sarcomas with prominent eosinophilic cytoplasm from sarcomatoid mesotheliomas.[264]

DIAGNOSIS

Mesotheliomas of the tunica vaginalis have the same immunohistochemical profile as pleural and peritoneal mesotheliomas.[348] These tumors are positive for CK7, calretinin, WT-1, D2-40, thrombomodulin, vimentin, EMA, and CK5/6. They are negative for BerEP4, CK20, and CEA.[347,348] Immunohistochemistry for cytokeratin is positive in both epithelial and spindle components (**Fig. 87**).

Peritoneal mesotheliomas sometimes present first in tunica vaginalis, mimicking a primary lesion.[349] Mesothelioma of tunica vaginalis also can be a component of simultaneous mesotheliomas arising in the pleura and peritoneum.[350]

Ultrastructural examination shows long, branching microvilli, cytoplasmic microfilaments, and desmosomes.[334] **Box 16** lists the markers for mesothelioma.

PROGNOSIS

Benign cystic mesotheliomas usually follow a benign course but can be recurrent. Well-differentiated papillary mesotheliomas usually behave in a benign fashion. Although they are considered to have low malignant potential, some have proved to be aggressive.[264,342,344,346]

Malignant mesotheliomas can recur, usually within the first 2 years of follow-up.[351] Thirty-nine percent of recurrences are local. Metastasis to inguinal and retroperitoneal lymph nodes and abdominal peritoneum, lung, mediastinum, bone, and brain occurs in 56% to 65% of recurrences.[265,336,342] Poor prognosis is predicted by invasion of adjacent structures and metastasis. Treatment is orchiectomy with scrotectomy and RPLND when indicated.[110,265] Follow-up should be long term because these patients

Fig. 85. Epithelioid me-sothelioma with clefted spaces showing papillary growths (original magni-fication ×200).

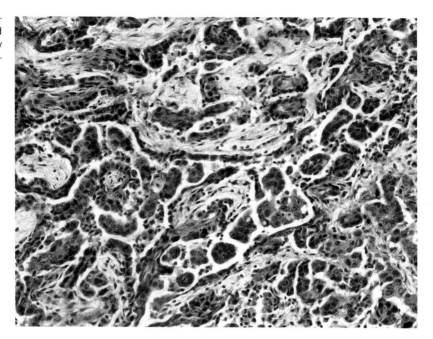

can develop late recurrences or develop mesotheli-omas at other sites.[264]

SARCOMAS

OVERVIEW

Sarcomas occur in the spermatic cord, epididy-mis, and scrotum and are histologically similar to soft tissue sarcomas elsewhere in the body. Most childhood sarcomas are rhabdomyosarco-mas; liposarcoma is the most common sarcoma in adults. Other sarcomas that occur in the testis and paratestis include leiomyosarcoma and angio-sarcoma. The following section briefly discusses paratesticular liposarcoma, rhabdomyosarcoma, and angiosarcoma as examples of sarcoma of the paratesticular region.

Fig. 86. Biphasic meso-thelioma with spindle cell/sarcomatoid and epi-thelial components (orig-inal magnification ×100).

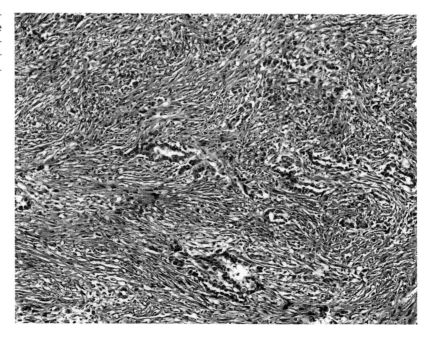

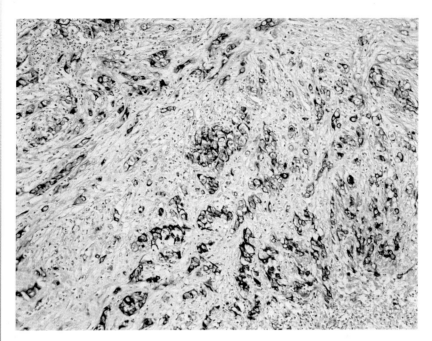

Fig. 87. AE1/AE3 immunostain positivity in a sarcomatoid mesothelioma (original magnification ×100).

PARATESTICULAR LIPOSARCOMA

OVERVIEW

Paratesticular liposarcoma is a rare tumor.[352] Paratesticular liposarcoma usually is difficult to diagnose preoperatively and often is mistaken for hernia, lipoma, or hydrocele. It usually presents

Box 16
Markers for mesothelioma
Mesothelioma is positive for
CK7
Calretinin
WT-1
D2-40
Thrombomodulin
Vimentin
EMA
CAM5.2
CK5/6
Mesothelioma is negative for
Leu-M1
Ber-EP4
B72.3
CEA

as a painless scrotal swelling that grows slowly over a variable period of time ranging from months to years.[353] Occasionally, this tumor presents as a previously stable mass that increases rapidly in size.[353] The reported age at presentation ranges from 16.5 to 85 years; the average patient age at presentation is 55 years.[354] Although most authorities believe that liposarcomas arise from mesenchymal cells, liposarcomas sometimes are associated pathologically with lipoma of the spermatic cord, suggesting the possibility of malignant degeneration.[355] Histologically, most liposarcomas reported in the groin area are well differentiated, and they tend to be predominantly lipoma-like.[353] They must be differentiated from the much more common benign lipoma.

DIAGNOSIS

The diagnosis of liposarcoma is based primarily on the presence of atypical cells with large, hyperchromatic nuclei. These cells can be identified either within fibrous septa or in the fat. Careful evaluation is necessary, because these cells can be present in small numbers or very focal. Another important feature is the marked variation in adipocyte size. Some tumors also contain lipoblasts, although these are not essential for the diagnosis (**Fig. 88**).[353] Liposarcoma may undergo low-grade or high-grade dedifferentiation.[353,356] The biologic behavior is correlated with tumor histology.

Fig. 88. High-power view of a well-differentiated liposarcoma with lipoblasts (*bottom right*) (original magnification ×400).

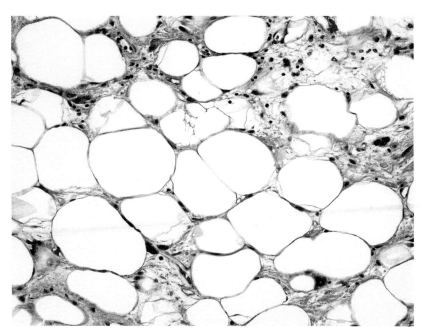

PROGNOSIS

Low-grade, well-differentiated liposarcomas have a favorable prognosis, but tumors with multiple recurrences or metastases are likely to be high grade.[357] Long-term follow-up of 10 cases of well-differentiated liposarcoma reported by Montgomery and Fisher[353] showed no metastasis; however, they reported that these tumors can be locally aggressive and that there were recurrences, often after a long period of latency, in more than half the cases. Weiss and Rao[356] also reported that 11 of 14 patients who had well-differentiated liposarcoma in the groin area had recurrences, with the first recurrence at a median of 5 years. Liposarcomas tend to spread primarily by local extension. Hematogenous and lymphatic spread usually is a late event involving high-grade tumors.[354] Adequate local resection provides the best chance of eradicating this disease.[358,359] Radical orchiectomy with wide local excision is the recommended treatment. Retroperitoneal lymphadenectomy does not seem to offer any additional therapeutic benefit. Adjuvant radiation can be useful in high-grade tumors or in recurrent liposarcoma.[354] Regardless of initial therapy, the risk of local recurrence and subsequent increase in grade should be kept in mind, and long-term follow-up is advised.[354]

RHABDOMYOSARCOMA

OVERVIEW

Most rhabdomyosarcomas are the embryonal subtype, which has a spindle cell variant. Other types such as alveolar and mixed alveolar/embryonal rhabdomyosarcoma are less common. Pleomorphic rhabdomyosarcoma is rare and is seen in older patients. Embryonal rhabdomyosarcoma usually is found in children under the age of 15 years but also has been reported in young adults. It is found most commonly in the head and neck region and in the genitourinary tract.[79,360] In the testis and paratestis, the tumor most commonly affects the spermatic cord. Patients present with a scrotal mass.[361] Grossly, the tumor has a smooth texture with a gray-white, lobulated cut surface and often has a myxoid appearance.

Histologically, embryonal carcinoma can be cellular with myxoid areas. Also seen is a spindle cell–type of embryonal rhabdomyosarcoma with cellular areas of large "strapshaped" or "racketshaped" spindle cells with eosinophilic cytoplasm (**Fig. 89**). Increased mitotic activity with bizarre and pleomorphic nuclei may be seen.[362] The neoplastic cells are positive for myogenin, myo-D1, muscle-specific actin, desmin, and vimentin (**Fig. 90**):

The differential diagnosis includes other small blue cell tumors.

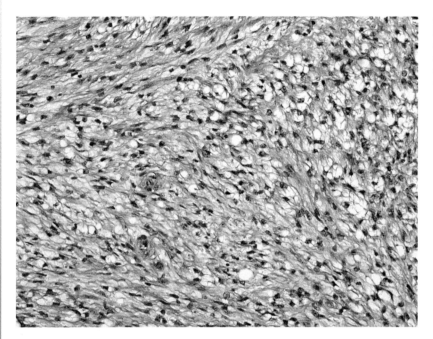

Fig. 89. Spindle-cell embryonal rhabdomyosarcoma with fascicular arrangement of spindle cells (original magnification ×200).

The treatment consists of surgery and chemotherapy.

The prognosis depends on the patient's age and the tumor stage.[71,79,360,363,364]

PRIMARY TESTICULAR ANGIOSARCOMA

OVERVIEW

Primary testicular angiosarcoma is a very rare entity. Only a handful of cases have been described in the literature. Most cases have not been associated with antecedent radiotherapy or prior exposure to arsenic, thorium dioxide, or vinyl chloride, but some cases may have been associated with a chronic history of hydrocele.[365–369]

These neoplasms present as sizeable, painless, hemorrhagic masses, typically in the testicular parenchyma or epididymis (**Fig. 91**).

They share most of the histopathologic features of other deep soft tissue angiosarcomas and

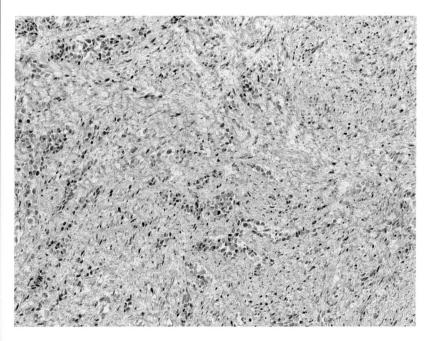

Fig. 90. Nuclear myogenin staining of embryonal rhabdomyosarcoma (original magnification ×100).

Fig. 91. Gross image of bisected testis showing angiosarcoma forming a hemorrhagic mass in the paratestis that is displacing the surrounding testicular parenchyma.

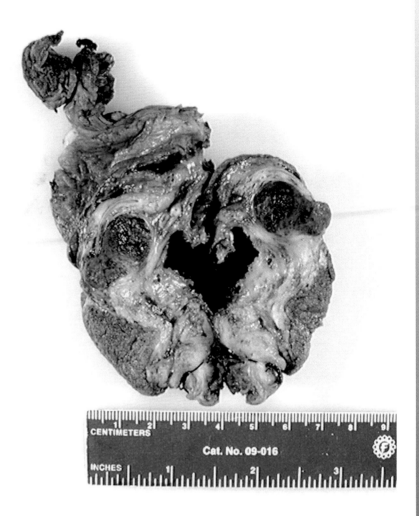

therefore may pose considerable diagnostic difficulty, particularly those with a solid pattern and epithelioid cytologic features. Most of the cases of primary testicular angiosarcomas show the classic architectural pattern (**Fig. 92**).[369] Focal solid patterns have been seen in at least some cases.

Immunohistochemical studies may be helpful, and more than one endothelial marker and at least one cytokeratin marker should be used to solidify the diagnosis of testicular angiosarcoma. Factor VIII–related antigen is positive. The other positive immunohistochemical markers are *Ulex Europaeus* lectin, CD31, and CD34.[365–368]

Because of the limited follow-up, the behavior of this entity is uncertain, but the prognosis for these patients may be better than the generally poor prognosis for deep soft tissue and visceral angiosarcomas.[365–369]

PAPILLARY CYSTADENOMA OF THE EPIDIDYMIS

OVERVIEW

Papillary cystadenoma is a classic but rare lesion of the epididymis with cysts and papillary growth formations.

CLINICAL FEATURES

Papillary cystadenoma of the epididymis is the only benign epithelial tumor of the epididymis.[370] This tumor is rare: fewer than 100 cases have been described in the literature. There is no age predominance; cases have been reported in patients between the ages of 16 and 81 years. There is no predilection for a specific race. This benign tumor is seen in about 17% of patients who have

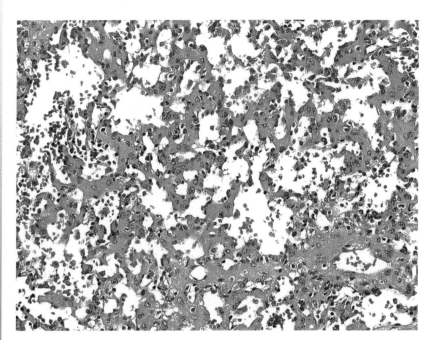

Fig. 92. Classical histologic pattern of an angiosarcoma with irregular interconnecting vascular channels lined by cells with hyperchromatic nuclei (original magnification ×200). Note the tumor cells with typical cytology of plump hyperchromatic, tufted endothelial cells with scant amphophilic cytoplasm.

von Hippel-Lindau (VHL) disease,[371] which also includes retinal, spinal, and cerebellar hemangioblastomas, renal cysts and carcinomas, pheochromocytomas, and solid organ cysts. Patients present painful or nonpainful intrascrotal masses and sometimes with infertility.

In females, the counterpart of papillary cystadenoma of the epididymis is represented by papillary tumors of the broad ligament and peritoneum. These tumors usually are solid, although they may have distinct cystic spaces. Distinctive clinical and pathologic features were described by Price.[372]

GROSS FEATURES

Papillary cystadenomas can have a solid or cystic appearance and typically occur in the head of epididymis. The tumors can grow up to 6.0 cm in diameter.

MICROSCOPIC FEATURES

Microscopic examination reveals dilated efferent ductules filled with eosinophilic colloidlike luminal fluid. Some areas show papillary infoldings projecting into cystic spaces lined by cuboidal epithelium with clear cytoplasm. The intervening stroma is vascular. Nuclear size can vary somewhat, and one or two small nucleoli are present (**Figs. 93** and **94**).

DIFFERENTIAL DIAGNOSIS

The distinction between cystadenoma and adenocarcinomas of the epididymis can be difficult. A high nuclear grade and high proliferation index together with invasive growth and the presence of necrosis are features most consistent with adenocarcinoma. None of these features have been described in cystadenoma. The finding of adenocarcinoma of the epididymis requires a metastatic workup because of the rarity of primary epididymal adenocarcinomas.[373]

Clear cell papillary cystadenoma is histologically similar to renal cell carcinoma. In reported cases clear cell papillary cystadenoma of the epididymis has been confused with metastatic renal cell carcinoma.[374] The differential diagnosis is complicated further because both renal cell carcinoma and papillary cystadenoma of the epididymis are known to develop in VHL disease. Lectin histochemistry studies are helpful in distinguishing papillary cystadenoma, which stains for soybean agglutinin, from metastatic renal cell carcinoma.[375] Allelic loss of the *VHL* gene, located on the short arm of chromosome 3, has been demonstrated in all benign papillary tumors (eg, papillary cystadenoma of the broad ligament, endometrioid cystadenoma of the broad ligament, papillary cystadenomas of the epididymis, papillary tumor of the retroperitoneum) developing in patients who have VHL disease.[376] Several hypoxia-inducible genes, including platelet-derived growth factor,

Fig. 93. Papillary cystadenoma of the epididy-
mis showing dilated
efferent ductules with
papillary infoldings and
fibrovascular cores pro-
jecting into cystic spaces
lined by cuboidal epithe-
lium with clear cytoplasm
(original magnification
×40). Some dilated tu-
bules have eosinophilic
colloidlike luminal fluid.

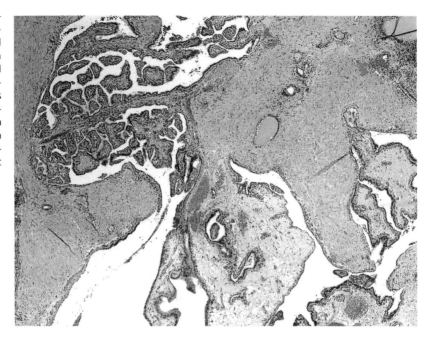

basic fibroblast growth factor, erythropoietin, and
vascular endothelial growth factor, are regulated
by protein encoded by the *VHL* gene.[377] Overexpression of vascular endothelial growth factor
has been demonstrated in tumors associated
with VHL disease and may explain the cyst formation and vascularized stroma present in these
tumors.[377]

Both seminoma and papillary cystadenoma of
the epididymis are characterized by clear cell
cytoplasmic alteration. Other neoplasms with clear
cell change are the clear cell type of renal cell carcinoma, clear cell adenocarcinoma of the urethra
and bladder, and well-differentiated adenocarcinoma of the prostate. Knowledge of the neoplastic
entities displaying clear cell change in the

Fig. 94. Papillary cystadenoma of the epididy-
mis with fibrovascular
cores lined by bland cells
with small, basally ori-
ented nuclei and delicate
clear cytoplasm (original
magnification ×100).

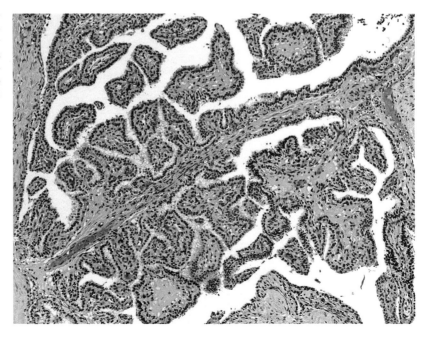

genitourinary tract aids in the differential diagnosis of these conditions.[378]

DIAGNOSIS

The tumor cells are strongly reactive for low and high molecular weight cytokeratin (CAM5.2 and CK903, respectively), CD10, and vimentin and are S-100 negative.

PROGNOSIS

Treatment is local excision. Prognosis is good in patients who do not have VHL disease.

EPIDIDYMAL ADENOCARCINOMA

OVERVIEW

Epididymal adenocarcinoma is an exceedingly rare tumor that occurs in adults. The tumor is centered on the epididymis and may have a solid or cystic growth. The size ranges up to 14 cm. The tumor rarely infiltrates the testicular parenchyma.

Microscopically, the cells can have sheetlike destructive growth or form tubules and papillae. The cytoplasm is pale, eosinophilic, amphophilic to clear and contains glycogen. These carcinomas may show very little nuclear atypia or mitosis.

Immunohistochemically, these tumors are positive for CD10, cytokeratins, and luminal EMA; they are negative for WT1.

Epididymal adenocarcinoma can metastasize to the retroperitoneum. The overall mortality rate is 50%.[11,267,279]

MELANOTIC NEUROECTODERMAL TUMOR OF INFANCY (RETINAL ANLAGE TUMOR)

OVERVIEW

Melanotic neuroectodermal tumor occurs in infancy or childhood (typically in infants less than 1 year old). This tumor usually is epididymal but, rarely, can occur in the testis or paratestis. It is similar to tumor of the same name occurring in the jaw. Urinary catecholamine metabolites may be increased.

Grossly, the tumor is a well-demarcated, white nodule with areas of dark pigmentation. Microscopically, the tumor has two types of cells: large, epithelioid cells with melanin pigment and nests of small neuroblastic cells.

Immunohistochemically, the large cells are positive for cytokeratin and HMB45, and both cell types are positive for NSE and CD57 (Leu7).

Most tumors are benign, but a few cases have metastasized to regional lymph nodes.[11]

DESMOPLASTIC SMALL ROUND CELL TUMOR

OVERVIEW

Desmoplastic small round cell tumor is a rare primary tumor in the paratesticular location and occurring most often near the epididymis in young men.

Grossly, it is a firm gray-white to tan tumor with a size range of 3 to 4 cm.

Microscopically, it is composed of small, uniform blue cells arranged in nests and cords, sometimes showing pseudorosette and tubule formation in a dense fibrotic stroma. Immunohistochemically, the cells are cytokeratin, desmin, and NSE positive.

Intra-abdominal desmoplastic small round cell tumors are aggressive, but patient prognosis and survival are better for tumors in the paratesticular region.[11,305,379]

REFERENCES

1. Jemal A, et al. Cancer statistics, 2008. CA Cancer J Clin 2008;58(2):71–96.
2. Tummala MK, Hussain A. Recent developments in germ cell tumors of the testes. Curr Opin Oncol 2008;20(3):287–93.
3. Reuter VE. Origins and molecular biology of testicular germ cell tumors. Mod Pathol 2005; 18(Suppl 2):S51–60.
4. Pettersson A, et al. Age at surgery for undescended testis and risk of testicular cancer. N Engl J Med 2007;356(18):1835–41.
5. Skakkebaek NE. Possible carcinoma-in-situ of the testis. Lancet 1972;2(7776):516–7.
6. Karellas ME, Damjanov I, Holzbeierlein JM. ITGCN of the testis, contralateral testicular biopsy and bilateral testicular cancer. Urol Clin North Am 2007;34(2):119–25 [abstract vii].
7. Skakkebaek NE. Carcinoma in situ of the testis: frequency and relationship to invasive germ cell tumours in infertile men. Histopathology 2002; 41(3A):5–18.
8. Sonne SB, et al. Testicular dysgenesis syndrome and the origin of carcinoma in situ testis. Int J Androl 2008;31(2):275–87.
9. McIntyre A, et al. Genes, chromosomes and the development of testicular germ cell tumors of adolescents and adults. Genes Chromosomes Cancer 2008;47(7):547–57.
10. Young RH. Testicular tumors—some new and a few perennial problems. Arch Pathol Lab Med 2008; 132(4):548–64.

11. Ulbright TM. Testicular and paratesticular tumors. In: Mills S, editor. Sternberg's diagnostic surgical pathology. Philadelphia: Lippincott Williams & Wilkins; 2004. p. 2167–232.

12. Skakkebaek NE. Carcinoma in situ of the testis: frequency and relationship to invasive germ cell tumours in infertile men. Histopathology 1978;2(3): 157–70.

13. von Hochstetter AR, Hedinger CE. The differential diagnosis of testicular germ cell tumors in theory and practice. A critical analysis of two major systems of classifiction and review of 389 cases. Virchows Arch A Pathol Anat Histol 1982;396(3):247–77.

14. Ulbright TM, AMB, Young RH. Atlas of tumor pathology: tumors of the testis, adenexa, spermatic cord and scrotum. 3rd edition. Washington, DC: Armed Forces Institute of Pathology; 1999.

15. Jacobsen Gk, BH, Olsen J, et al. Testcular germ cell tumors in Denmark 1976–1980. Pathology of 1058 consecutive cases. Acta Radiol Oncol 1984; 23:239–47.

16. Ulbright TM, Amin MB, Young RH. Third seriesIn: Atlas of tumor pathology: tumors of the testis, adenexa, spermatic cord and scrotum. Washington, DC: Armed Forces Institute of Pathology; 1999.

17. Eble JN, S G, Epstein JI, Sesterhenn IA, editors. World Health Organization classification of tumors, pathology and gentics. Tumors of the urinary system and male genital organs. Lyon, France: IARC Press; 2004.

18. Damjanov I, et al. Cribriform and sclerosing seminoma devoid of lymphoid infiltrates. Arch Pathol Lab Med 1980;104(10):527–30.

19. Ulbright TM, Young RH. Seminoma with tubular, microcystic, and related patterns: a study of 28 cases of unusual morphologic variants that often cause confusion with yolk sac tumor. Am J Surg Pathol 2005;29(4):500–5.

20. Ulbright TM. Germ cell tumors of the gonads: a selective review emphasizing problems in differential diagnosis, newly appreciated, and controversial issues. Mod Pathol 2005;18(Suppl 2):S61–79.

21. Young RH, Finlayson N, Scully RE. Tubular seminoma. Report of a case. Arch Pathol Lab Med 1989;113(4): 414–6.

22. Jacobsen GK, v.d MH, Specht L, et al. Histopathological features in stage I seminoma treated with orchiectomy only. J Urol Pathol 2003;3:85–94.

23. Mostofi FK, I S. Pathology of germ cell tumors of testes. Prog Clin Biol Res 1985;203:1–34.

24. Henley JD, Young RH, Ulbright TM. Malignant Sertoli cell tumors of the testis: a study of 13 examples of a neoplasm frequently misinterpreted as seminoma. Am J Surg Pathol 2002;26(5):541–50.

25. Jones TD, et al. OCT4: A sensitive and specific biomarker for intratubular germ cell neoplasia of the testis. Clin Cancer Res 2004;10(24):8544–7.

26. Looijenga LH, et al. POU5F1 (OCT3/4) identifies cells with pluripotent potential in human germ cell tumors. Cancer Res 2003;63(9):2244–50.

27. Kraggerud SM, et al. Spermatocytic seminoma as compared to classical seminoma: an immunohistochemical and DNA flow cytometric study. Apmis 1999;107(3):297–302.

28. Iczkowski KA, et al. Trials of new germ cell immunohistochemical stains in 93 extragonadal and metastatic germ cell tumors. Hum Pathol 2008;39(2): 275–81.

29. Lau SK, Weiss LM, Chu PG. D2-40 immunohistochemistry in the differential diagnosis of seminoma and embryonal carcinoma: a comparative immunohistochemical study with KIT (CD117) and CD30. Mod Pathol 2007;20(3):320–5.

30. Tickoo SK, et al. Testicular seminoma: a clinicopathologic and immunohistochemical study of 105 cases with special reference to seminomas with atypical features. Int J Surg Pathol 2002;10(1):23–32.

31. Denk H, et al. Intermediate filaments and desmosomal plaque proteins in testicular seminomas and non-seminomatous germ cell tumours as revealed by immunohistochemistry. Virchows Arch A Pathol Anat Histopathol 1987;410(4):295–307.

32. Eglen DE, Ulbright TM. The differential diagnosis of yolk sac tumor and seminoma. Usefulness of cytokeratin, alpha-fetoprotein, and alpha-1-antitrypsin immunoperoxidase reactions. Am J Clin Pathol 1987;88(3):328–32.

33. Bosl GJ, Motzer RJ. Testicular germ-cell cancer. N Engl J Med 1997;337(4):242–53.

34. Marks LB, et al. Testicular seminoma: clinical and pathological features that may predict para-aortic lymph node metastases. J Urol 1990;143(3):524–7.

35. Masson P. Etude sur le seminome. Rev Canad Biol 1946;5:361–87.

36. Talerman A. Spermatocytic seminoma: clinicopathological study of 22 cases. Cancer 1980;45(8): 2169–76.

37. Burke A, Mostofi FK. Spermatocytic seminoma: a clinicopathologic study study of 79 cases. J Urol Pathol 1993;1:21–32.

38. Tickoo S, Amin AB, Cramer HM, et al. The testis, paratesticular structures, and male external genitalia. In: Silverberg S, Delellis RA, Frable WJ, editors. Priciples and practice of surgical pathology and cytopathology. Philadelphia: Churchill Livingstone; 2006. p. 1731–89.

39. Bergner DM, Duck GB, Rao M. Bilateral sequential spermatocytic seminoma. J Urol 1980;124(4):565.

40. Leocadio DE, Stein BS. A case of synchronous bilateral spermatocytic seminoma. Urol Oncol 2008; 26(2):202–3.

41. Scully RE. Spermatocytic seminoma of the testis. A report of 3 cases and review of the literature. Cancer 1961;14:788–94.

42. Tumours of the testis and paratesticular tissue. In: Eble JN, Sauder G, Epstein JI, Sesterhenn IA, editors. World Health Organization Classification of tumors, pathology and gentics. Tumors of the urinary system and male genital organs. Lyon, France: IARC Press; 2004. p. 218–78.

43. Dundr P, et al. Anaplastic variant of spermatocytic seminoma. Pathol Res Pract 2007;203(8):621–4.

44. Albores-Saavedra J, et al. Anaplastic variant of spermatocytic seminoma. Hum Pathol 1996;27(7): 650–5.

45. Skakkebaek NE, et al. Carcinoma-in-situ of the testis: possible origin from gonocytes and precursor of all types of germ cell tumours except spermatocytoma. Int J Androl 1987;10(1):19–28.

46. Cummings OW, et al. Spermatocytic seminoma: an immunohistochemical study. Hum Pathol 1994; 25(1):54–9.

47. Dekker I, et al. Placental-like alkaline phosphatase and DNA flow cytometry in spermatocytic seminoma. Cancer 1992;69(4):993–6.

48. Decaussin M, et al [Spermatocytic seminoma. A clinicopathological and immunohistochemical study of 7 cases]. Ann Pathol 2004;24(2):161–6 [in French].

49. Zeeman AM, et al. VASA is a specific marker for both normal and malignant human germ cells. Lab Invest 2002;82(2):159–66.

50. Rosai J, Khodadoust K, Silber I. Spermatocytic seminoma. II. Ultrastructural study. Cancer 1969; 24(1):103–16.

51. Talerman A, Fu YS, Okagaki T. Spermatocytic seminoma. Ultrastructural and microspectrophotometric observations. Lab Invest 1984;51(3): 343–9.

52. Matoska J, Ondrus D, Hornak M. Metastatic spermatocytic seminoma. A case report with light microscopic, ultrastructural, and immunohistochemical findings. Cancer 1988;62(6):1197–201.

53. Steiner H, et al. Metastatic spermatocytic seminoma—an extremely rare disease: Part 2. Eur Urol 2006;49(2): 408–9.

54. Matoska J, Talerman A. Spermatocytic seminoma associated with rhabdomyosarcoma. Am J Clin Pathol 1990;94(1):89–95.

55. Floyd C, et al. Spermatocytic seminoma with associated sarcoma of the testis. Cancer 1988;61(2): 409–14.

56. Robinson A, Bainbridge T, Kollmannsberger C. A spermatocytic seminoma with rhabdomyosarcoma transformation and extensive metastases. Am J Clin Oncol 2007;30(4):440–1.

57. Bishop EF, et al. Apoptosis in spermatocytic and usual seminomas: a light microscopic and immunohistochemical study. Mod Pathol 2007;20(10): 1036–44.

58. True LD, et al. Spermatocytic seminoma of testis with sarcomatous transformation. Am J Surg Pathol 1988;12(10):806.

59. Bahrami A, Ro JY, Ayala AG. An overview of testicular germ cell tumors. Arch Pathol Lab Med 2007; 131(8):1267–80.

60. Aschim EL, et al. Risk factors for testicular cancer—differences between pure non-seminoma and mixed seminoma/non-seminoma? Int J Androl 2006;29(4):458–67.

61. Ulbright TM. The most common, clinically significant misdiagnoses in testicular tumor pathology, and how to avoid them. Adv Anat Pathol 2008; 15(1):18–27.

62. Emerson RE, Ulbright TM. The use of immunohistochemistry in the differential diagnosis of tumors of the testis and paratestis. Semin Diagn Pathol 2005;22(1):33–50.

63. de Jong J, Looijenga LH. Stem cell marker OCT3/4 in tumor biology and germ cell tumor diagnostics: history and future. Crit Rev Oncog 2006;12(3–4): 171–203.

64. Vugrin D, et al. Embryonal carcinoma of the testis. Cancer 1988;61(11):2348–52.

65. Ataergin S, et al. Outcome of patients with stage II and III nonseminomatous germ cell tumors: results of a single center. Indian J Cancer 2007;44(1): 6–11.

66. Perlman EJ, et al. Genetic analysis of childhood endodermal sinus tumors by comparative genomic hybridization. J Pediatr Hematol Oncol 2000; 22(2):100–5.

67. Kanto S, et al. Clinical features of testicular tumors in children. Int J Urol 2004;11(10):890–3.

68. Murphy FL, et al. Testicular and paratesticular pathology in infants and children: the histopathological experience of a tertiary paediatric unit over a 17 year period. Pediatr Surg Int 2007; 23(9):867–72.

69. Talerman A. Germ cell tumours. Ann Pathol 1985; 5(3):145–57.

70. Levy DA, Kay R, Elder JS. Neonatal testis tumors: a review of the Prepubertal Testis Tumor Registry. J Urol 1994;151(3):715–7.

71. Young RH. Sex cord-stromal tumors of the ovary and testis: their similarities and differences with consideration of selected problems. Mod Pathol 2005;18(Suppl 2):S81–98.

72. Talerman A. Endodermal sinus (yolk sac) tumor elements in testicular germ-cell tumors in adults: comparison of prospective and retrospective studies. Cancer 1980;46(5):1213–7.

73. Ulbright TM, Gersell DJ. Rete testis hyperplasia with hyaline globule formation. A lesion simulating yolk sac tumor. Am J Surg Pathol 1991;15(1): 66–74.

74. Palmer PE, Safaii H, Wolfe HJ. Alpha1-antitrypsin and alpha-fetoprotein. Protein markers in endodermal sinus (yolk sac) tumors. Am J Clin Pathol 1976; 65(4):575–82.

75. Ramalingam P, et al. The use of cytokeratin 7 and EMA in differentiating ovarian yolk sac tumors from endometrioid and clear cell carcinomas. Am J Surg Pathol 2004;28(11):1499–505.

76. Jung SM, et al. Expression of OCT4 in the primary germ cell tumors and thymoma in the mediastinum. Appl Immunohistochem Mol Morphol 2006;14(3): 273–5.

77. Zynger DL, et al. Glypican 3: a novel marker in testicular germ cell tumors. Am J Surg Pathol 2006; 30(12):1570–5.

78. Talerman A, Haije WG. Alpha-fetoprotein and germ cell tumors: a possible role of yolk sac tumor in production of alpha-fetoprotein. Cancer 1974;34(5):1722–6.

79. Oottamasathien S, et al. Testicular tumours in children: a single-institutional experience. BJU Int 2007;99(5):1123–6.

80. Pectasides D, Farmakis D, Pectasides M. The management of stage I nonseminomatous testicular germ cell tumors. Oncology 2006;71(3–4):151–8.

81. Trobs RB, et al. Surgery in infants and children with testicular and paratesticular tumours: a single centre experience over a 25-year-period. Klin Padiatr 2007;219(3):146–51.

82. Grady RW, Ross JH, Kay R. Patterns of metastatic spread in prepubertal yolk sac tumor of the testis. J Urol 1995;153(4):1259–61.

83. Klepp O, et al. Prognostic factors in clinical stage I nonseminomatous germ cell tumors of the testis: multivariate analysis of a prospective multicenter study. Swedish-Norwegian Testicular Cancer Group. J Clin Oncol 1990;8(3):509–18.

84. Walsh TJ, et al. Incidence of testicular germ cell cancers in U.S. children: SEER program experience 1973 to 2000. Urology 2006;68(2):402–5 [discussion 405].

85. Grady RW, Ross JH, Kay R. Epidemiological features of testicular teratoma in a prepubertal population. J Urol 1997;158(3 Pt 2):1191–2.

86. Brosman SA. Testicular tumors in prepubertal children. Urology 1979;13(6):581–8.

87. Schneider DT, et al. Genetic analysis of childhood germ cell tumors with comparative genomic hybridization. Klin Padiatr 2001;213(4):204–11.

88. Leibovitch I, et al. Adult primary pure teratoma of the testis. The Indiana experience. Cancer 1995; 75(9):2244–50.

89. Simmonds PD, et al. Primary pure teratoma of the testis. J Urol 1996;155(3):939–42.

90. Beeker A, et al. Retroperitoneal mature teratoma after orchidectomy for a stage IB pure embryonal testicular carcinoma. Int J Clin Oncol 2008;13(1):71–3.

91. Comiter CV, et al. Prognostic features of teratomas with malignant transformation: a clinicopathological study of 21 cases. J Urol 1998;159(3):859–63.

92. Aguirre P, Scully RE. Primitive neuroectodermal tumor of the testis. Report of a case. Arch Pathol Lab Med 1983;107(12):643–5.

93. Michael H, et al. Primitive neuroectodermal tumors arising in testicular germ cell neoplasms. Am J Surg Pathol 1997;21(8):896–904.

94. Serrano-Olmo J, et al. Neuroblastoma as a prominent component of a mixed germ cell tumor of testis. Cancer 1993;72(11):3271–6.

95. Ganjoo KN, et al. Germ cell tumor associated primitive neuroectodermal tumors. J Urol 2001;165(5): 1514–6.

96. Michael H, et al. Nephroblastoma-like tumors in patients with testicular germ cell tumors. Am J Surg Pathol 1998;22(9):1107–14.

97. Motzer RJ, et al. Teratoma with malignant transformation: diverse malignant histologies arising in men with germ cell tumors. J Urol 1998;159(1):133–8.

98. Ulbright TM, et al. The development of non-germ cell malignancies within germ cell tumors. A clinicopathologic study of 11 cases. Cancer 1984; 54(9):1824–33.

99. Ulbright TM, et al. Spindle cell tumors resected from male patients with germ cell tumors. A clinicopathologic study of 14 cases. Cancer 1990;65(1): 148–56.

100. Ritchey ML, et al. Development of nongerm cell malignancies in nonseminomatous germ cell tumors. J Urol 1985;134(1):146–9.

101. Michael H, et al. The pathology of late recurrence of testicular germ cell tumors. Am J Surg Pathol 2000;24(2):257–73.

102. Ahmed T, Bosl GJ, Hajdu SI. Teratoma with malignant transformation in germ cell tumors in men. Cancer 1985;56(4):860–3.

103. Burt AD, et al. Dermoid cyst of the testis. Scott Med J 1987;32(5):146–8.

104. Ulbright TM, Srigley JR. Dermoid cyst of the testis: a study of five postpubertal cases, including a pilomatrixoma-like variant, with evidence supporting its separate classification from mature testicular teratoma. Am J Surg Pathol 2001; 25(6):788–93.

105. Price EB Jr. Epidermoid cysts of the testis: a clinical and pathologic analysis of 69 cases from the Testicular Tumor Registry. J Urol 1969;102(6):708–13.

106. Shah KH, Maxted WC, Chun B. Epidermoid cysts of the testis: a report of three cases and an analysis of 141 cases from the world literature. Cancer 1981;47(3):577–82.

107. Rushton HG, et al. Testicular sparing surgery for prepubertal teratoma of the testis: a clinical and pathological study. J Urol 1990;144(3):726–30.

108. Miettinen M, Virtanen I, Talerman A. Intermediate filament proteins in human testis and testicular germ-cell tumors. Am J Pathol 1985;120(3):402–10.

109. Harms D, et al. Pathology and molecular biology of teratomas in childhood and adolescence. Klin Padiatr 2006;218(6):296–302.

110. Levin HS. Neoplasms of the testis. In: Zhou M, Magi-Galluzzi C, editors. Series foundations in diagnostic pathology. Philadelphia: Elsevier; 2007. p. 534–622.

111. Kernek KM, et al. Identical allelic losses in mature teratoma and other histologic components of malignant mixed germ cell tumors of the testis. Am J Pathol 2003;163(6):2477–84.

112. Spiess PE, et al. Malignant transformation of testicular teratoma: a chemoresistant phenotype. Urol Oncol 2008. Epub ahead of print.

113. Cheng L, et al. Interphase fluorescence in situ hybridization analysis of chromosome 12p abnormalities is useful for distinguishing epidermoid cysts of the testis from pure mature teratoma. Clin Cancer Res 2006;12(19):5668–72.

114. Walsh C, Rushton HG. Diagnosis and management of teratomas and epidermoid cysts. Urol Clin North Am 2000;27(3):509–18.

115. Umar SA, MacLennan GT. Epidermoid cyst of the testis. J Urol 2008;180(1):335.

116. Manivel JC, et al. Intratubular germ cell neoplasia in testicular teratomas and epidermoid cysts. Correlation with prognosis and possible biologic significance. Cancer 1989;64(3):715–20.

117. Dieckmann KP, Loy V. Epidermoid cyst of the testis: a review of clinical and histogenetic considerations. Br J Urol 1994;73(4):436–41.

118. Sesterhenn Ia, C M, Davis CJ, et al. Testicular teratomas in adults. Histopathology 2002;41(Suppl 1):24.

119. Nistal M, Paniagua R. Primary neuroectodermal tumour of the testis. Histopathology 1985;9(12):1351–9.

120. Chang WC, et al. Choriocarcinoma with pulmonary metastasis: report of a case of successful treatment with serial FDG-PET follow-up. J Reprod Med 2007;52(5):450–2.

121. Ulbright TM. Germ cell neoplasms of the testis. Am J Surg Pathol 1993;17(11):1075–91.

122. Henry SC, Walsh PC, Rotner MB. Choriocarcinoma of the testis. J Urol 1974;112(1):105–8.

123. Iyomasa S, et al. Primary choriocarcinoma of the jejunum: report of a case. Surg Today 2003;33(12):948–51.

124. Mamelak AN, Withers GJ, Wang X. Choriocarcinoma brain metastasis in a patient with viable intrauterine pregnancy. Case report. J Neurosurg 2002;97(2):477–81.

125. Vegh GL, et al. Primary pulmonary choriocarcinoma: a case report. J Reprod Med 2008;53(5):369–72.

126. Rosenblatt GS, Walsh CJ, Chung S. Metastatic testis tumor presenting as gastrointestinal hemorrhage. J Urol 2000;164(5):1655.

127. Mosharafa AA, et al. Histology in mixed germ cell tumors. Is there a favorite pairing? J Urol 2004;171(4):1471–3.

128. Ro JY, et al. Testicular germ cell tumors. Clinically relevant pathologic findings. Pathol Annu 1991;26(Pt 2):59–87.

129. Jones TD, et al. OCT4 staining in testicular tumors: a sensitive and specific marker for seminoma and embryonal carcinoma. Am J Surg Pathol 2004;28(7):935–40.

130. Zynger DL, et al. Expression of glypican 3 in ovarian and extragonadal germ cell tumors. Am J Clin Pathol 2008;130(2):224–30.

131. De Backer A, et al. Influence of tumor site and histology on long-term survival in 193 children with extracranial germ cell tumors. Eur J Pediatr Surg 2008;18(1):1–6.

132. Park DS, et al. Histologic type, staging, and distribution of germ cell tumors in Korean adults. Urol Oncol 2008.

133. Sheinfeld J, Motzer RJ. Stage I testicular cancer management and necessity for surgical expertise. J Clin Oncol 2008;26(18):2934–6.

134. Sogani PC, et al. Clinical stage I testis cancer: long-term outcome of patients on surveillance. J Urol 1998;159(3):855–8.

135. Shintaku I, et al. Survival of metastatic germ cell cancer patients assessed by international germ cell consensus classification in Japan. Jpn J Clin Oncol 2008;38(4):281–7.

136. Berney DM, et al. Malignant germ cell tumours in the elderly: a histopathological review of 50 cases in men aged 60 years or over. Mod Pathol 2008;21(1):54–9.

137. Huddart R, Kataja V. Mixed or non-seminomatous germ-cell tumors: ESMO clinical recommendations for diagnosis, treatment and follow-up. Ann Oncol 2008;19(Suppl 2):ii52–4.

138. Mostofi FK, Sesterhenn IA, Davis CJ Jr. Immunopathology of germ cell tumors of the testis. Semin Diagn Pathol 1987;4(4):320–41.

139. Rustin GJ, et al. Consensus statement on circulating tumour markers and staging patients with germ cell tumours. Prog Clin Biol Res 1990;357:277–84.

140. Sesterhenn IA, et al. Prognosis and other clinical correlates of pathologic review in stage I and II testicular carcinoma: a report from the Testicular Cancer Intergroup Study. J Clin Oncol 1992;10(1):69–78.

141. Brawn PN. The characteristics of embryonal carcinoma cells in teratocarcinomas. Cancer 1987;59(12):2042–6.

142. Freedman LS, et al. Histopathology in the prediction of relapse of patients with stage I testicular teratoma treated by orchidectomy alone. Lancet 1987;2(8554):294–8.

143. Hesketh PJ, Krane RJ. Prognostic assessment in nonseminomatous testicular cancer: implications for therapy. J Urol 1990;144(1):1–9.

144. Fung CY, et al. Stage I nonseminomatous germ cell testicular tumor: prediction of metastatic potential by primary histopathology. J Clin Oncol 1988; 6(9):1467–73.

145. Balzer BL, Ulbright TM. Spontaneous regression of testicular germ cell tumors: an analysis of 42 cases. Am J Surg Pathol 2006;30(7):858–65.

146. Bar W, Hedinger C. Comparison of histologic types of primary testicular germ cell tumors with their metastases: consequences for the WHO and the British nomenclatures? Virchows Arch A Pathol Anat Histol 1976;370(1):41–54.

147. Berdjis CC, Mostofi FK. Carcinoid tumors of the testis. J Urol 1977;118(5):777–82.

148. Zavala-Pompa A, et al. Primary carcinoid tumor of testis. Immunohistochemical, ultrastructural, and DNA flow cytometric study of three cases with a review of the literature. Cancer 1993;72(5):1726–32.

149. Ordonez NG, Ayala AG. Primary malignant carcinoid of the testis. Arch Pathol Lab Med 1982;106(10):539.

150. Reyes A, et al. Neuroendocrine carcinomas (carcinoid tumor) of the testis. A clinicopathologic and immunohistochemical study of ten cases. Am J Clin Pathol 2003;120(2):182–7.

151. Abbosh PH, et al. Germ cell origin of testicular carcinoid tumors. Clin Cancer Res 2008;14(5):1393–6.

152. Kato N, et al. Primary carcinoid tumor of the testis: immunohistochemical, ultrastructural and FISH analysis with review of the literature. Pathol Int 2003;53(10):680–5.

153. Son HY, et al. Primary carcinoid tumor of the bilateral testis associated with carcinoid syndrome. Int J Urol 2004;11(11):1041–3.

154. Hayashi T, et al. Primary carcinoid of the testis associated with carcinoid syndrome. Int J Urol 2001;8(9):522–4.

155. Kim HJ, et al. Primary carcinoid tumor of the testis: immunohistochemical, ultrastructural and DNA flow cytometric study of two cases. J Korean Med Sci 1999;14(1):57–62.

156. Talerman A, et al. Primary carcinoid tumor of the testis: case report, ultrastructure and review of the literature. Cancer 1978;42(6):2696–706.

157. Blumberg JM, Sedberry S, Kazmi SO. Bilateral asynchronous metastatic carcinoid tumor of the testis. Urology 2005;65(1):174.

158. Danikas D, et al. Testicular metastasis from ileal carcinoid: report of a case. Dis Colon Rectum 2001;44(9):1365–6.

159. Hosking DH, et al. Primary carcinoid of the testis with metastases. J Urol 1981;125(2):255–6.

160. Kaufman JJ, Waisman J. Primary carcinoid tumor of testis with metastasis. Urology 1985;25(5):534–6.

161. Shimura S, et al [Primary carcinoid tumor of the testis with metastasis to the upper vertebrae. Report of a case]. Nippon Hinyokika Gakkai Zasshi 1991; 82(7):1157–60 [in Japanese].

162. Sullivan JL, Packer JT, Bryant M. Primary malignant carcinoid of the testis. Arch Pathol Lab Med 1981; 105(10):515–7.

163. Abrahamsson J, et al. Multiple lymph node metastases in a boy with primary testicular carcinoid, despite negative preoperative imaging procedures. J Pediatr Surg 2005;40(11):e19–21.

164. Talerman A, Roth LM. Recent advances in the pathology and classification of gonadal neoplasms composed of germ cells and sex cord derivatives. Int J Gynecol Pathol 2007;26(3):313–21.

165. Scully RE. Gonadoblastoma; a gonadal tumor related to the dysgerminoma (seminoma) and capable of sex-hormone production. Cancer 1953; 6(3):455–63.

166. Scully RE. Gonadoblastoma. A review of 74 cases. Cancer 1970;25(6):1340–56.

167. Hoei-Hansen CE, et al. New evidence for the origin of intracranial germ cell tumours from primordial germ cells: expression of pluripotency and cell differentiation markers. J Pathol 2006;209(1):25–33.

168. Talerman A. Gonadoblastoma and dysgerminoma in two siblings with dysgenetic gonads. Obstet Gynecol 1971;38(3):416–26.

169. Young RH. A brief history of the pathology of the gonads. Mod Pathol 2005;18(Suppl 2):S3–17.

170. Cheville JC. Classification and pathology of testicular germ cell and sex cord-stromal tumors. Urol Clin North Am 1999;26(3):595–609.

171. Coleman JF, MacLennan GT. Gonadoblastoma. J Urol 2006;175(6):2300.

172. Cools M, et al. Germ cell tumors in the intersex gonad: old paths, new directions, moving frontiers. Endocr Rev 2006;27(5):468–84.

173. Pohl HG, et al. Prepubertal testis tumors: actual prevalence rate of histological types. J Urol 2004; 172(6 Pt 1):2370–2.

174. Sugita Y, et al. Testicular and paratesticular tumours in children: 30 years' experience. Aust N Z J Surg 1999;69(7):505–8.

175. Siti Aishah MA, Chandran R, Tahir H. Bilateral pure gonadoblastoma in a 46 XY individual—a case report. Med J Malaysia 1991;46(4):384–7.

176. Lo KW, et al. Gonadoblastoma in patient with Turner's syndrome. J Obstet Gynaecol Res 1996; 22(1):35–41.

177. Li Y, et al. Testis-specific protein Y-encoded gene is expressed in early and late stages of

gonadoblastoma and testicular carcinoma in situ. Urol Oncol 2007;25(2):141–6.

178. Slowikowska-Hilczer J, Szarras-Czapnik M, Kula K. Testicular pathology in 46,XY dysgenetic male pseudohermaphroditism: an approach to pathogenesis of testis cancer. J Androl 2001;22(5):781–92.

179. Seraj IM, et al. Malignant teratoma arising in a dysgenetic gonad. Gynecol Oncol 1993;50(2):254–8.

180. Talerman A, Dlemarre JF. Gonadoblastoma associated with embryonal carcinoma in an anatomically normal man. J Urol 1975;113(3):355–9.

181. Talerman A, Haije WG, Baggerman L. Serum alphafetoprotein (AFP) in diagnosis and management of endodermal sinus (yolk sac) tumor and mixed germ cell tumor of the ovary. Cancer 1978; 41(1):272–8.

182. Cheng L, et al. OCT4: biological functions and clinical applications as a marker of germ cell neoplasia. J Pathol 2007;211(1):1–9.

183. Kommoss F, et al. Inhibin expression in ovarian tumors and tumor-like lesions: an immunohistochemical study. Mod Pathol 1998;11(7):656–64.

184. Kim I, Young RH, Scully RE. Leydig cell tumors of the testis. A clinicopathological analysis of 40 cases and review of the literature. Am J Surg Pathol 1985;9(3):177–92.

185. Sesterhenn I, Mostofi FK, Davis CJ. Testicular tumours in infants and children. In: Jones W, editor. Advances in biosciences germ cell tumours II. Oxford: Pergamon Press; 1986. p. 173–84.

186. Dilworth JP, Farrow GM, Oesterling JE. Non-germ cell tumors of testis. Urology 1991;37(5):399–417.

187. Al-Agha OM, Axiotis CA. An in-depth look at Leydig cell tumor of the testis. Arch Pathol Lab Med 2007; 131(2):311–7.

188. Mineur P, et al. Feminizing testicular Leydig cell tumor: hormonal profile before and after unilateral orchidectomy. J Clin Endocrinol Metab 1987;64(4):686–91.

189. Billings SD, Roth LM, Ulbright TM. Microcystic Leydig cell tumors mimicking yolk sac tumor: a report of four cases. Am J Surg Pathol 1999; 23(5):546–51.

190. Ulbright TM, et al. Leydig cell tumors of the testis with unusual features: adipose differentiation, calcification with ossification, and spindle-shaped tumor cells. Am J Surg Pathol 2002;26(11):1424–33.

191. Ashley RA, et al. Clinical and pathological features associated with the testicular tumor of the adrenogenital syndrome. J Urol 2007;177(2):546–9 [discussion 549].

192. Miettinen M, et al. Cellular differentiation in ovarian sex-cord-stromal and germ-cell tumors studied with antibodies to intermediate-filament proteins. Am J Surg Pathol 1985;9(9):640–51.

193. Sohval AR, et al. Ultrastructure of feminizing testicular Leydig cell tumors. Ultrastruct Pathol 1982; 3(4):335–45.

194. Sohval AR, et al. Electron microscopy of a feminizing Leydig cell tumor of the testis. Hum Pathol 1977;8(6):621–34.

195. Kay S, et al. Interstitial-cell tumor of the testis. Tissue culture and ultrastructural studies. Am J Clin Pathol 1975;63(3):366–76.

196. Giannarini G, et al. Long-term followup after elective testis sparing surgery for Leydig cell tumors: a single center experience. J Urol 2007;178(3 Pt 1): 872–6 quiz, 1129.

197. Henderson CG, et al. Enucleation for prepubertal Leydig cell tumor. J Urol 2006;176(2):703–5.

198. Cheville JC, et al. Leydig cell tumor of the testis: a clinicopathologic, DNA content, and MIB-1 comparison of nonmetastasizing and metastasizing tumors. Am J Surg Pathol 1998;22(11):1361–7.

199. Grem JL, et al. Metastatic Leydig cell tumor of the testis. Report of three cases and review of the literature. Cancer 1986;58(9):2116–9.

200. Gulbahce HE, et al. Metastatic Leydig cell tumor with sarcomatoid differentiation. Arch Pathol Lab Med 1999;123(11):1104–7.

201. Richmond I, et al. Sarcomatoid Leydig cell tumour of testis. Histopathology 1995;27(6):578–80.

202. Nicoletto MO, et al. Sertoli cell tumor: a rare case in an elderly patient. Eur J Gynaecol Oncol 2006; 27(1):86–7.

203. Talon I, et al. Sertoli cell tumor of the testis in children: reevaluation of a rarely encountered tumor. J Pediatr Hematol Oncol 2005;27(9):491–4.

204. Young RH, Koelliker DD, Scully RE. Sertoli cell tumors of the testis, not otherwise specified: a clinicopathologic analysis of 60 cases. Am J Surg Pathol 1998;22(6):709–21.

205. Weitzner S, Gropp A. Sertoli cell tumor of testis in childhood. Am J Dis Child 1974;128(4):541–3.

206. Young RH, Talerman A. Testicular tumors other than germ cell tumors. Semin Diagn Pathol 1987;4(4): 342–60.

207. Talerman A. Malignant Sertoli cell tumor of the testis. Cancer 1971;28(2):446–55.

208. Kaplan GW, et al. Gonadal stromal tumors: a report of the Prepubertal Testicular Tumor Registry. J Urol 1986;136(1 Pt 2):300–2.

209. Thomas JC, Ross JH, Kay R. Stromal testis tumors in children: a report from the Prepubertal Testis Tumor Registry. J Urol 2001;166(6):2338–40.

210. Kratzer SS, et al. Large cell calcifying Sertoli cell tumor of the testis: contrasting features of six malignant and six benign tumors and a review of the literature. Am J Surg Pathol 1997;21(11): 1271–80.

211. Abbas F, Bashir NW, Hussainy AS. Sclerosing Sertoli cell tumor of the testis. J Coll Physicians Surg Pak 2005;15(7):437–8.

212. Wilson DM, et al. Testicular tumors with Peutz-Jeghers syndrome. Cancer 1986;57(11):2238–40.

213. Verdorfer I, et al. Molecular-cytogenetic characterisation of sex cord-stromal tumours: CGH analysis in sertoli cell tumours of the testis. Virchows Arch 2007;450(4):425–31.

214. Nielsen K, Jacobsen GK. Malignant Sertoli cell tumour of the testis. An immunohistochemical study and a review of the literature. Apmis 1988;96(8):755–60.

215. Kommoss F, et al. Inhibin-alpha CD99, HEA125, PLAP, and chromogranin immunoreactivity in testicular neoplasms and the androgen insensitivity syndrome. Hum Pathol 2000;31(9):1055–61.

216. Vidal-Jimenez A. New immunohistochemical markers in testicular tumors. Anal Quant Cytol Histol 2007;29(6):377.

217. Rosvoll RV, Woodard JR. Malignant Sertoli cell tumor of the testis. Cancer 1968;22(1):8–13.

218. Proppe KH, Scully RE. Large-cell calcifying Sertoli cell tumor of the testis. Am J Clin Pathol 1980;74(5):607–19.

219. Cano-Valdez AM, Chanona-Vilchis J, Dominguez-Malagon H. Large cell calcifying Sertoli cell tumor of the testis: a clinicopathological, immunohistochemical, and ultrastructural study of two cases. Ultrastruct Pathol 1999;23(4):259–65.

220. Plata C, et al. Large cell calcifying Sertoli cell tumour of the testis. Histopathology 1995;26(3):255–9.

221. Perez-Atayde AR, et al. Large-cell calcifying sertoli cell tumor of the testis. An ultrastructural, immunocytochemical, and biochemical study. Cancer 1983;51(12):2287–92.

222. Al-Bozom IA, et al. Granulosa cell tumor of the adult type: a case report and review of the literature of a very rare testicular tumor. Arch Pathol Lab Med 2000;124(10):1525–8.

223. Gaylis FD, et al. Granulosa cell tumor of the adult testis: ultrastructural and ultrasonographic characteristics. J Urol 1989;141(1):126–7.

224. Talerman A. Pure granulosa cell tumour of the testis. Report of a case and review of the literature. Appl Pathol 1985;3(3):117–22.

225. Hammerich KH, et al. Malignant advanced granulosa cell tumor of the adult testis: case report and review of the literature. Hum Pathol 2008;39(5):701–9.

226. Nistal M, et al. Testicular granulosa cell tumor of the adult type. Arch Pathol Lab Med 1992;116(3):284–7.

227. Morgan DR, Brame KG. Granulosa cell tumour of the testis displaying immunoreactivity for inhibin. BJU Int 1999;83(6):731–2.

228. Jimenez-Quintero LP, et al. Granulosa cell tumor of the adult testis: a clinicopathologic study of seven cases and a review of the literature. Hum Pathol 1993;24(10):1120–5.

229. Matoska J, Ondrus D, Talerman A. Malignant granulosa cell tumor of the testis associated with gynecomastia and long survival. Cancer 1992;69(7):1769–72.

230. Domeniconi RF, et al. Immunolocalization of aquaporins 1, 2 and 7 in rete testis, efferent ducts, epididymis and vas deferens of adult dog. Cell Tissue Res 2008;332(2):329–35.

231. Shukla AR, et al. Juvenile granulosa cell tumor of the testis: contemporary clinical management and pathological diagnosis. J Urol 2004;171(5):1900–2.

232. Yikilmaz A, Lee EY. MRI findings of bilateral juvenile granulosa cell tumor of the testis in a newborn presenting as intraabdominal masses. Pediatr Radiol 2007;37(10):1031–4.

233. Lawrence WD, Young RH, Scully RE. Juvenile granulosa cell tumor of the infantile testis. A report of 14 cases. Am J Surg Pathol 1985;9(2):87–94.

234. Alexiev BA, Alaish SM, Sun CC. Testicular juvenile granulosa cell tumor in a newborn: case report and review of the literature. Int J Surg Pathol 2007;15(3):321–5.

235. Nistal M, Redondo E, Paniagua R. Juvenile granulosa cell tumor of the testis. Arch Pathol Lab Med 1988;112(11):1129–32.

236. Chan JK, Chan VS, Mak KL. Congenital juvenile granulosa cell tumour of the testis: report of a case showing extensive degenerative changes. Histopathology 1990;17(1):75–80.

237. Tanaka Y, et al. Testicular juvenile granulosa cell tumor in an infant with X/XY mosaicism clinically diagnosed as true hermaphroditism. Am J Surg Pathol 1994;18(3):316–22.

238. Groisman GM, et al. Juvenile granulosa cell tumor of the testis: a comparative immunohistochemical study with normal infantile gonads. Pediatr Pathol 1993;13(4):389–400.

239. Pinto MM. Juvenile granulosa cell tumor of the infant testis: case report with ultrastructural observations. Pediatr Pathol 1985;4(3–4):277–89.

240. Garrett JE, et al. Cystic testicular lesions in the pediatric population. J Urol 2000;163(3):928–36.

241. Raju U, et al. Congenital testicular juvenile granulosa cell tumor in a neonate with X/XY mosaicism. Am J Surg Pathol 1986;10(8):577–83.

242. Young RH, Lawrence WD, Scully RE. Juvenile granulosa cell tumor—another neoplasm associated with abnormal chromosomes and ambiguous genitalia. A report of three cases. Am J Surg Pathol 1985;9(10):737–43.

243. Belville WD, et al. Benign testis tumors. J Urol 1982;128(6):1198–200.

244. Deveci MS, et al. Testicular (gonadal stromal) fibroma: case report and review of the literature. Pathol Int 2002;52(4):326–30.

245. Mostofi FK. Classification of tumors of testis. Ann Clin Lab Sci 1979;9(6):455–61.

246. Nistal M, Martinez-Garcia C, Paniagua R. Testicular fibroma. J Urol 1992;147(6):1617–9.

247. de Pinieux G, et al. Testicular fibroma of gonadal stromal origin with minor sex cord elements: clinicopathologic and immunohistochemical study of 2 cases. Arch Pathol Lab Med 1999;123(5):391–4.

248. Parveen T, Fleischmann J, Petrelli M. Benign fibrous tumor of the tunica vaginalis testis. Report of a case with light, electron microscopic, and immunocytochemical study, and review of the literature. Arch Pathol Lab Med 1992;116(3):277–80.

249. Sadowski EA, et al. Fibroma of the testicular tunics: an unusual extratesticular intrascrotal mass. J Ultrasound Med 2001;20(11):1245–8.

250. Val-Bernal JF, et al. Primary pure intratesticular fibrosarcoma. Pathol Int 1999;49(2):185–9.

251. Frates MC, et al. Solid extratesticular masses evaluated with sonography: pathologic correlation. Radiology 1997;204(1):43–6.

252. Renshaw AA, Gordon M, Corless CL. Immunohistochemistry of unclassified sex cord-stromal tumors of the testis with a predominance of spindle cells. Mod Pathol 1997;10(7):693–700.

253. Magro G, et al. Incompletely differentiated (unclassified) sex cord/gonadal stromal tumor of the testis with a "pure" spindle cell component: report of a case with diagnostic and histogenetic considerations. Pathol Res Pract 2007;203(10):759–62.

254. Perito PE, et al. Sertoli-Leydig cell testicular tumor: case report and review of sex cord/gonadal stromal tumor histogenesis. J Urol 1992;148(3):883–5.

255. Miettinen M, Salo J, Virtanen I. Testicular stromal tumor: ultrastructural, immunohistochemical, and gel electrophoretic evidence of epithelial differentiation. Ultrastruct Pathol 1986;10(6):515–28.

256. Greco MA, et al. Testicular stromal tumor with myofilaments: ultrastructural comparison with normal gonadal stroma. Hum Pathol 1984;15(3):238–43.

257. Lawrence W, Young RH, Scully RE. Sex cord-stromal tumors. In: Talerman A, Roth LM, editors. Pathology of the testis and its adnexa. New York: Churchill Livingstone; 1986. p. 67–92.

258. Kumaravelu PG, et al. Malignant undifferentiated sex cord-stromal testis tumor with brain metastasis: case report. Urol Oncol 2008;26(1):53–5.

259. Kajo K, et al. Cystic dysplasia of the rete testis. Case report. Apmis 2005;113(10):720–3.

260. Nanni L, et al. Cystic dysplasia of the rete testis associated to cryptorchidism: a case report. Arch Ital Urol Androl 2005;77(4):199–201.

261. Landry JL, et al [Cystic dysplasia of the rete testis and ipsilateral kidney agenesis in children]. Arch Pediatr 1999;6(4):416–20 [in French].

262. Nistal M, Regadera J, Paniagua R. Cystic dysplasia of the testis. Light and electron microscopic study of three cases. Arch Pathol Lab Med 1984;108(7):579–83.

263. Bouron-Dal Soglio D, et al. Bilateral cystic dysplasia of the rete testis with renal adysplasia. Pediatr Dev Pathol 2006;9(2):157–60.

264. Ulbright T, Amin MB, Young RH. Miscellaneous primary tumors of the testis, adnexa and spermatic cord. In: Tumors of the testis, adnexa, spermatic cord, and scrotum. Washington (DC): Armed Forces Institute of Pathology; 1999. p. 235–90.

265. Srigley JR, Hartwick RW. Tumors and cysts of the paratesticular region. Pathol Annu 1990;25(Pt 2):51–108.

266. Hartwick RW, et al. Adenomatous hyperplasia of the rete testis. A clinicopathologic study of nine cases. Am J Surg Pathol 1991;15(4):350–7.

267. Amin MB. Selected other problematic testicular and paratesticular lesions: rete testis neoplasms and pseudotumors, mesothelial lesions and secondary tumors. Mod Pathol 2005;18(Suppl 2):S131–45.

268. Jones EC, Murray SK, Young RH. Cysts and epithelial proliferations of the testicular collecting system (including rete testis). Semin Diagn Pathol 2000;17(4):270–93.

269. Sinclair AM, et al. Sertoliform cystadenoma of the rete testis. Pathol Int 2006;56(9):568–9.

270. Jones M, Young RH. Sertoliform rete cystadenoma: a report of two cases. J Urol Pathol 1997;7:47–53.

271. Orozco RE, Murphy WM. Carcinoma of the rete testis: case report and review of the literature. J Urol 1993;150(3):974–7.

272. Nochomovitz LE, Orenstein JM. Adenocarcinoma of the rete testis: consolidation and analysis of 31 reported cases with a review of the literature. J Urol Pathol 1994;2:1–37.

273. Mehra BR, et al. Adenocarcinoma of the rete testis with uncommon presentation as haematocele. Singapore Med J 2007;48(12):e311–3.

274. Nakagawa T, et al. Primary adenocarcinoma of the rete testis with preceding diagnosis of pulmonary metastases. Int J Urol 2006;13(12):1532–5.

275. Rubegni P, et al. Cutaneous metastases from adenocarcinoma of the rete testis. J Cutan Pathol 2006;33(2):181–4.

276. Sogni F, et al. Primary adenocarcinoma of the rete testis: diagnostic problems and therapeutic dilemmas. Scand J Urol Nephrol 2008;42(1):83–5.

277. Nochomovitz LE, Orenstein JM. Adenocarcinoma of the rete testis. Case report, ultrastructural observations, and clinicopathologic correlates. Am J Surg Pathol 1984;8(8):625–34.

278. Menon PK, et al. A case of carcinoma rete testis: histomorphological, immunohistochemical and ultrastructural findings and review of literature. Indian J Cancer 2002;39(3):106–11.

279. Jones MA, Young RH, Scully RE. Adenocarcinoma of the epididymis: a report of four cases and review of the literature. Am J Surg Pathol 1997;21(12):1474–80.

280. Al-Abbadi MA, et al. Primary testicular and para-testicular lymphoma: a retrospective clinicopatho-logic study of 34 cases with emphasis on differential diagnosis. Arch Pathol Lab Med 2007; 131(7):1040–6.

281. Ferry JA, et al. Malignant lymphoma of the testis, epididymis, and spermatic cord. A clinicopatho-logic study of 69 cases with immunophenotypic analysis. Am J Surg Pathol 1994;18(4):376–90.

282. Sussman EB, et al. Malignant lymphoma of the tes-tis: a clinicopathologic study of 37 cases. J Urol 1977;118(6):1004–7.

283. Paladugu RR, Bearman RM, Rappaport H. Malig-nant lymphoma with primary manifestation in the gonad: a clinicopathologic study of 38 patients. Cancer 1980;45(3):561–71.

284. Zucca E, et al. Patterns of outcome and prognos-tic factors in primary large-cell lymphoma of the testis in a survey by the International Extranodal Lymphoma Study Group. J Clin Oncol 2003; 21(1):20–7.

285. Zietman AL, et al. The management and outcome of stage IAE nonHodgkin's lymphoma of the testis. J Urol 1996;155(3):943–6.

286. Finn LS, et al. Primary follicular lymphoma of the testis in childhood. Cancer 1999;85(7):1626–35.

287. Pakzad K, et al. Follicular large cell lymphoma local-ized to the testis in children. J Urol 2002;168(1):225–8.

288. Dalle JH, et al. Testicular disease in childhood B-cell non-Hodgkin's lymphoma: the French Soci-ety of Pediatric Oncology experience. J Clin Oncol 2001;19(9):2397–403.

289. Zouhair A, et al. Outcome and patterns of failure in testicular lymphoma: a multicenter Rare Cancer Network study. Int J Radiat Oncol Biol Phys 2002; 52(3):652–6.

290. Lagrange JL, et al. Non-Hodgkin's lymphoma of the testis: a retrospective study of 84 patients treated in the French anticancer centres. Ann Oncol 2001;12(9):1313–9.

291. Mazzu D, Jeffrey RB Jr, Ralls PW. Lymphoma and leukemia involving the testicles: findings on gray-scale and color Doppler sonography. AJR Am J Roentgenol 1995;164(3):645–7.

292. Goodman JD, et al. Testicular lymphoma: sono-graphic findings. Urol Radiol 1985;7(1):25–7.

293. Ferry JA, Young RH, Scully RE. Testicular and epididymal plasmacytoma: a report of 7 cases, including three that were the initial manifestation of plasma cell myeloma. Am J Surg Pathol 1997; 21(5):590–8.

294. Vega F, Medeiros LJ, Abruzzo LV. Primary parates-ticular lymphoma: a report of 2 cases and review of

literature. Arch Pathol Lab Med 2001;125(3): 428–32.

295. Oppenheim PI, Cohen S, Anders KH. Testicular plasmacytoma. A case report with immunohisto-chemical studies and literature review. Arch Pathol Lab Med 1991;115(6):629–32.

296. Iizumi T, et al. Plasmacytoma of the testis. Urol Int 1995;55(4):218–21.

297. Ferry JA, Srigley JR, Young RH. Granulocytic sarcoma of the testis: a report of two cases of a neoplasm prone to misinterpretation. Mod Pathol 1997;10(4):320–5.

298. Ferry J, Ulbright TM, Young RH. Anaplastic large-cell lymphoma presenting in the testis: a lesion that may be confused with embryonal carcinoma. J Urol Pathol 1997;5:139–47.

299. Root M, et al. Burkitt's lymphoma of the testicle: report of 2 cases occurring in elderly patients. J Urol 1990;144(5):1239–41.

300. Wilkins BS, Williamson JM, O'Brien CJ. Morpholog-ical and immunohistological study of testicular lymphomas. Histopathology 1989;15(2):147–56.

301. Chan JK, et al. Aggressive T/natural killer cell lymphoma presenting as testicular tumor. Cancer 1996;77(6):1198–205.

302. Seliem RM, et al. Classical Hodgkin's lymphoma presenting as a testicular mass: report of a case. Int J Surg Pathol 2007;15(2):207–12.

303. Bacon CM, et al. Primary follicular lymphoma of the testis and epididymis in adults. Am J Surg Pathol 2007;31(7):1050–8.

304. Economopoulos T, et al. Primary granulocytic sarcoma of the testis. Leukemia 1994;8(1): 199–200.

305. Henley JD, Ferry J, Ulbright TM. Miscellaneous rare paratesticular tumors. Semin Diagn Pathol 2000; 17(4):319–39.

306. Ulbright TM, Young RH. Primary mucinous tumors of the testis and paratestis: a report of nine cases. Am J Surg Pathol 2003;27(9):1221–8.

307. Young RH, Scully RE. Testicular and paratesticular tumors and tumor-like lesions of ovarian common epithelial and Mullerian types. A report of four cases and review of the literature. Am J Clin Pathol 1986;86(2):146–52.

308. McClure RF, et al. Serous borderline tumor of the paratestis: a report of seven cases. Am J Surg Pathol 2001;25(3):373–8.

309. Jones MA, et al. Paratesticular serous papillary car-cinoma. A report of six cases. Am J Surg Pathol 1995;19(12):1359–65.

310. Remmele W, et al. Serous papillary cystic tumor of borderline malignancy with focal carcinoma arising in testis: case report with immunohistochemical and ultrastructural observations. Hum Pathol 1992;23(1):75–9.

311. Young RH, Rosenberg AE, Clement PB. Mucin deposits within inguinal hernia sacs: a presenting finding of low-grade mucinous cystic tumors of the appendix. A report of two cases and a review of the literature. Mod Pathol 1997;10(12): 1228–32.

312. Almagro UA. Metastatic tumors involving testis. Urology 1988;32(4):357–60.

313. Emerson RE, Ulbright TM. Morphological approach to tumours of the testis and paratestis. J Clin Pathol 2007;60(8):866–80.

314. Grignon DJ, Shum DT, Hayman WP. Metastatic tumours of the testes. Can J Surg 1986;29(5): 359–61.

315. Meares EM Jr, Ho TL. Metastatic carcinomas involving the testis: a review. J Urol 1973;109(4): 653–5.

316. Price EB Jr, Mostofi FK. Secondary carcinoma of the testis. Cancer 1957;10(3):592–5.

317. Tiltman AJ. Metastatic tumours in the testis. Histopathology 1979;3(1):31–7.

318. Datta MW, Ulbright TM, Young RH. Renal cell carcinoma metastatic to the testis and its adnexa: a report of five cases including three that accounted for the initial clinical presentation. Int J Surg Pathol 2001;9(1):49–56.

319. Lyngdorf P, Nielsen K. Prostatic cancer with metastasis to the testis. Urol Int 1987;42(1):77–8.

320. Moskovitz B, Kerner H, Richter Levin D. Testicular metastasis from carcinoma of the prostate. Urol Int 1987;42(1):79–80.

321. Haupt HM, et al. Metastatic carcinoma involving the testis. Clinical and pathologic distinction from primary testicular neoplasms. Cancer 1984;54(4): 709–14.

322. Delahunt B, et al. Immunohistochemical evidence for mesothelial origin of paratesticular adenomatoid tumour. Histopathology 2000;36(2):109–15.

323. Eble JN, Sauder G, Epstein JI, et al. World Health Organization classification of tumors, pathology and genetics. Tumors of the urinary system. Lyon (France): IACR Press; 2004.

324. Stephenson TJ, Mills PM. Adenomatoid tumours: an immunohistochemical and ultrastructural appraisal of their histogenesis. J Pathol 1986; 148(4):327–35.

325. Schwartz EJ, Longacre TA. Adenomatoid tumors of the female and male genital tracts express WT1. Int J Gynecol Pathol 2004;23(2):123–8.

326. Gokce G, et al. Adenomatoid tumors of testis and epididymis: a report of two cases. Int Urol Nephrol 2001;32(4):677–80.

327. Kolgesiz AI, et al. Adenomatoid tumor of the tunica vaginalis testis: a special maneuver in diagnosis by ultrasonography. J Ultrasound Med 2003;22(3): 303–5.

328. Piccin A, et al. Adenomatoid tumor of the testis in a patient on imatinib therapy for chronic myeloid leukemia. Leuk Lymphoma 2006;47(7):1394–6.

329. Williams SB, et al. Adenomatoid tumor of the testes. Urology 2004;63(4):779–81.

330. Tammela TL, et al. Intrascrotal adenomatoid tumors. J Urol 1991;146(1):61–5.

331. Nogales FF, et al. Adenomatoid tumors of the uterus: an analysis of 60 cases. Int J Gynecol Pathol 2002;21(1):34–40.

332. Lane TM, et al. Benign cystic mesothelioma of the tunica vaginalis. BJU Int 1999;84(4):533–4.

333. Tobioka H, et al. Multicystic mesothelioma of the spermatic cord. Histopathology 1995;27(5): 479–81.

334. Mikuz G, Hopfel-Kreiner I. Papillary mesothelioma of the tunica vaginalis propria testis. Case report and ultrastructural study. Virchows Arch A Pathol Anat Histol 1982;396(2):231–8.

335. Chetty R. Well differentiated (benign) papillary mesothelioma of the tunica vaginalis. J Clin Pathol 1992;45(11):1029–30.

336. Perez-Ordonez B, Srigley JR. Mesothelial lesions of the paratesticular region. Semin Diagn Pathol 2000;17(4):294–306.

337. Churg A. Paratesticular mesothelial proliferations. Semin Diagn Pathol 2003;20(4):272–8.

338. Menut P, et al [Bilateral malignant mesothelioma of the tunica vaginalis testis. Apropos of a case]. Prog Urol 1996;6(4):587–9 [in French].

339. Pelzer A, et al. Synchronous bilateral malignant mesothelioma of tunica vaginalis testis: early diagnosis. Urology 2004;64(5):1031.

340. Chollet Y, et al. Well-differentiated papillary mesothelioma of the tunica vaginalis testis: imaging on Tc-99m heat-denatured red blood cell scintigraphy. Clin Nucl Med 2008;33(4):282–4.

341. Fujisaki M, et al. Case of mesothelioma of the tunica vaginalis testis with characteristic findings on ultrasonography and magnetic resonance imaging. Int J Urol 2000;7(11):427–30.

342. Jones MA, Young RH, Scully RE. Malignant mesothelioma of the tunica vaginalis. A clinicopathologic analysis of 11 cases with review of the literature. Am J Surg Pathol 1995;19(7):815–25.

343. Machlenkin S, Diment J, Kashtan H. Benign cystic mesothelioma of the peritoneum. Isr Med Assoc J 2006;8(7):511–2.

344. Butnor KJ, et al. Well-differentiated papillary mesothelioma. Am J Surg Pathol 2001;25(10):1304–9.

345. Xiao SY, Rizzo P, Carbone M. Benign papillary mesothelioma of the tunica vaginalis testis. Arch Pathol Lab Med 2000;124(1):143–7.

346. Burrig KF, Pfitzer P, Hort W. Well-differentiated papillary mesothelioma of the peritoneum: a borderline mesothelioma. Report of two cases and review of

literature. Virchows Arch A Pathol Anat Histopathol 1990;417(5):443–7.

347. Ordonez NG. The diagnostic utility of immunohisto-chemistry and electron microscopy in distinguishing between peritoneal mesotheliomas and serous carcinomas: a comparative study. Mod Pathol 2006;19(1):34–48.

348. Winstanley AM, et al. The immunohistochemical profile of malignant mesotheliomas of the tunica vaginalis: a study of 20 cases. Am J Surg Pathol 2006;30(1):1–6.

349. Aggarwal M, et al. Malignant peritoneal mesothelioma in an inguinal hernial sac: an unusual presentation. Indian J Cancer 2000;37(2–3):91–4.

350. Ascoli V, et al. Concomitant malignant mesothelioma of the pleura, peritoneum, and tunica vaginalis testis. Diagn Cytopathol 1996;14(3):243–8.

351. Plas E, Riedl CR, Pfluger H. Malignant mesothelioma of the tunica vaginalis testis: review of the literature and assessment of prognostic parameters. Cancer 1998;83(12):2437–46.

352. Blitzer PH, et al. Treatment of malignant tumors of the spermatic cord: a study of 10 cases and a review of the literature. J Urol 1981;126(5):611–4.

353. Montgomery E, Fisher C. Paratesticular liposarcoma: a clinicopathologic study. Am J Surg Pathol 2003;27(1):40–7.

354. Schwartz SL, et al. Liposarcoma of the spermatic cord: report of 6 cases and review of the literature. J Urol 1995;153(1):154–7.

355. Beccia DJ, Krane RJ, Olsson CA. Clinical management of non-testicular intrascrotal tumors. J Urol 1976;116(4):476–9.

356. Weiss SW, Rao VK. Well-differentiated liposarcoma (atypical lipoma) of deep soft tissue of the extremities, retroperitoneum, and miscellaneous sites. A follow-up study of 92 cases with analysis of the incidence of "dedifferentiation". Am J Surg Pathol 1992;16(11):1051–8.

357. Henricks WH, et al. Dedifferentiated liposarcoma: a clinicopathological analysis of 155 cases with a proposal for an expanded definition of dedifferentiation. Am J Surg Pathol 1997;21(3):271–81.

358. Cardenosa G, et al. Spermatic cord sarcomas: sonographic and CT features. Urol Radiol 1990;12(3):163–7.

359. Milner SM, Hawthorn IE, Morgans BT. Liposarcoma of the cord presenting at vasectomy counselling. J R Army Med Corps 1989;135(2):86–7.

360. McLean TW, Castellino SM. Pediatric genitourinary tumors. Curr Opin Oncol 2008;20(3):315–20.

361. Skoog SJ. Benign and malignant pediatric scrotal masses. Pediatr Clin North Am 1997;44(5):1229–50.

362. Rao CR, et al. Adult paratesticular sarcomas: a report of eight cases. J Surg Oncol 1994;56(2):89–93.

363. Coleman J, et al. Adult spermatic cord sarcomas: management and results. Ann Surg Oncol 2003;10(6):669–75.

364. Crist WM, et al. Intergroup rhabdomyosarcoma study-IV: results for patients with nonmetastatic disease. J Clin Oncol 2001;19(12):3091–102.

365. Chiu LS, et al. Angiosarcoma of the scrotum after treatment of cancer of the rectum. Clin Exp Dermatol 2006;31(5):706–7.

366. Hayn MH, Bastacky S, Franks ME. Epididymal angiosarcoma. Urology 2007;69(3):576, e5–7.

367. Masera A, Ovcak Z, Mikuz G. Angiosarcoma of the testis. Virchows Arch 1999;434(4):351–3.

368. Steele GS, et al. Angiosarcoma arising in a testicular teratoma. J Urol 2000;163(6):1872–3.

369. Armah HB, Rao UN, Parwani AV. Primary angiosarcoma of the testis: report of a rare entity and review of the literature. Diagn Pathol 2007;2:23.

370. Elsasser E. Tumors of the epididymis. Recent Results Cancer Res 1977;(60):163–75.

371. Lamiell JM, Salazar FG, Hsia YE. von Hippel-Lindau disease affecting 43 members of a single kindred. Medicine (Baltimore) 1989;68(1):1–29.

372. Price EB Jr. Papillary cystadenoma of the epididymis. A clinicopathologic analysis of 20 cases. Arch Pathol 1971;91(5):456–70.

373. Ganem JP, Jhaveri FM, Marroum MC. Primary adenocarcinoma of the epididymis: case report and review of the literature. Urology 1998;52(5):904–8.

374. Gilcrease MZ, et al. Somatic von Hippel-Lindau mutation in clear cell papillary cystadenoma of the epididymis. Hum Pathol 1995;26(12):1341–6.

375. Kragel PJ, et al. Papillary cystadenoma of the epididymis. A report of three cases with lectin histochemistry. Arch Pathol Lab Med 1990;114(7):672–5.

376. Shen T, et al. Allelic deletion of VHL gene detected in papillary tumors of the broad ligament, epididymis, and retroperitoneum in von Hippel-Lindau disease patients. Int J Surg Pathol 2000;8(3):207–12.

377. Leung SY, et al. Expression of vascular endothelial growth factor in von Hippel-Lindau syndrome-associated papillary cystadenoma of the epididymis. Hum Pathol 1998;29(11):1322–4.

378. Humphrey PA. Clear cell neoplasms of the urinary tract and male reproductive system. Semin Diagn Pathol 1997;14(4):240–52.

379. Roganovich J, et al. Paratesticular desmoplastic small round cell tumor: case report and review of the literature. J Surg Oncol 1999;71(4):269–72.

BENIGN DISEASES AND NEOPLASMS OF THE PENIS

Matthew J. Wasco, MD[a], Rajal B. Shah, MD[a,b,*]

KEYWORDS

• Penis • Precancerous lesions • Squamous cell carcinoma • Penile neoplasia

ABSTRACT

Penile diseases consist of a wide spectrum of benign and malignant conditions for which careful histopathological examination remains the cornerstone of diagnosis, prognosis, and management, most notably for penile carcinoma. From an epidemiologic standpoint, penile carcinoma remains primarily a disease of developing countries. Environmental factors, notably human papillomavirus infection (HPV), have played a much more important role than genetic factors in understanding the pathogenesis of penile carcinoma. Several new histologic entities for penile neoplasms with distinct outcomes and clinical behavior have been proposed in recent years. This article provides a handy, yet comprehensive, review of benign diseases and neoplastic conditions of the penis with emphasis on clinical findings, key pathologic features with representative images, and ancillary techniques to aid in differential diagnoses

ANATOMY OF THE PENIS

Anatomy plays a key role in staging and understanding neoplasms of the penis. Certain types of tumor are more likely to occur in specific anatomic sites. There are three parts to the penis: the body, or shaft, which makes up the central portion of the structure; the anterior portion which includes the glans, coronal sulcus, and foreskin (prepuce); and the posterior portion, also known as the root. The glans is an extension of the urethral corpus spongiosum and is demarcated from the shaft by the slightly elevated, circumferential corona and adjacent coronal sulcus, where the foreskin is attached (**Fig. 1**). The glans is the most common site for penile malignancies.[1,2]

HISTOLOGY OF THE PENIS

The different anatomic areas of the penis also differ in their histologic makeup. Much of the penile urethra is covered by urothelium, but toward the glans and the urethral meatus, the epithelium transitions to a stratified, nonkeratinizing squamous epithelium which covers the entire glans. Beneath the epithelium is a loose connective tissue layer, the lamina propria, which serves to separate the mucosa from the corpus spongiosum, and is usually approximately 1 to 3 mm in thickness. In the glans, however, the lamina propria may be very thin or merge abruptly with the underlying corpus spongiosum, an important feature to recognize for the purposes of staging invasive neoplasms (**Fig. 2**).[1,2] The corpus spongiosum is a highly vascular structure composed of specialized erectile tissue including numerous anastomosing venous sinuses and peripheral nerves. Between the corpus spongiosum and underlying corpus cavernosa is a dense, fibroelastic layer, the tunica albuginea, which is a barrier to spread of malignancies (see **Fig. 1**).

[a] Department of Pathology, University of Michigan, 1500 East Medical Center Drive, 2G332 UH, Ann Arbor, MI 48109, USA
[b] Department of Urology, University of Michigan, 1500 East Medical Center Drive, 2G332 UH, Ann Arbor, MI 48109, USA
* Corresponding author. Department of Pathology, University of Michigan, 1500 East Medical Center Drive, 2G332 UH, Ann Arbor, MI 48109, USA
E-mail address: rajshah@umich.edu (R.B. Shah).

Surgical Pathology 2 (2009) 161–197
doi:10.1016/j.path.2008.07.007

> ### Key Pathologic Features
> #### PRECANCEROUS LESIONS, PENIS
>
> Gross findings
>
> > Irregular or discrete, moist, and erythematous or scaly plaques
> >
> > Low grade lesions present as white patches (leukoplakia)
>
> Microscopic findings
>
> > Graded according to proportion of atypical cells occupying the epithelial thickness and degree of cytologic atypia. LGSIL, PeIN I have mild atypia, confined to the lower third, while HGSIL, PeIN II/III have moderate to severe cytologic atypia involving 2/3 thickness of the epithelium. The surface is often hyperkeratotic. The nuclei are enlarged, pleomorphic, and hyperchromatic, with irregular nuclear membranes. Koilocytic atypia is frequently prominent in warty or basaloid subtypes associated with HPV infection.
> >
> > PeIN associated with squamous differentiation has preferential association with LSA and is not associated with HPV infection.

The foreskin in uncircumcised individuals covers the glans as a double membrane. It contains five histologic layers. Opposing the glans is the inner mucosal epithelium which is similar to that of the glans. Beneath this epithelium are lamina propria, a double layer of smooth muscle fibers known as the dartos muscle, the dermis, and finally the epidermis, a keratinizing squamous epithelium containing rare adnexal structures, which is continuous with the epithelium of the body. The histology of the body includes squamous epithelium with underlying dermis and dartos muscle and adipose tissue. Beneath the adipose tissue is Buck's fascia, containing blood vessels and nerves, and the tunica albuginea, which encases the corpora cavernosa and spongiosum (**Fig. 3**). Corpus spongiosum encases the urethra.

PRECANCEROUS SQUAMOUS AND RELATED LESIONS

OVERVIEW

The terminology used in describing and classifying preneoplastic squamous lesions of the penis is confusing and varied. Numerous designations have been previously proposed: squamous intraepithelial lesion, low- (LGSIL) and high-grade (HGSIL); mild, moderate, and severe dysplasia, with or without HPV changes;[2,3] penile intraepithelial neoplasia (PeIN) I, II, and III; and carcinoma in situ (CIS) have been used with similar significance (**Table 1**). Other terms that have been used previously include erythroplasia of Queyrat (for lesions of the glans and foreskin) and Bowen's disease (for lesions involving the body/shaft), both of which refer to CIS. We prefer the terminology of LGSIL, HGSIL, or PeIN I, II, and III. In part, difficulty in classification is based on the histologic overlap between benign and premalignant conditions. HPV DNA is expressed in the majority (70%–100%) of premalignant squamous lesions, many of which are subclinical, and is believed to play a key role in progression to penile carcinoma.[3–5] However, some premalignant lesions of the penis, including lichen sclerosus et atrophicus (LSA), are not associated with HPV.[6] A recent proposal has been made to characterize preneoplastic squamous lesions based on their etiology. This proposal classifies lesions with HPV-associated atypia as either warty or basaloid type, depending on their morphology. Alternately, non-HPV-associated intraepithelial lesions are associated with differentiated squamous atypia, have preferential association with LSA, and are termed "simplex" or "differentiated" type. Simplex squamous atypia is associated with squamous cell carcinoma (SCC) but many lesions do not progress to malignancy.[6]

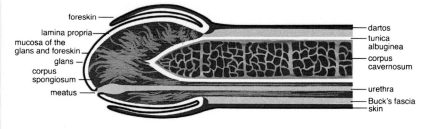

Fig. 1. Diagrammatic representation of the anatomy of the penis: cut section view. (*Adapted from* Young RH, Srigley JR, Amin MB, et al. Tumors of the prostate gland, seminal vesicles, male urethra, and penis. In: Atlas of tumor pathology. Washington, DC: AFIP; 2000. *From* Shah RB, Amin MB. Diseases of the penis, urethra, and scrotum. In: Zhou M, Magi-Galluzzi C, editors. Genitourinary pathology. Philadelphia: Churchill Livingstone Elsevier; 2007. p. 419; with permission.)

Fig. 2. Glans penis: histologic features. Low power view of a section of the glans penis, demonstrating three histologic levels: nonkeratinizing squamous epithelium, lamina propria, and corpus spongiosum with richly vascular erectile tissue. Note separation between the lamina propria and spongiosum is abrupt.

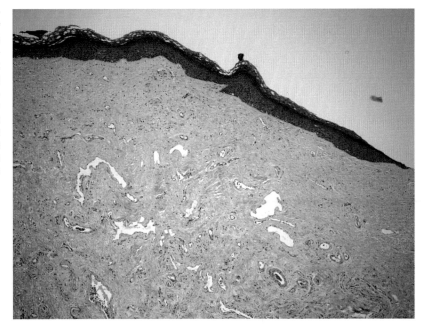

Fig. 3. Diagrammatic representation of the cross-sectional anatomy of the body (shaft) of the penis. The dartos (D) is closely attached to the skin (S); Buck's fascia (BF) covers the inferior of the urethra (U); the corpus spongiosum (CS) and the urethra are located in the groove between the corpora cavernosa (CC) and Buck's fascia. The tunica albuginea (A) encases the corpora cavernosa. (*Adapted from* Young RH, Srigley JR, Amin MB, et al. Tumors of the prostate gland, seminal vesicles, male urethra, and penis. In: Atlas of tumor pathology. Washington, DC: AFIP; 2000. *From* Shah RB, Amin MB. Diseases of the penis, urethra, and scrotum. In: Zhou M, Magi-Galluzzi C, editors. Genitourinary pathology. Philadelphia: Churchill Livingstone Elsevier; 2007. p. 419; with permission.)

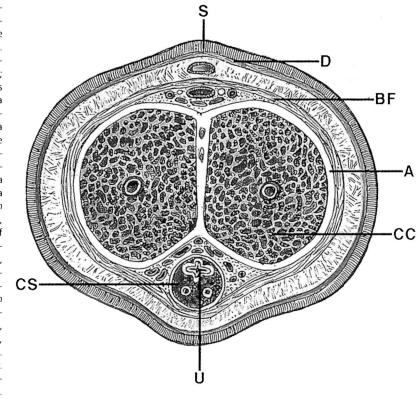

Table 1
WHO histologic classification of tumors of the penis

Malignant epithelial tumors of the penis
 SCC
 Basaloid carcinoma
 Warty (condylomatous) carcinoma
 Verrucous carcinoma
 Papillary carcinoma, NOS
 Sarcomatous carcinoma
 Mixed carcinomas
 Adenosquamous carcinoma
Paget's disease
Merkel cell carcinoma
Small cell carcinoma of neuroendocrine type
Sebaceous carcinoma
Clear cell carcinoma
Basal cell carcinoma

Precursor lesions
Intraepithelial neoplasia grade III
Bowen Disease
Erythroplasia of Queyrat
Melanocytic tumors
Melanocytic nevi
Melanoma
Mesenchymal tumors
Hematopoietic tumors
Secondary tumors

Data from Eble JN, Sauter G, Epstein JI, et al, (eds). Pathology and genetics, tumors of the urinary system and male genital organs. Lyon, France: World Health Organization, International Agency for Research on Cancer, 2004:280.

Clinical and Gross Features

Preneoplastic squamous lesions are most commonly seen in the sixth decade of life, at a later age than in cases of bowenoid papulosis. Grossly, they can appear as moist, scaly plaques or erythematous areas (**Fig. 4**), often adjacent to areas of SCC.[6] Lower grade lesions can present as areas of leukoplakia (white patches).

Microscopic Features

The microscopic features of preneoplastic squamous lesions range from a histologic picture difficult to distinguish from benign conditions to full-thickness, severe atypia. In general, PeIN has cytologic atypia and transformation of the basal cell layer. The atypia includes varying degrees of nuclear hyperchromasia and pleomorphism, along with loss of normal polarity and mitotic figures. LGSIL have mild atypia, confined to the lower third of the epithelium, whereas HGSIL atypia affects 2/3 of the epithelium or has moderate to severe cytologic atypia (**Fig. 5**).[3] Koilocytic atypia is frequently prominent. Full-thickness atypia of the epithelium is referred to as in situ carcinoma.

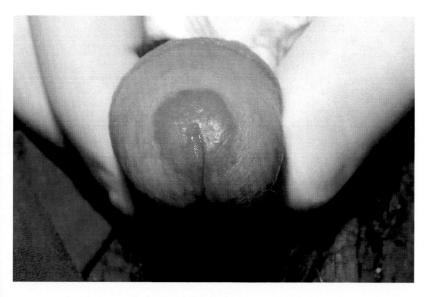

Fig. 4. Bowen's disease: clinical features. An irregular, moist, erythematous flat lesion involves the urethral meatus and the mucosa of the glans penis. (*Courtesy of* Kenneth Angermeier, M.D., Cleveland Clinic, Cleveland OH; with permission.)

Fig. 5. High-grade SIL (PeIN III): microscopic features. Squamous epithelium demonstrates prominent hyperkeratosis, parakeratosis, acanthosis, and full-thickness, high-grade cytologic atypia with basaloid features. Focal koilocytic atypia is seen.

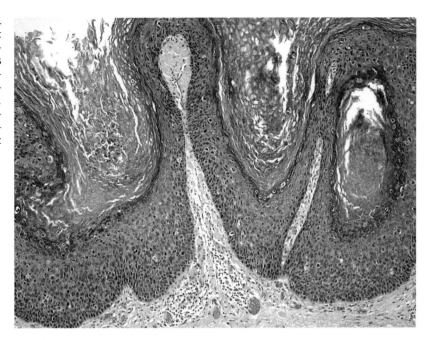

Squamous intraepithelial atypia is also classified, similar to SCC, based on the architectural and cytologic features. Differentiated squamous penile intraepithelial lesion, or "simplex" intraepithelial atypia, has preferential association with lichen sclerosus and may be difficult to distinguish from background squamous hyperplasia.[6] This lesion is generally not associated with HPV. Other premalignant lesions can be classified as warty or basaloid. These lesions are associated with HPV and have definable features.[3,7] Warty squamous intraepithelial lesions are condylomatous, with koilocytic atypia, whereas basaloid lesions have increased nuclear-to-cytoplasmic ratios and a basaloid cytologic phenotype (see **Fig. 5**). HPV-associated warty or basaloid lesions are generally high grade, as opposed to simplex atypia that is generally low grade.

Differential Diagnosis

Bowenoid papulosis significantly overlaps histologically with squamous intraepithelial neoplasia, although clinical differences can help in making the distinction, which are summarized in **Table 2**.

Table 2
Comparison between PeIN III and bowenoid papulosis

Feature	PeIN III (Includes BD & EQ)	Bowenoid Papulosis
Site	Glans, prepuce (EQ), shaft (BD)	Shaft
Age	4th – 6th decade	3rd – 4th decade
Lesion	Scaly (BD) or erythematous plaque (EQ)	Papules
Maturation	–	+
Sweat gland involvement	–	+
Pilosebaceous involvement	+/–	–
Precancerous potential	5% – 10%	–
Spontaneous regression	–	+
HPV	+	+

Abbreviations: BD, Bowen's disease; EQ, erythroplasia of Queyrat.
Data from Young RH, Srigley JR, Amin MB, et al. Tumors of the prostate gland, seminal vesicles, male urethra, and penis. In: Atlas of tumor pathology. Washington, DC: AFIP; 2000.

Differential Diagnosis
PRECANCEROUS LESIONS, PENIS

- Bowenoid papulosis
- Condyloma
- Zoon's balanitis (clinical presentation)
- Urothelial CIS

Pitfalls
PRECANCEROUS LESIONS, PENIS

! Many preneoplastic squamous lesions of the penis have overlapping histologic features with benign conditions. As a result, confident diagnosis may depend on clinical presentation and presence of an adjacent invasive carcinoma.

! HSGIL has significant overlap with bowenoid papulosis histologically, although clinical presentation usually helps in making the distinction.

! High-grade squamous precursor lesions may be confused with urothelial CIS or other primary malignancies such as Paget disease. Careful attention to histologic details and adjacent mucosal changes can usually resolve this problem.

Clinically, erythroplasia of Queyrat can mimic Zoon's balanitis, however histologically the presence of benign squamous epithelium with a thickened band of plasma cells and chronic inflammatory cells distinguishes the latter condition. In lesions involving the glans, particularly around the urethral meatus, the differential diagnosis can include urothelial CIS extending from the urethra to the glans. Careful attention to histologic detail and adjacent mucosa can usually resolve this problem. Lesions which do not fit the criteria above and cannot be definitively classified as preneoplastic are often classified as squamous hyperplasia. These lesions demonstrate acanthosis (flat or papillary) and variable hyperkeratosis but with normal maturation and minimal cytologic atypia. Squamous hyperplasia can also be associated with SCC, further evidence of the difficulty in distinguishing benign from malignant conditions.

Prognosis and Therapy

The main therapeutic consideration with preneoplastic and in situ neoplastic lesions of the penis is the small but real risk of progression to invasive carcinoma. Approximately 5% to 10% of untreated high-grade precursor lesions are estimated to progress to invasive carcinoma, and the risk is higher in those patients who cannot clear HPV infection.[2,6–9] In lesions associated with HPV infection, the individual may clear the infection and reduce their risk of malignant transformation. Clinically, however, it is usually impossible to tell which patients will clear the infection and which will have persistence. There is a higher risk of persistence and progression in immunosuppressed or older patients.[7,8] Because of this, these lesions are best considered as preneoplastic and treated with either wide excision with clear margins or topical chemotherapy. Some lesions can be difficult to clear as margins can be indistinct or lesions may extend deep into adnexal structures.

LICHEN SCLEROSUS ET ATROPHICUS

Clinical and Gross Features

LSA is also known as balanitis xerotica obliterans, and is the corresponding lesion in males to that of vulvar LSA in women. Most commonly seen in the third to fifth decade of life, although also affecting the extremes of life, it affects the glans penis or

Key Pathologic Features
LICHEN SCLEROSUS ET ATROPHICUS

Gross findings

White-gray, flat, irregular geographic atrophic areas involving the foreskin or glans, especially perimeatal region. Phimosis or urethral strictures are common clinical presentations.

Microscopic findings

Atrophy of squamous epithelium with hyperkeratosis. The rete ridges are flat. In early lesions lamina propria demonstrates edema and chronic inflammation and in later cases a characteristic band of eosinophilic fibrosis, frequently with vacuolar interface dermatitis. The lesion is superficial, 3 to 4mm in depth.

Preferential association with PeIN of differentiated type that is not associated with HPV infection. It also has association with SCC.

foreskin and presents as a gray-white atrophic area, frequently presenting clinically with phimosis or narrowing of the urethral meatus (**Fig. 6**). It overlaps with penile intraepithelial neoplasia of simplex or differentiated type and can coexist with an adjacent penile SCC.[6,8] It is not associated with HPV.[10]

Microscopic Features

LSA is characterized by a thin, atrophic squamous epithelium overlying an acellular, hyalinized, and fibrotic superficial dermis with a band of variable chronic inflammation (**Fig. 7**). Early lesions show more inflammation and less hyalinization. The squamous epithelium is often hyperkeratotic but rete ridges are generally lost to varying degrees. Hyperplastic variants exist. Variable differentiated squamous atypia can be present in lesions associated with differentiated-type squamous PeIN.[6]

Differential Diagnosis

LSA is generally histologically distinct in well-developed cases, although certain lesions,

Differential Diagnosis
LICHEN SCLEROSUS ET ATROPHICUS

- Zoon's balanitis
- Lichen planus
- Stromal amyloid deposition
- Squamous hyperplasia

particularly early ones with a prominent band of inflammatory cells, can be confused with inflammatory conditions such as dermatitis, lichen planus, and Zoon's balanitis. Zoon's balanitis is a lesion with increased plasma cells. In these cases, the presence of stromal hyalinization is an important factor. Rarely, the stromal hyalinization can resemble amyloid deposition, which can occur in this site.[11]

Prognosis and Therapy

LSA has been suggested as one of the etiologic factors for SCC, because of its frequent association with it and the overlap with differentiated (simplex) intraepithelial neoplasia.[6,10,12] The condition can, however, have many significant complications of its own, including phimosis and urethral stricture. Thus, early diagnosis and treatment to prevent these complications is clinically relevant. The treatment varies from topical corticosteroids and laser therapy in early cases to meatoplasty and urethroplasty in severe cases.[13]

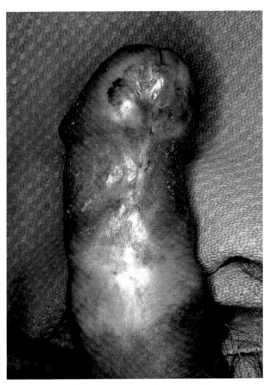

Fig. 6. LSA: clinical features. A gray-white irregular atrophic appearing lesion involves the perimeatal area of the glans penis. (*Courtesy of* Lori Lowe, MD, Ann Arbor, MI.)

Pitfalls
LICHEN SCLEROSUS ET ATROPHICUS

! Lesions associated with PeIN of differentiated or simplex type can be deceptively bland, and can overlap histologically. Careful attention and knowledge about such associations is important.

! Some lesions, particularly early ones, may have a prominent inflammatory component and mimic other inflammatory conditions such as lichen planus or Zoon's balanitis. Knowledge about the clinical presentation and histologic details usually provide separation from such conditions.

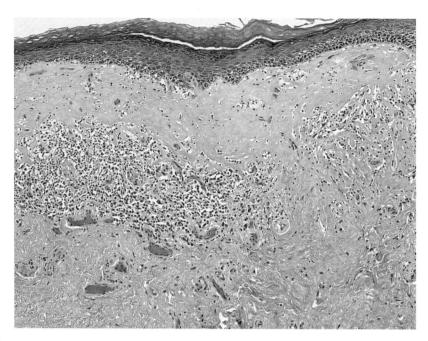

Fig. 7. LSA: microscopic features. The lamina propria is edematous with characteristic eosinophilic band of hyalinization. The overlying epithelium demonstrates hyperkeratosis, atrophy, and loss of rete ridges.

BOWENOID PAPULOSIS

Clinical and Gross Features

Bowenoid papulosis is an HPV-related condition that presents at an average age of 30 years. Grossly, solitary or multiple red papules, resembling warts, are seen usually on the shaft of the penis but occasionally on the glans or foreskin.[14] HPV association with oncogenic high-risk types 16 and 18 has been reported.[15]

Key Features
BOWENOID PAPULOSIS

Gross findings

Solitary or multiple small red nodules or papules, resembling warts, usually seen on the shaft of the penis.

Microscopic findings

Histologic features are essentially similar to usual PeIN II/III (HGSIL). In general, a more spotty distribution of atypical cells and greater maturation of keratinocytes than HGSIL.

Immunohistochemical features

Oncogenic HPV DNA, most commonly type 16, but types 18 or 33 to 35 have also been reported.

Microscopic Features

Bowenoid papulosis microscopically can be indistinguishable from HSGIL. In general, there is a more spotty distribution of atypical cells and greater maturation of keratinocytes (**Fig. 8**).[14]

Differential Diagnosis

Diagnosis of bowenoid papulosis is made purely on clinicopathological basis. Young people presenting with multiple lesions and spotty cytologic atypia are typical for this condition. One report indicates that P16 protein expression is less common in bowenoid papulosis, although this is not specific.[16]

Prognosis and Therapy

Malignant transformation is rare and many lesions spontaneously regress. Recent reports suggest good response with immunomodulatory treatments. In view of the oncogenic potential of high-risk HPV infections (types 16 and 18), regardless of treatment used, all patients with bowenoid

Differential Diagnosis
BOWENOID PAPULOSIS

- PeIN (Bowen's disease)
- SCC
- Condyloma

Pitfalls

BOWENOID PAPULOSIS

! Histologically overlaps with PeIN, high grade, and can be impossible to separate on the basis of microscopy alone. Young patients presenting with multiple lesions and spotty cytologic atypia are typical of bowenoid papulosis.

! Bowenoid papulosis is HPV associated and requires close clinical follow-up of the patient and sexual partners.

papulosis and their sexual partners should be included in long-term follow-up and regularly examined for malignant transformation.[17]

MALIGNANT NEOPLASMS

Penile malignancies represent less than 1% of malignancies in the western, developed world, with an age-adjusted incidence rate of 0.3 to 1.0 cases per 100,000 population.[2,18] In developing countries the incidence is much higher. It can be as high as 10% of malignancies in some countries, including Brazil, Paraguay, Mexico, Jamaica, Haiti, and parts of Africa (Uganda).[19,20] Much of this difference is thought to be attributable to environmental factors. Epithelial tumors (carcinomas) make up over 95% of cases of penile malignancy, and encompass a wide range of subtypes of SCC

as well as other malignancies more typical of other skin sites.[2,21]

SQUAMOUS CELL CARCINOMA, USUAL TYPE

Overview

The majority of SCC of the penis resemble SCC of other sites in the body. Approximately one-third of cases, however, can be classified under a specific subtype of penile SCC and are described here under specific subtype headings.

Etiology

SCC of the penis has been linked to multiple environmental factors, including smoking, HPV infection, and ultraviolet irradiation; and co-existing conditions such as phimosis, LSA, and other chronic inflammatory conditions.[10,18,20–22] Neonatal circumcision has been recently associated with a three-fold decreased risk of carcinoma.[5,23] An interesting hypothesis is that foreskin length may be related to risk for development of SCC; in particular a long foreskin. Patients with a long foreskin (such as one that completely covers the glans penis) develop phimosis at a far higher rate.[24]

Association with HPV Infection

HPV infection is increasingly recognized as having a major role in the development of penile SCC through progression of HPV-associated penile intraepithelial lesions that are usually positive for HPV DNA. Risk depends in part on the subtype of HPV, with HPV 16 as the currently recognized

Fig. 8. Bowenoid papulosis: microscopic features. In bowenoid papulosis, squamous epithelium demonstrates cytologic atypia, similar to that seen in squamous intraepithelial neoplasia. However, it is spotty in distribution and still demonstrates surface maturation.

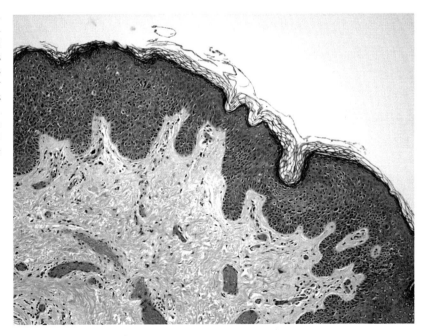

Key Pathologic Features
SQUAMOUS CELL CARCINOMA, USUAL TYPE

Gross findings

Depending on the growth pattern, the lesions range from an exophytic and cauliflower-like appearance to flat, slightly elevated, or deeply ulcerated. Adjacent mucosa is usually erythematous or has leukoplakia suggestive of precancerous changes.

Microscopic findings

The majority of squamous carcinomas are similar to their counterparts in other organs and exhibit usual, non-papillary differentiation, and range of differentiation from good to moderate to poor. Characteristic features include keratinizing nests of squamous cells with variable atypia surrounded by reactive fibrous stroma.

Superficially invasive tumors are usually well differentiated and deep tumors are often poorly differentiated.

Adjacent squamous epithelium may show changes of PeIN with koilocytic atypia or differentiated squamous intraepithelial atypia associated with or without LSA.

most frequent subtype.[5,23] HPV infection, however, is present in only one-third of carcinomas, in particular those with warty or basaloid features. Conventional, keratinizing SCC has less of an association.[4,7,9] This has led to various proposals which suggest that there are two pathways leading toward development of penile SCC; one associated with HPV infection, and one unrelated.[9]

Clinical and Gross Features

Clinically, the most common presenting feature is an exophytic, fungating, or ulcerating mass, although a flat erythematous lesion may also be present (**Fig. 9**). The majority of lesions arise in the mucosa of the glans (75%–80%), with the foreskin mucosa as the next most common site (15%).[8] The shaft and external skin of the foreskin are rarely primary sites. Tumors often have adjacent precancerous lesions, either leukoplakia (white and thickened) or erythema (often moist) (see **Fig. 9**). In uncircumcised patients, phimosis may effectively act to mask an underlying lesion of either the mucosal layer of the foreskin or the glans, and delay the clinical presentation. Patients with this type of neoplasm occasionally present with metastatic disease. The mean age of patients with SCC is 60.[18,25]

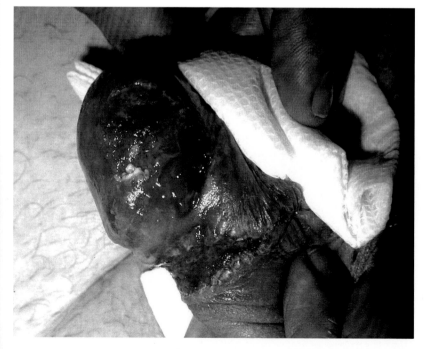

Fig. 9. Squamous carcinoma, usual type: clinical features. An ulcerated red or tan tumor involves the glans. Surrounding mucosa is flat, moist, and erythematous, and demonstrates histologic changes of PeIN. (*Courtesy of* Cheryl T. Lee, University of Michigan, Ann Arbor, MI; with permission.)

Gross Tumor Growth Patterns

The growth patterns of penile SCC fall under three main categories, which are important in terms of prognosis (**Fig. 10**). These patterns include:[26]

Superficial spreading: generally flat, white, plaque-like lesions with horizontal growth

Vertical: generally a large and ulcerated mass which spreads deeply into underlying tissue, highly associated with lymph node metastasis

Verruciform, which includes multiple separately classified histologic subtypes characterized by well-differentiated neoplastic cells and a low rate of metastasis. Verruciform tumors most commonly involve the glans but also involve the foreskin and coronal sulcus.

Superficial spreading is the most common, seen in approximately 40% of cases (**Fig. 11**), followed by vertical (30%), and verruciform (20%). Approximately 10% to 15% of lesions fall under multiple categories of growth pattern.[26]

Microscopic Features

The majority (at least 60%) of penile SCC demonstrate similar histologic features to those of other sites in the body.[27] Within this spectrum, the tumors can range from well to poorly differentiated but usually do not have the significant papillary growth more typical of the special histologic subtypes. Of note, poorly differentiated, non-keratinizing SCC are rare entities at this site.[8] Characteristic histologic features include keratinizing nests of squamous cells with variable cytologic atypia and fibrous stroma surrounding the deeper, invasive portions (**Fig. 12**). Tumors that invade more deeply tend to be more poorly differentiated than the well-differentiated superficial tumors. When invasion is present, it can be in the form of individual cells, or as cords or sheets of cells, extending into the lamina propria or corpus spongiosum. Adjacent squamous epithelium can be dysplastic with viral cytopathic changes suggestive of HPV infection or show changes typical of a pre-existing preneoplastic lesion such as hyperplasia, or an atrophic epidermis with underlying hyalinized stroma suggestive of LSA.

Differential Diagnosis

The differential diagnosis of penile SCC includes non-neoplastic entities as well as the variants of SCC. An important diagnostic consideration in many well-differentiated and superficial tumors is pseudoepitheliomatous hyperplasia, a benign, non-invasive epithelial proliferation that can resemble invasive disease architecturally. In particular, pseudoepitheliomatous hyperplasia can demonstrate acanthotic, thickened epithelium with long and irregularly shaped rete ridges (**Fig. 13**). When cut tangentially, these rete ridges can appear as detached, infiltrating nests. Features that favor a diagnosis of carcinoma over

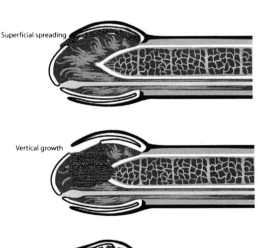

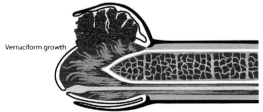

Fig. 10. Squamous carcinoma of the penis: diagrammatic representation of the growth patterns. (*From* Shah RB, Amin MB. Disorders of the penis, urethra, and scrotum. In: Zhou M, Magi-Galluzzi C, editors. Genitourinary pathology. Philadelphia: Churchill Livingstone Elsevier; 2007:442; with permission.)

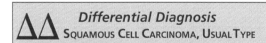

△△ **Differential Diagnosis**
SQUAMOUS CELL CARCINOMA, USUAL TYPE

- Pseudoepitheliomatous hyperplasia
- SCC with verruciform growth pattern (verrucous, papillary, and warty subtypes)
- Basaloid SCC
- Urothelial carcinoma
- Amelanotic melanoma

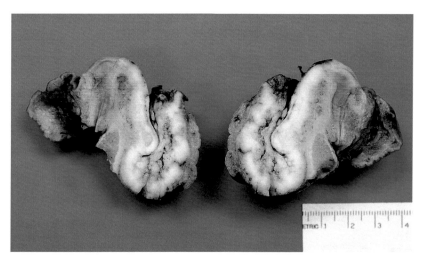

Fig. 11. SCC, growth pattern. A cross section of the tumor in **Fig. 9**, demonstrating a superficial spreading pattern of invasion of tumor into the underlying tissue.

this entity include disorderly maturation, nuclear atypia and eosinophilia, and paradoxical keratinizing differentiation near the interface with stroma. The presence of nests of squamous cells deep within the wall, such as into the corpus or dartos muscle, suggests carcinoma. Desmoplasia usually is evidence of invasive carcinoma. Pseudoepitheliomatous hyperplasia is often seen in association with underlying pathologic conditions such as granular cell tumor.[28] While rare, some non-verrucous carcinomas may demonstrate pseudohyperplastic features; particularly on small or superficial biopsies.[29] Tumors with this morphology are often

associated with adjacent lichen sclerosus. Differentiation from benign conditions may also be accomplished by the presence of adjacent premalignant changes, including LSA or PeIN. An important consideration is that small biopsies may not represent the whole lesion, and may not reflect important prognostic information.[30]

When SCC is poorly differentiated, it may be confused with urothelial carcinoma or, rarely, amelanotic melanoma. The location is often helpful in differentiation from urothelial carcinoma, which has its epicenter in the urethra; as is the coexistence of urothelial CIS. Melanoma should not

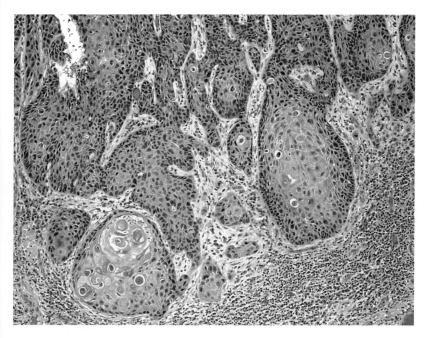

Fig. 12. Squamous carcinoma: microscopic features. Low power view of invasive, well- to moderately-differentiated squamous carcinoma. Invasive nests demonstrate cytologic atypia, paradoxical maturation, and pronounced stromal desmoplasia.

Fig. 13. Pseudoepithelio-matous hyperplasia: microscopic features. Low power view of the mucosa demonstrates downward proliferation of squamous nests with focal keratinization. However, the proliferating nests are superficial, mature without cytologic atypia, and lack a desmoplastic response.

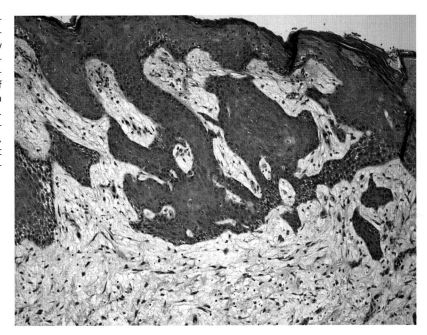

demonstrate keratinization, which most penile SCC will have at least focally. In certain cases, immunostaining is definitive in making the diagnosis. Melanoma-associated stains (such as S100, HMB-45, and Melan-A) will usually be helpful, whereas carcinomas will stain for keratin.

Prognosis and Therapy

The prognosis of SCC largely depends on pathologic stage as determined based on level of invasion into underlying tissue (pT) as well as lymph node status (**Table 3**). The primary site of the tumor can be a factor, as tumors of the foreskin carry

Table 3
Tumor, Node, Metastasis (TNM) classification of carcinomas of the penis

TNM classification			
T Primary tumor	M Distant metastasis		
TX Primary tumor cannot be assessed	MX Distant metastasis cannot be assessed		
T0 No evidence of primary tumor	M0 No distant metastasis		
Tis CIS	M1 Distant metastasis		
Ta Non-invasive verrucous carcinoma	Stage grouping		
T1 Tumor invades subepithelial connective	Stage 0	Tis	N0	M0
tissue		Ta	N0	M0
T2 Tumor invades corpus spongiosum or	Stage I	T1	N0	M0
cavernosum	Stage II	T1	N1	M0
T3 Tumor invades urethra or prostate		T2	N0,N1	M0
T4 Tumor invades other adjacent structures	Stage III	T1,T2	N2	M0
N Regional lymph nodes		T3	N0,N1,N2	M0
NX Regional lymph nodes cannot be assessed	Stage IV	T4	Any N	M0
N0 No regional lymph node metastasis		Any T	N3	M0
N1 Metastasis in a single superficial inguinal		Any T	Any N	M1
lymph node				
N2 Metastasis in multiple or bilateral				
superficial inguinal lymph nodes				
N3 Metastasis in deep inguinal or pelvic lymph				
node(s), unilateral or bilateral				

Data from American Joint Committee on Cancer. AJCC cancer staging manual, 6th edition, New York: Springer; 2002:303–8.

a better prognosis. In part, this is due to more frequent superficial tumors, and detection at an earlier stage.[8] Of various pathologic parameters, histologic type, grade, and vascular invasion have been most strongly correlated with final outcome.[31]

Lymph node involvement is a key prognostic factor, with inguinal nodes being the primary site of involvement.[18,32] Superficial lymph nodes are generally the first site of metastasis, followed by deep groin and pelvic nodes, and then retroperitoneal nodes. Only rarely will tumors demonstrate "skip" metastasis of spreading beyond this recurring pattern. Distant metastasis occurs late to sites such as liver, lung, and bone.[2] Generally, it is safe to assume that superficially invasive (pT1), well-differentiated tumors are not at significant risk for lymph node metastasis. Tumors with a vertical growth pattern are more likely to metastasize than those with a superficial spreading growth pattern (82% versus 42%), and they have a higher mortality (67% versus 10%).[26,31]

Due to its prognostic importance, it is important to accurately and consistently measure the depth of invasion in each case. Measurement is taken from the basement membrane of the adjacent squamous epithelium down to the deepest point of invasion. For exophytic, verrucous tumors depth is measured from the nonkeratinized surface. Depth of invasion of more than 4 to 6 mm or invasion into the corpus spongiosum (or pathologic stage T2 or greater) is considered to put the patient at increased risk for metastasis.[2] A prognostic index system has been devised by Cubilla and colleagues[33] which includes a numerical index for histologic grade (1–3) as well as depth of invasion (1–3, with 1 corresponding to lamina propria). Tumors with a total index of 1–3 are generally associated with no mortality, while those with an index of 5–6 have a high metastatic rate and high mortality.

Other prognostic factors have been studied but not rigorously applied in most cases.[34] Molecular studies such as expression of p53 are associated with increased risk for metastasis and disease progression.[35] Another study has demonstrated an association of improved survival with tissue eosinophilia.[36]

Surgery is the mainstay of treatment. Superficially invasive tumors can be treated with local resection (partial penectomy in many cases).[21,37] Deeply invasive tumors require more extensive surgery (total penectomy) along with inguinal lymph node dissection.[19,25,38] Currently, radiation therapy does not play a significant role in patient care. Following surgery, most patients are closely followed to detect recurrence as early as possible.[18,37,39]

SQUAMOUS CELL CARCINOMA VARIANTS

Several recent works have identified many variants of SCC with unique clinical and prognostic implications.

Verruciform Growth Patterns

SCC with verruciform growth patterns, either condylomatous or noncondylomatous, can be classified differently from "ordinary" SCC. Noncondylomatous tumors include verrucous and papillary carcinomas, while condylomatous tumors include warty carcinoma as well as the non-invasive giant condyloma (**Table 4**).

Clinical and Gross Features

Verrucous Carcinoma

Verrucous carcinomas are generally large cauliflower-like tumors, often ulcerated, averaging 3cm, which have often been present for years (average 56 months). They are slow-growing tumors which invade in a pushing fashion and do not metastasize.[40,41] On cross section, they are often seen to burrow through normal tissues (**Fig. 14**). Frequency is difficult to assess, in part due to variable classification in the past, but they make up approximately 20% of verruciform tumors (3%–

Key Pathologic Features
SQUAMOUS CELL CARCINOMA VARIANTS WITH VERRUCIFORM GROWTH PATTERN

Verrucous carcinoma

Gross findings

Cauliflower-like, frequently ulcerated gray-white mass that burrows deeply into normal tissues.

Microscopic findings

Very well differentiated SCC with prominent papillomatosis, acanthosis, and hyperkeratosis. The papillae do not contain fibrovascular cores and show broad-based regular bulbous infiltration into soft tissues. Minimal cytologic atypia. No koilocytic changes.

Papillary carcinoma, not otherwise specified (NOS)

Gross findings

Large, cauliflower-like or papillary mass. On cut sections tumor demonstrates invasion into lamina propria or corpus spongiosum, however, infiltration into cavernosa is uncommon.

Microscopic findings

Well- to moderately-differentiated, hyperkeratotic lesions with irregular, complex papillae with or without fibrovascular cores are typical. Obvious cytologic atypia with base of the lesion demonstrating characteristic jagged, irregular infiltration into soft tissues. Koilocytic atypia absent.

Warty carcinoma

Gross findings

A cauliflower-like, firm, white-gray granular mass measuring up to 8cm (average 4cm). The cut surface demonstrates deep invasion into lamina propria and corpus spongiosum, but the cavernosa is rarely involved.

Microscopic findings

Hyper-parakeratotic arborizing papillomatous growth with central fibrovascular cores. Prominent koilocytic atypia. Base of the tumor shows irregular, deep infiltration into soft tissues.

13% of penile cancers).[8] The glans and coronal sulcus are the most frequent sites of involvement, usually including the preputial skin. They are not related to HPV infection.[42]

Carcinoma Cuniculatum
Carcinoma cuniculatum is a recently described low-grade verruciform penile neoplasm. It affects the glans of older men (mean age 77 years) with extension to the coronal sulcus or foreskin. Grossly, on the surface they can resemble other penile verruciform lesions, but on the cut surface irregular narrow sinus tracts extend down to deep anatomic structures.[43]

Papillary Carcinoma, NOS
Papillary carcinoma accounts for approximately 15% of penile cancers and the most common subtype of verruciform tumor.[27] It commonly presents around the age of 60 years and involves the glans or foreskin with a large, cauliflower-like mass. It resembles verrucous carcinoma grossly except at the deep aspect, where it has an irregular border and often deeply infiltrates into the dartos muscle and corpus spongiosum, with occasional extension into the corpus cavernosum.

Warty Carcinoma
Warty carcinomas are verruciform tumors, low to intermediate grade. In particular, they resemble condyloma due to HPV association and corresponding cytomorphologic features.[25] Warty carcinomas make up approximately 20% to 35% of verruciform tumors (6%–10% of penile cancers). Grossly, they are also large and cauliflower-like, white and granular. On the cut surface, they can demonstrate both exophytic and endophytic growth patterns, with typically a jagged or serrated appearance at the base. Multiple sites can be involved, although the glans is the most common site. Warty carcinomas generally involve only the lamina propria and corpus spongiosum, and are unlikely to involve the corpus cavernosum.[44]

Microscopic Features

Verrucous Carcinoma
Verrucous carcinoma is a very well differentiated squamous carcinoma. Superficial biopsies may not be recognizable as malignant. An exophytic, papillary growth pattern without papillary fibrovascular cores is present along with hyperkeratosis and acanthosis. The base of the lesion is characterized by broad-based infiltration (**Fig. 15**), often accompanied, or even obscured, by a dense lymphocytic inflammatory infiltrate. The neoplastic cells are very well differentiated and only minimally atypical, without significant koilocytic change.[40] Rare mitotic figures may be present, generally at the base of the lesion. Up to 5% of verrucous carcinomas can have foci of traditional SCC.[8]

Table 4
Comparison of verruciform neoplasms

	Giant Condyloma	Warty Carcinoma	Verrucous Carcinoma	Papillary Carcinoma
Papillae	Arborizing, non-undulating, rounded	Long and undulating, condylomatous, complex	Straight with keratin cysts	Variable, complex
Fibrovascular cores	Prominent	Prominent	Rare	Present
Invasive borders	None	Irregular and jagged	Regular, broad, and pushing	Irregular and jagged
Differentiation	Well-differentiated	Well- to moderately-differentiated	Well-differentiated	Well- to moderately-differentiated
Koilocytic atypia	Present at surface	Prominent and diffuse	Absent	Absent or very focal
HPV association	Type 6–11	Type 16	Usually absent	Absent
Metastasis	No	Yes	No	Yes

Data from Young RH, Srigley JR, Amin MB, et al. Tumors of the prostate gland, seminal vesicles, male urethra, and penis. In: Atlas of tumor pathology. Washington, DC: AFIP; 2000.

Carcinoma Cuniculatum

Carcinoma cuniculatum can resemble other verruciform carcinomas. The distinguishing feature is the growth pattern, with irregular and narrow sinus tracts extending deep beneath the surface to adjacent anatomic structures. These sinus tracts can be contiguous with deep, dilated keratin-filled cysts. Some cases may have high histologic grade or microscopically infiltrative borders.[43]

Papillary Carcinoma, NOS Type

Papillary carcinomas are also well to moderately differentiated with irregular, complex papillae. Central fibrovascular cores may or may not be present. HPV-associated, koilocytic changes are absent to differentiate it from warty carcinoma, but cytologic atypia is generally prominent and beyond that seen in verrucous carcinoma (**Fig. 16** A, B). At the base, irregularly infiltrating nests are present. Irregular

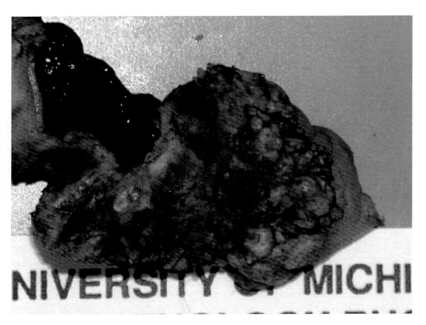

Fig. 14. Verrucous carcinoma: clinical features. A large cauliflower-like, gray-white mass involves the skin.

Fig. 15. Verrucous carcinoma: microscopic features. Low power view of the mass shows prominent papillomatosis, hyperkeratosis, and acanthosis. The interface between the tumor and stroma is relatively sharp with broad bulbous pattern of infiltration. The epithelium is well differentiated and without evidence of HPV-related atypia.

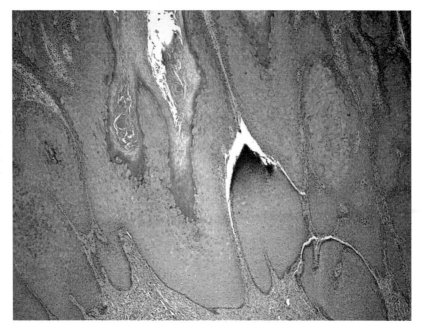

wide areas of keratinization, referred to as "keratin lakes" are frequently present.[8]

Warty Carcinomas

Warty carcinomas are hyperparakeratotic lesions, with arborizing papillomatous growth. The papillae contain fibrovascular cores and are long and undulating with rounded or tapered tips (**Fig. 17A, B**). The most important feature is HPV-associated koilocytic atypia, which is invariably present.[25,44] The basal layer and interface with the stroma is often irregular, and may contain intraepithelial abscesses (**Fig. 17B**).

Differential Diagnosis

Squamous carcinomas with verruciform growth pattern are often confused with each other and importantly with benign conditions including giant condyloma or viral verruca.[42] Verrucous carcinomas do not have the koilocytic atypia that is seen in giant condyloma or warty carcinomas,

---

Pitfalls
SQUAMOUS CELL CARCINOMA VARIANTS WITH VERRUCIFORM GROWTH PATTERN

! Squamous carcinomas with verruciform growth pattern are often confused with each other and, importantly, with benign conditions including giant condyloma or viral verruca. Verrucous carcinomas do not have the koilocytic atypia that is seen in giant condyloma or warty carcinomas, lack fibrovascular cores, and do not have the cytologic atypia or irregular, invasive front of papillary carcinomas, NOS.

! It may be difficult or impossible to distinguish verrucous carcinoma from squamous hyperplasia and papillary SCC unless the entire lesion, in particular the base, is sampled.

! Verrucous, papillary, and warty subtypes can often coexist with conventional SCC. The grade, stage, and prognosis of such tumors depends on the component of traditional SCC.

! Warty subtype can also coexist with an aggressive basaloid subtype of squamous carcinoma. Careful analysis of the entire tumor is necessary before diagnosis of these entities is made.

Differential Diagnosis
SQUAMOUS CELL CARCINOMA VARIANTS WITH VERRUCIFORM GROWTH PATTERN

- SCC, usual type
- Squamous hyperplasia
- Condyloma including giant condyloma
- Pseudoepitheliomatous hyperplasia

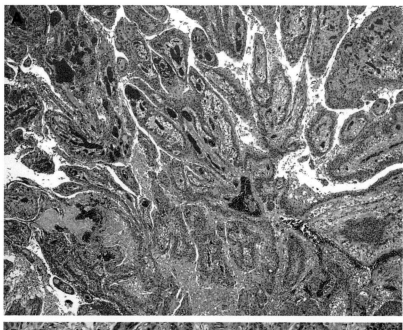

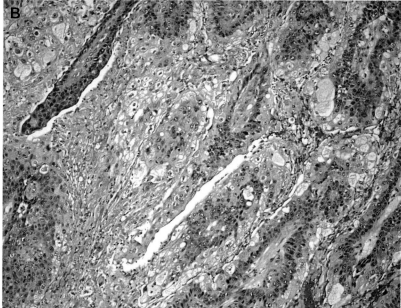

Fig. 16. (*A*) Papillary carcinoma, NOS type: microscopic features. Tumor demonstrates irregular papillary growth pattern with prominent fibrovascular cores. The interface between the tumor and stroma is jagged. (*B*) Papillary carcinoma, NOS type: microscopic features. Note prominent wide areas of keratinization between papillae and absence of koilocytic changes at higher magnification.

lack fibrovascular cores, and do not have the cytologic atypia or irregular, invasive front of papillary carcinomas, NOS. It may be difficult or impossible to distinguish verrucous carcinoma from squamous hyperplasia and papillary SCC unless the entire lesion, in particular the base, is sampled. Warty carcinomas combine the koilocytic atypia seen in giant condyloma with an irregular, infiltrative base. Papillary and warty carcinomas can both be deeply invasive with an irregular base, and are differentiated based on the HPV-like changes seen in warty carcinoma. Typical SCCs not falling under one of these three subtypes generally do not have prominent papillary features.

Fig. 17. (*A*) Warty carcinoma: microscopic features. Low power view demonstrates undulating, complex, hyperkeratotic papillary growth with prominent koilocytic atypia. (*B*) Warty carcinoma: microscopic features. High power view shows an irregular interface between tumor and underlying stroma.

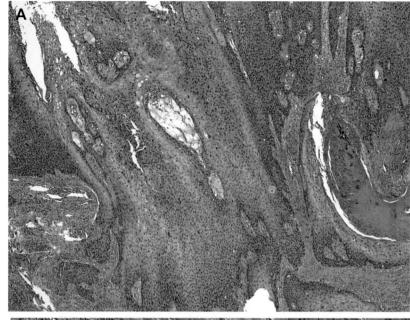

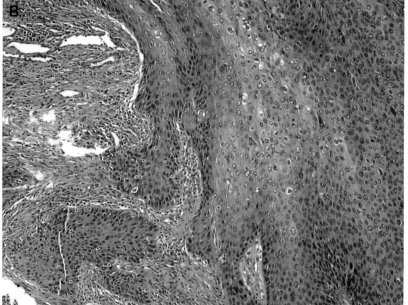

The morphologic features that are helpful in separating these tumors are summarized in **Table 4** and **Fig. 18**.

Prognosis and Therapy

Verrucous Carcinomas

Verrucous carcinomas are locally aggressive but are not biologically aggressive and do not metastasize, although they may have foci of more traditional SCC. In this situation, the behavior is determined by the traditional SCC. Treatment with wide excision (partial penectomy) is usually adequate, although tumors may recur due to incomplete resection or multicentricity.[21,40] Radiation therapy is not a recommended treatment for this entity due to reports of subsequent anaplastic transformation.[45]

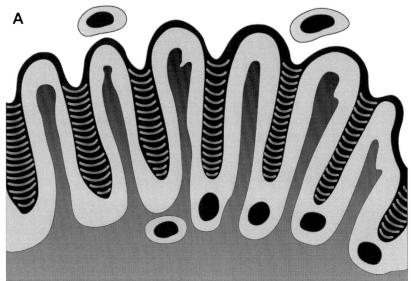

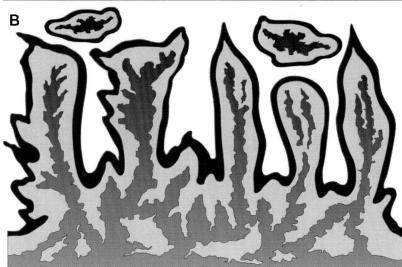

Fig. 18. Tumors with verruciform growth pattern: diagrammatic comparison of the histologic differences. (*A*) Verrucous carcinoma: regular papillae with broad bulbous base and prominent hyperkeratosis (red). Keratinized cysts are prominent (seen at the base). (*B*) Papillary carcinoma, NOS type: papillae are more irregular than (*A*), many with fibrovascular cores. Infiltration is seen at the base and koilocytosis is absent.

Papillary Carcinomas

Papillary carcinomas are deeply invasive, but are less likely than warty carcinomas or traditional SCCs to develop lymph node metastasis. The five-year survival rate is approximately 90%, and surgery is the mainstay of treatment.[8]

Carcinoma Cuniculatum

Carcinoma cuniculatum, despite its deep invasion, has not been associated with lymph node metastasis. The growth pattern reflects its deep extension into underlying tissue and necessity for wide resection.[43]

Warty Carcinomas

Warty carcinomas can be deeply invasive and, when invasive, are often associated with lymph node metastasis. One large series demonstrated inguinal lymph node metastasis in 2 out of 11 tumors. In general, however, warty carcinomas have an improved survival and are less aggressive than usual-type SCC.[25,44]

Fig. 18. (*C*) Giant condyloma: arborescent hyperkeratotic papillae with broad bases and koilocytosis (indicated by white dots) at the surface. (*D*) Warty (condylomatous) carcinoma: papillae are more irregular than in (*C*), koilocytosis is diffuse, and the interface between tumor and stroma is irregular. (*Reproduced from* Figure 10–31, Young RH, Srigley JR, Amin MB, et al. Tumors of the prostate gland, seminal vesicles, male urethra, and penis. In: Atlas of tumor pathology. Washington, DC: AFIP; 2000; p. 424 and *reproduced from* Figure 8–10, S Shah RB, Amin MB. Diseases of the penis, urethra, and scrotum. In: Zhou M, Magi-Galluzzi C, editors. Genitourinary pathology. Philadelphia: Churchill Livingstone Elsevier; 2007: 429; with permission.)

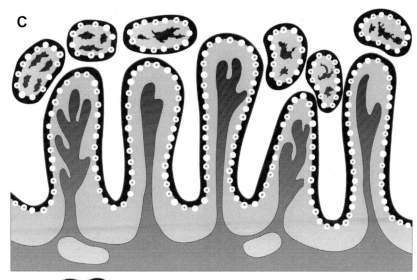

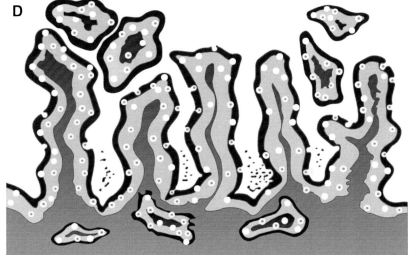

BASALOID CARCINOMA

Clinical and Gross Features

Basaloid carcinoma is an aggressive subtype which accounts for 5% to 10% of penile SCCs and is highly associated with HPV.[9,27] Clinically, it most commonly arises in the glans near the urethral meatus and presents in patients with an average age of 52.[46] Basaloid carcinomas are usually flat and ulcerated, and often deeply infiltrative with associated inguinal lymph node enlargement. It may be the sole lesion or it may be present along with basaloid CIS or conventional or warty SCC.[2]

Microscopic Features

Basaloid carcinoma consists of tightly packed nests of basaloid cells, often with central,

comedo-like necrosis.[46] Cytologically, the cells are smaller with less cytoplasm, hyperchromatic nuclei, and inconspicuous nucleoli, with frequent mitotic figures and apoptotic bodies, resembling a starry-sky appearance. The periphery of the nests can demonstrate palisading, and the center may often have abrupt central keratinization (**Fig. 19**). Perineural invasion and angiolymphatic invasion are frequently seen.

Differential Diagnosis

Basaloid carcinoma can be distinguished from basal cell carcinoma by the site of the primary lesion, as basal cell carcinoma generally occurs on the shaft. It also generally does not have the prominent peripheral palisading of basal cell carcinoma, and often has comedo-type necrosis and

Key Pathologic Features
BASALOID SQUAMOUS CELL CARCINOMA

Gross findings

Flat, ulcerated, firm gray-white mass. Cut sections demonstrate deep infiltration into underlying soft tissues.

Microscopic findings

Nests of monotonous small basaloid tumor cells with scant cytoplasm, oval to round, hyperchromatic nuclei, and inconspicuous nucleoli. Brisk mitotic rate and apoptotic bodies giving a starry sky pattern. Abrupt keratinization with central comedo-type necrosis is common.

Adjacent mucosa frequently demonstrates basaloid- or warty-type PeIN associated with HPV infection.

Differential Diagnosis
BASALOID SQUAMOUS CELL CARCINOMA

- Basal cell carcinoma
- SCC, usual type
- Urothelial carcinoma
- Small cell or neuroendocrine carcinoma

apoptotic tumor cells not usually seen in basal cell carcinoma. The site of many basaloid carcinomas, the area around the urethral meatus, can also be the site of urothelial carcinoma, which may have a similar morphologic appearance. Urothelial carcinomas, however, generally have their epicenter in the urethra as well as adjacent urothelial CIS or an area of more conventional urothelial carcinoma. Rarely, small cell neuroendocrine carcinoma can be present in the area and cause confusion with basaloid carcinoma. Usually, however, it is distinguished by the presence of nuclear molding, nuclear cytologic features, crushed or spindled nuclei, and mitotic rate. Presence of adjacent PeIN associated with HPV changes is often helpful in these differentials.

Pitfalls
BASALOID SQUAMOUS CELL CARCINOMA

! Correct diagnosis of basaloid SCC is important as it as an aggressive neoplasm with a mortality rate of over 50% at 5 years. Basal cell carcinoma, a rare primary skin neoplasm more commonly present in the shaft of the penis, lack high mitotic activity and comedo-type necrosis.

! Basaloid carcinoma may coexist with other types of squamous carcinoma such as warty carcinoma. The prognosis in this situation depends on the component of basaloid carcinoma.

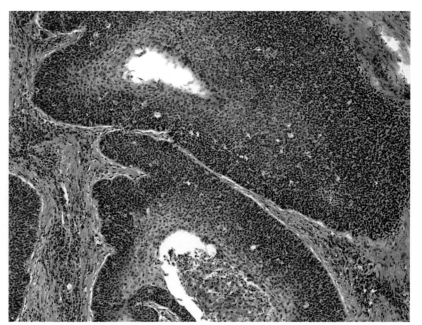

Fig. 19. Basaloid carcinoma: microscopic features. Medium power view demonstrates nodules of tumor cells with relatively monotonus hypercromatic basaloid cells. In the center, tumor shows focal, comedo-type necrosis, and abrupt keratinization. There are a high number of apoptotic tumor cells, giving a starry sky pattern.

Prognosis and Treatment

In comparison to usual squamous carcinomas, basaloid squamous carcinomas tend to have higher histologic grade, a deeper invasion of the penile anatomic layers, and higher mortality. It is one of the aggressive variants of squamous carcinoma, with a high rate of inguinal lymph node metastasis and mortality of 59% at 5 years.[46]

SARCOMATOID (SPINDLE CELL) CARCINOMA

Clinical and Gross Features

Sarcomatoid carcinoma represents 1% to 3% of penile cancers, and can be seen as a dedifferentiation of a typical SCC, either as a consequence of radiation therapy or de novo.[27,45] It occurs in patients with an average age of 60 years and usually presents on the glans or mucosal side of the foreskin. It can be exophytic or ulcerated. Deep invasion is seen on cross section.

Microscopic Features

Microscopically, the tumors are often biphasic with variable mixture of spindle cell and epithelioid components. The spindle cell component may resemble virtually any type of sarcoma, including fibrosarcoma or leiomyosarcoma in addition to osteogenic or cartilaginous differentiation. A typical, differentiated squamous component may be present only focally or as an in situ component.[47,48]

Differential Diagnosis

When an epithelial component is not present or is only focal, sarcomatoid carcinoma can be confused with a sarcoma or melanoma. Tumors demonstrating focal presence of squamous carcinoma or in situ component suggest the diagnosis of sarcomatoid carcinoma. The diagnosis is made in the absence of typical squamous carcinoma if there is a prior history of pure SCC. Pseudoangiomatoid areas are seen in SCC and may not necessarily represent angiosarcoma. In difficult cases, immunohistochemical staining panels should include broad-spectrum keratins including high molecu-lar weight keratin, melanoma markers (S100, HMB-45, Melan-A), desmin, muscle specific actin and CD31. A caveat is that focal keratin immunoreactivity is seen in cases of epithelioid angiosarcoma, although CD31 staining should be strongly positive in these cases.

Prognosis and Treatment

Sarcomatoid carcinomas are associated with a high rate of regional lymph node metastasis and carry a bad prognosis. Recurrence is common, with a mortality rate of 60%.[47]

ADENOSQUAMOUS CARCINOMA

Occasionally, SCC may be associated with glandular differentiation, although the squamous component usually predominates in these tumors.[49] Gross features are usually similar to conventional SCC and most of these tumors involve the glans. Possible explanations for the histogenesis of these tumors are embryologically misplaced perimeatal glands or metaplastic mucinous glands. Immunohistochemistry may be helpful in that carcinoembryonic antigen (CEA) may stain the glandular component.[50] This entity should be distinguished from SCCs that secondarily involve periurethral glands, which can be accomplished by noting the morphologically benign nature of the glands.

RARE PRIMARY EPITHELIAL CARCINOMAS

PSEUDOHYPERPLASTIC CARCINOMA

Cubilla and colleagues[29] recently described a rare subtype of non-verruciform and very well differentiated SCC with pseudohyperplastic features demonstrating excellent prognosis. These tumors can be multicentric and preferentially involve the inner surface of the foreskin. Histologically, keratinizing nests of SCC are present with minimal atypia (**Fig. 20**). LSA was present in background epithelium in all cases, suggesting its preneoplastic role. Pseudoepitheliomatous hyperplasia was the principal differential diagnosis in superficial biopsies and is discussed in the section of SCC, usual type.

MIXED CARCINOMAS

Approximately one fourth of penile carcinomas demonstrate a mixture of the subtypes discussed here. The most common pattern is that of a typical verrucous carcinoma with focal areas of moderate to high-grade squamous carcinoma, referred to as hybrid verrucous carcinomas. The worst pattern defines the prognosis, and increases the risk of metastasis. Similarly, when areas of basaloid carcinoma are present within a SCC, usual type there is a higher incidence of groin lymph node metastasis. Other reported combinations have included mixtures of basaloid and warty carcinoma (adenobasaloid) and squamous and neuroendocrine carcinoma.[8,30]

CLEAR CELL CARCINOMA

Liegl and Regauer recently described a rare penile tumor with a poor prognosis, commonly associated with inguinal lymph node metastasis. The tumor is composed of large clear cells with intracytoplasmic PAS-positive material (**Fig. 21**). The tumors also stain for EMA, CEA, and MUC-1. Angiolymphatic invasion is common. Although HPV-associated cytologic changes are not seen, these tumors are positive for HPV 16 DNA.[51]

BASAL CELL CARCINOMA

Basal cell carcinoma of the penis commonly arises on the shaft, and has a similar behavior to those of other body sites. It is rare, and usually only superficially invasive with limited metastatic potential.[52,53] The importance in acknowledging its existence is so that it is not confused with basaloid carcinoma, which is far more aggressive and usually involves the glans.

EXTRAMAMMARY PAGET DISEASE

Clinical and Gross Features

Paget disease may exist in isolation on the penis or also be present on the scrotum, with the glans being a common site. Clinically, it presents as a red, moist plaque which may be eroded or scaly (**Fig. 22**). It may be misdiagnosed clinically as eczema or dermatitis, which may delay therapy.[54] Paget disease of the genital area may be a consequence of epidermotropic spread from an underlying colorectal, urogenital, or cutaneous

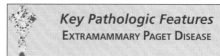

Key Pathologic Features
EXTRAMAMMARY PAGET DISEASE

Gross findings

   The lesion appears as an irregular erythematous or eczematous scaly lesion.

Microscopic findings

   Characterized by isolated or clusters of atypical large cells with abundant vacuolated cytoplasm, scattered within the epidermis. Underlying invasive carcinoma may be present.

Histochemistry

   Mucin stains positive

Immunohistochemical Features

   CEA, EMA and MUC 5AC positive. S-100, HMB 45 and Melan-A negative.

adnexal malignancy.[55] However, an underlying malignancy is not identified in many cases, and some view it as an epidermotropic spread from an underlying apocrine adnexal carcinoma.[56]

Microscopic Features

Histologically, there is an intraepithelial proliferation of scattered, or clusters of, large atypical cells with abundant pale, granular, and vacuolated cytoplasm in conjunction with or without an invasive

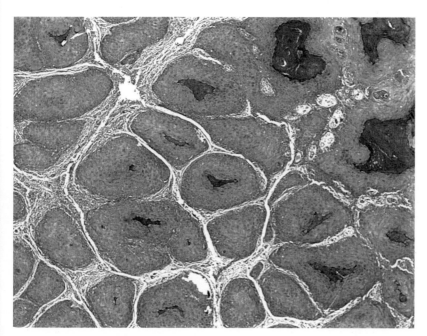

Fig. 20. Pseudohyperplastic carcinoma: microscopic features. Low power view demonstrates nests of well-differentiated carcinoma proliferating downwards involving the lamina propria. Surface nests show keratinization and mimic pseudoepitheliomatous hyperplasia. (*Courtesy of* M. Amin, MD, Los Angeles, CA.)

dermal component. Nucleoli are generally prominent (**Fig. 23**).

Differential Diagnosis

Primary extramammary Paget disease should be distinguished from pagetoid spread of urothelial carcinoma.[55] Other cancers which may demonstrate pagetoid spread include prostate carcinoma.[57] Proper clinical background is important to work up the case. Rarely, Bowen's disease may have a pagetoid growth pattern; however typical full-thickness cytologic atypia is present at least focally in most cases (**Fig. 24**). Superficial spreading malignant melanoma may mimic Paget disease. Immunohistochemical stains may aid in the differential in difficult cases. Paget tumor cells express CEA, EMA, and low molecular

Fig. 21. (*A*). Clear cell carcinoma: microscopic features. Large nests of high grade epithelioid tumor cells are seen with predominantly clear cytoplasm, without evidence of keratinization. (*B*). PAS stain demonstrates globules of PAS-positive eosinophilic material within the cytoplasm of the cells, characteristic of clear cell carcinoma. (*Courtesy of* S. Regauer, MD, Graz, Austria.)

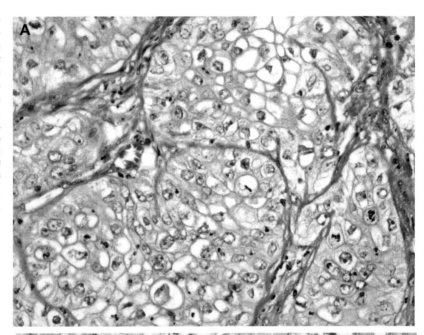

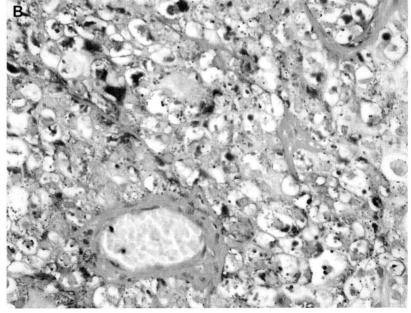

- Eczema or dermatitis (clinical)
- Bowen's disease (HGSIL, PeIN)
- Urothelial CIS
- Benign mucinous metaplasia
- Pagetoid dyskeratosis
- Mucinous syringometaplasia

weight cytokeratin, and are negative for S100. They will also express mucin. If it is associated with prostate cancer, a PSA can help to confirm this.[8]

Entities that have rarely been reported to be confused with Paget disease include benign mucinous metaplasia, pagetoid dyskeratosis, and mucinous syringometaplasia. SCC can also have mucinous metaplasia. Benign mucinous metaplasia is usually distinguished by the mucinous cells replacing the squamous epithelium, rather than infiltrating it as in Paget's disease.[58] Pagetoid dyskeratosis is usually an incidental finding, associated with phimosis, and consists of pale keratinocytes within the epithelium resembling Paget cells.[59] Clinical information can be important in

making the diagnosis or associating the lesion with another primary site.

Prognosis and Therapy

Wide surgical excision of involved skin, with negative surgical margins, is the mainstay of therapy.[60] Topical chemotherapy can also be used (5-FU). Invasion to the subcutaneous tissue is associated with adverse prognosis, including metastatic disease.[60] Evolution of the associated malignancy, if present, is also a key to defining prognosis.[56]

Pitfalls
PAGET DISEASE

! Paget disease may be clinically misdiagnosed as eczema or dermatitis, which may delay therapy.

! It may be a consequence of epidermotropic spread from an underlying colorectal, urogenital, or cutaneous adnexal malignancy, which should always be ruled out with appropriate work up and with knowledge of clinical background.

! Superficial spreading malignant melanoma could be an important mimic. Immunohistochemical stains in difficult cases can resolve the diagnosis.

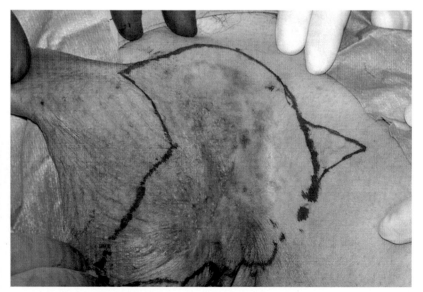

Fig. 22. Extramammary Paget disease of scrotum: clinical features. An irregular eczematous, scaly, erythematous lesion involves the scrotum, portion of penis, and extends to other parts of the genital skin. (*Courtesy of* K. Angermeier, MD, Cleveland, OH.)

Fig. 23. Extramammary Paget disease of penis: microscopic features. Low power view demonstrates intraepidermal proliferation of large atypical cells with abundant vacuolated cytoplasm scattered throughout the epidermis.

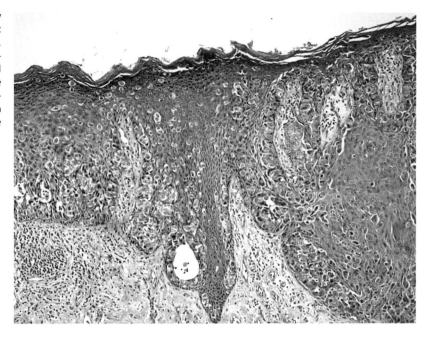

RARE TUMORS OF THE PENIS

MELANOMA

Primary melanomas of the penis are rare, and usually affect white males between the ages of 50 and 70. Most occur in the glans, with an additional 10% involving the prepuce and a lesser amount involving the shaft. Clinically they can present as papules, nodules, or ulcers that are blue, brown, red, or non-pigmented. Features are otherwise typical histologically of melanomas of other sites. Melanoma of the penis may be associated with prior ultraviolet radiation.[61]

MERKEL CELL AND SEBACEOUS CARCINOMA

Other rare epithelial tumors of the penis that have been reported include sebaceous carcinoma and Merkel cell carcinoma.[62,63] These neoplasms

Fig. 24. Pagetoid Bowen disease: microscopic features. Nests of relatively small-size atypical cells with scant pale cytoplasm are seen within the epidermis in a pagetoid growth pattern. In other areas of the lesion, full-thickness atypia of the squamous epithelium was present.

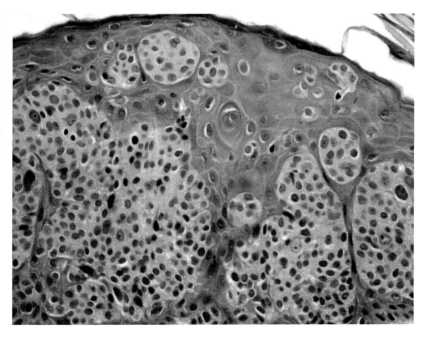

should have histologic features in keeping with those at other anatomic sites.

METASTATIC TUMORS

While metastasis to the penis is rare, it can often present with priapism. Primary sites of tumor are most commonly prostate and bladder.[64,65]

BENIGN TUMOR-LIKE LESIONS OF THE PENIS

CONDYLOMA

Clinical and Gross Features

The most common tumor-like condition of the penis is a benign lesion, condyloma. This lesion is associated with HPV infection, types 6 and 11.[7,42] Most patients are sexually active young men and are associated with sexual transmission, as they associate with HPV-related cervical lesions in women. Within the age range of 20 to 40 years, they are in up to 5% of men. Condyloma can be seen in children, and are often associated with sexual abuse. Grossly, these lesions can be multiple, flat or large, cauliflower-like and are commonly seen on the coronal sulcus (**Fig. 25**A). They can be seen on the fossa navicularis, meatus, shaft, and scrotal or perineal skin. Size ranges from millimeters to up to 10 cm in diameter.

Giant condyloma is a related lesion, also HPV associated, which is generally large (5–10 cm) and cauliflower-like. Another name which has been used in the past is Buschke-Lowenstein tumor, although many would likely now be classified as verrucous carcinomas.[42,66] Giant condyloma more commonly occur in a slightly older age range than common condyloma.

Microscopic Features

Condyloma has a papillary growth pattern with hyperkeratosis, generally with prominent fibrovascular cores. Koilocytic atypia is seen but generally limited to superficial cells (**Fig. 25**B). A flat growth pattern can also be present. Giant condyloma have similar histology although there can be slight atypia and increased cellularity. The base of the lesion can be expansile.[66]

Differential Diagnosis

Condyloma can often be distinguished clinically, but cytologic features usually do not rise to the level of findings in other preneoplastic squamous lesions. Occasionally, the koilocytic atypia is not prominent and the differential diagnosis with simple squamous papillomas is difficult. In situ hybridization or immunohistochemistry for HPV DNA can be helpful in these cases.

Giant condyloma must be distinguished from both verrucous and warty carcinomas. While many of these cases in the past have been considered as verrucous carcinomas due to their size and bulbous, expansile base, verrucous carcinomas do not show similar koilocytic atypia or the prominent papillary fibrovascular cores. Warty carcinomas also must be distinguished, and these tumors have an irregular, jagged base and more malignant cytologic features.

Key Pathologic Features
CONDYLOMA

Gross findings

  Multiple, papillary, warty, cauliflower-like lesions. Also can be small, flat lesions.

Microscopic findings

  Varying degree of papillomatosis, acanthosis, parakeratosis, and hyperkeratosis, with prominent to inconspicuous koilocytic atypia and cytoplasmic vacuolization, raisinoid nuclei and binucleation. True condyloma, including giant variants, should not have an irregular or infiltrative appearance.

Immunohistochemical features

  Most are positive for HPV 6 and 11 by in situ hybridization.

Differential Diagnosis
CONDYLOMA

- Verrucous carcinoma
- Warty carcinoma
- PeIN
- Squamous hyperplasia
- Verruciform xanthoma
- Bowenoid papulosis
- Pearly penile plaque (clinical)

Fig. 25. (*A*) Condyloma: clinical features. Multiple well-demarcated cauliflower-like lesions are seen involving the shaft of the penis. (*Courtesy of* K. Angermeier, MD, Cleveland, OH.) (*B*) Condyloma: microscopic features. Papillomatosis and acanthosis with well-developed fibrovascular cores. Note prominent koilocytic atypia of the surface epithelium.

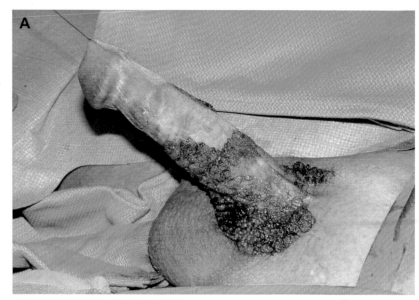

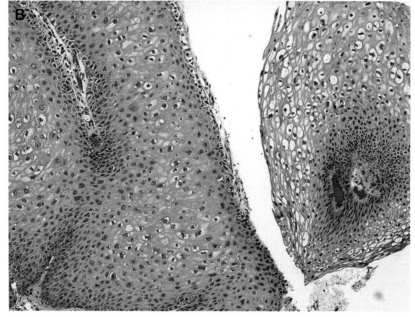

Prognosis and Therapy

Condyloma can be difficult to eradicate. Typical treatments include cryotherapy or topical immunomodulatory treatments, and thus many may not come to surgery and biopsy. Recurrence rate is high, and surgery may be necessary.[67]

VERRUCIFORM XANTHOMA

Verruciform xanthoma is a benign lesion which is most commonly seen in the oral mucosa, but which also occurs in the anogenital skin and can involve the penis.[68] The etiology is unknown, although its association in oral and genital areas raises the possibility of HPV association, although this has not been confirmed by molecular or immunohistochemical studies.[69]

Clinical and Gross Features

The lesion commonly presents as a solitary slow growing nodule, resembling a wart or cyst. They are polypoid, tan or yellow lesions.[68]

Pitfalls
Condyloma

! Condyloma, notably giant condyloma, may be confused with verruciform SCC, notably verrucous carcinoma or warty carcinoma. Careful analysis of cytologic features and specifically the base of the tumor with underlying stroma is important in making the distinction. Verrucous carcinomas lack koilocytic atypia and fibrovascular cores in papillae and have a broad-based invasive front. Warty carcinomas are characterized by deep irregular or jagged growth pattern.

! Flat condyloma also can mimic penile intraepithelial neoplasia. In condyloma, koilocytic atypia is restricted to the superficial layer.

Microscopic Features

Microscopically, the surface of the lesion can be verrucoid, papillary, or crater-like. The epidermis is acanthotic, papillomatous, and demonstrates hyper- and parakeratosis with an absent or decreased granular layer. No koilocytic atypia is seen. Immediately beneath the parakeratotic layer, at the junction with the stratum spinosum is a prominent neutrophilic infiltrate. The most characteristic finding is a population of foamy macrophages within the papillary dermis (**Fig. 26**). At the base of the lesion, an inflammatory infiltrate of lymphocytes and plasma cells is often present.

Differential Diagnosis

The main differential diagnosis is with other verrucous lesions, such as condyloma and verrucous carcinoma, neither of which should have a prominent population of foamy histiocytes. Verruciform xanthoma also does not have the koilocytic atypia of other lesions. The presence of the superficial neutrophilic infiltrate and other changes may suggest a fungal infection, which can be ruled out with appropriate tissue stains.

Prognosis and Therapy

Simple excision is all that is required in these cases.[68]

PEARLY PENILE PAPULES (HIRSUTOID PAPILLOMA)

These lesions are thought to be probable embryologic remnants of a copulative organ.

Clinical and Gross Features

Approximately 20% to 30% of males have these lesions, which consist of dome-shaped yellow-white papules on the corona or the frenulum of the penis.[70] They often resemble hair follicles.

Microscopic Features

Microscopic features include mild epithelial thickening associated with a central fibrovascular core, the histologic features of an angiofibroma.

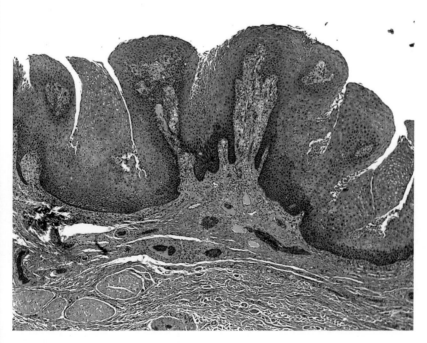

Fig. 26. Verruciform xanthoma: microscopic features. Low power view of a verrucoid lesion demonstrating papillary epithelial hyperplasia, hyperkeratosis, and parakeratosis and collection of characteristic stromal histiocytes with foamy cytoplasm between elongated rete ridges. (*Courtesy of* D. Fullen, MD, Ann Arbor, MI.)

Prognosis and Therapy

There is no propensity for malignant transformation and they do not require any treatment unless cosmetic removal is desired, usually with laser therapy.

ANGIOKERATOMA

While angiokeratoma is most commonly reported in the scrotum, it has rarely been reported to involve the glans or the shaft of the penis. These are benign lesions.[71]

Clinical, Gross, and Microscopic Features

It presents as one or more soft 1 to 4mm red papules, with histologic features including dilation of papillary dermal vasculature, often with thrombi. Hyperkeratosis is usually present along with elongation of the rete ridges around the dilated vasculature (**Fig. 27**).

NON-EPITHELIAL TUMORS OF THE PENIS: BENIGN LESIONS

PEYRONIE'S DISEASE

Peyronie's disease is associated in approximately 10% of cases with fibromatosis at other sites in the body, leading many to believe that the lesion itself is related to fibromatosis. Other theories include

Key Pathologic Features
PEYRONIE'S DISEASE

Gross findings

Characterized by gray-white firm fibrous tissue between the corpora cavernosa and tunica albuginea.

Microscopic findings

Appearance similar to that of fibromatosis at other sites, although it tends to be less cellular and more sclerotic. A perivascular lymphoid infiltrate is seen in early stages of disease. Rarely calcification or ossification in advanced lesions.

an inflammatory or fibrosing reactive pattern to conditions such as urethritis or trauma.[8]

Clinical and Gross Features

Peyronie's disease, in addition to the above associations, has also been associated with hypertension and diabetes. It generally occurs in men over the age of 40 and presents as a firm plaque or nodule on the dorsal surface of the erect penile shaft.[72,73] During erection, the plaque can cause pain and abnormal curvature. Grossly, a proliferation of fibrous tissue is seen, located

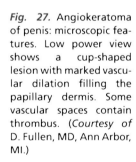

Fig. 27. Angiokeratoma of penis: microscopic features. Low power view shows a cup-shaped lesion with marked vascular dilation filling the papillary dermis. Some vascular spaces contain thrombus. (*Courtesy of* D. Fullen, MD, Ann Arbor, MI.)

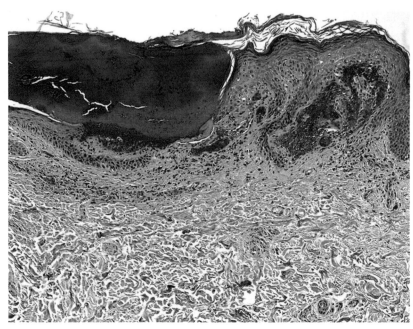

between the corpora cavernosa and the tunica albuginea.[74]

Microscopic Features

The histologic features are characterized by dense fibrosis, which varies in character depending on the age of the lesion. Early-stage lesions contain a loose type of fibrosis with corresponding inflammatory component, while later stages demonstrate dense hyalinizing fibrosis and occasional metaplastic bone and cartilage (**Fig. 28**).

Differential Diagnosis

In the appropriate clinical context, the diagnosis is fairly straightforward. Similar changes can be seen with non-specific inflammatory and scarring changes as a response to injury or other factors.

Prognosis and Therapy

Normal course of the disease is variable, with spontaneous resolution in the absence of treatment in up to one-third of patients. If treatment is necessary, it can take the form of surgery or other nonsurgical treatments including radiotherapy, steroids, or anti-inflammatory medications.[75]

SCLEROSING LIPOGRANULOMA

Clinical and Gross Features

Sclerosing lipogranuloma often involves the scrotum, but the penis is an important site of presentation. Published literature suggests that these lesions are associated with cosmetic (enlargement of genitalia), therapeutic injection, or topical use of oil-based substances including paraffin, silicone, or oil. Rare cases have been reported to be secondary to trauma and cold weather. They are usually seen in males under the age of 40 and present as tender, indurated plaques or masses. On gross examination, the specimens are usually fragmented but may be firm, yellow to gray-white, and have a cystic appearance.[76,77]

Microscopic Features

Microscopically, lipid vacuoles of varying sizes are seen embedded within a sclerotic fibrous stroma. The vacuoles do not have a cellular lining, but may be surrounded by multinucleated giant cells. A variable inflammatory response is also present, consisting of nodular or interspersed aggregates of inflammatory cells along with a histiocytic or foreign body-type granulomatous component (**Fig. 29**). Eosinophils may be present.

Differential Diagnosis

The histologic differential diagnosis may include signet-ring carcinoma, sclerosing liposarcoma, and adenomatoid tumor. However, distinction is usually straightforward. Vacuoles in sclerosing lipogranuloma are fatty, compared with mucin material in the signet-ring carcinomas. The presence of the multinucleated giant cells associated with vacuoles is helpful to separate them from sclerosing liposarcoma. The diagnosis may be confirmed

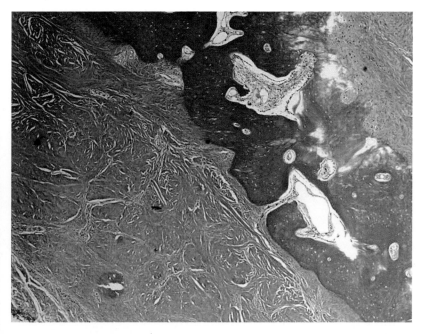

Fig. 28. Peyronie's disease: microscopic features. High power view demonstrates microscopic features of advanced Peyronie's disease. There is proliferation of spindle cells in the sclerotic and collagenized stroma. Metaplastic ossification is present.

Fig. 29. Sclerosing lipo-granuloma: microscopic features. There is a collection of multiple, variably sized vacuoles within dense sclerotic stroma. There is focal foreign body-type granulomatous response.

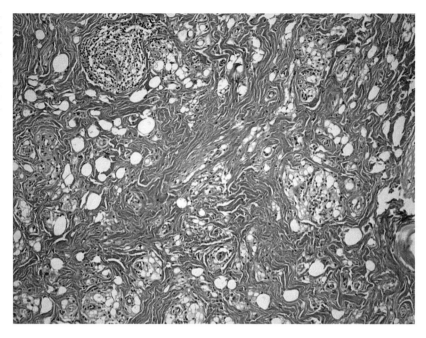

if necessary with lipid stains on frozen tissue (Oil red O). Osmium tetroxide fails to blacken the lipid, which is characteristic of paraffin hydrocarbons.

MESENCHYMAL TUMORS

PENILE MYOINTIMOMA

Penile myointimoma is a recently described lesion occurring in both children and adults. Lesions exclusively involve the corpus spongiosum and are clinically benign, ranging up to 2cm. Histology is similar in most cases, with a prominent fibro-intimal proliferation of stellate or spindled muscle cells involving the vasculature of the corpus spongiosum (**Fig. 30**).[78,79]

EPITHELIOID HEMANGIOMA

Epithelioid hemangioma is a rare entity, often confused with a malignant vascular tumor. It most commonly involves the shaft, generally dorsally, but can also be present in the glans. It presents as masses or with pain and tenderness. Microscopically, a proliferation of epithelioid endothelial cells is present in a nodular or lobular configuration, variably admixed with a mixed inflammatory infiltrate.[80] Hemangiomas of more common histologic type, including cavernous hemangioma and verrucous hemangioma, also can occur in the penis.[81,82]

GRANULAR CELL TUMOR

Granular cell tumors in the penis are similar to those of other locations, and can be present beneath an exuberant squamous proliferation which can mimic cancer clinically and microscopically. The key to the diagnosis is noting the infiltrating tumor cells with abundant granular eosinophilic cytoplasm and small nuclei. S100 is positive in the lesional cells.[28]

FIBROEPITHELIAL POLYPS

Fibroepithelial polyps are benign lesions that have commonly been associated with long-term use of condom catheters, and are often present for many months before diagnosis. They are polypoid, edematous stromal lesions with dilated vessels, prominent mesenchymal cells, and overlying keratinized squamous epithelium.[83]

OTHER RARE TUMORS

Other rare tumors reported include Glomus tumors, leiomyoma, and schwannoma.[84–86] Glomus tumor may present as painful nodule. Their microscopic features confirm to definitions provided at other body sites.

MALIGNANT NON-EPITHELIAL NEOPLASMS

SARCOMA

Sarcomas of the penis are rare but important entities. A broad spectrum of sarcomas occurs at this

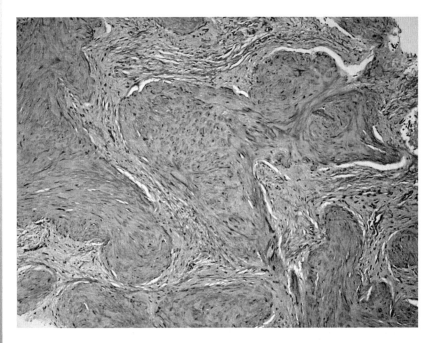

Fig. 30. Penile myointimoma: a prominent fibro-intimal proliferation of stellate or spindled muscle cells is seen involving the vasculature of the corpus spongiosum. (*Courtesy of* J. McKenney, MD, Stanford, CA.)

site. The most common are leiomyosarcoma and vascular tumors, notably angiosarcoma and Kaposi's sarcoma.[2,87,88] Histologic features are similar to those of other sites, and management is generally with wide excision and close clinical follow up.

REFERENCES

1. Cubilla AL, Piris A, Pfanni R, et al. Anatomic levels: important landmarks in penectomy specimens: a detailed anatomic and histologic study based on examination of 44 cases. Am J Surg Pathol 2001; 25(8):1091–4.

2. Young RH, Srigley JR, Amin MB, et al. Tumors of the prostate gland, seminal vesicles, male urethra, and penis. Atlas of Tumor Pathology Fascicle 28. 3rd edition. Washington, DC: AFIP; 2000.

3. Cubilla AL, Velazquez EF, Young RH. Epithelial lesions associated with invasive penile squamous cell carcinoma: a pathologic study of 288 cases. Int J Surg Pathol 2004;12(4):351–64.

4. Cupp MR, Malek RS, Goellner JR, et al. The detection of human papillomavirus deoxyribonucleic acid in intraepithelial, in situ, verrucous and invasive carcinoma of the penis. J Urol 1995;154(3): 1024–9.

5. Dillner J, von Krogh G, Horenblas S, et al. Etiology of squamous cell carcinoma of the penis. Scand J Urol Nephrol Suppl 2000;205:189–93.

6. Velazquez EF, Cubilla AL. Lichen sclerosus in 68 patients with squamous cell carcinoma of the penis: frequent atypias and correlation with special carcinoma variants suggests a precancerous role. Am J Surg Pathol 2003;27(11):1448–53.

7. Rubin MA, Kleter B, Zhou M, et al. Detection and typing of human papillomavirus DNA in penile carcinoma: evidence for multiple independent pathways of penile carcinogenesis. Am J Pathol 2001;159(4): 1211–8.

8. Shah RB, Amin MB. Diseases of the penis, urethra, and scrotum. In: Zhou M, Magi-Galluzzi C, editors. Genitourinary pathology. Philadelphia: Churchill Livingstone Elsevier; 2007. p. 419–76.

9. Gregoire L, Cubilla AL, Reuter VE, et al. Preferential association of human papillomavirus with high-grade histologic variants of penile-invasive squamous cell carcinoma. J Natl Cancer Inst 1995; 87(22):1705–9.

10. Perceau G, Derancourt C, Clavel C, et al. Lichen sclerosus is frequently present in penile squamous cell carcinomas but is not always associated with oncogenic human papillomavirus. Br J Dermatol 2003;148(5):934–8.

11. Ritter M, Nawab RA, Tannenbaum M, et al. Localized amyloidosis of the glans penis: a case report and literature review. J Cutan Pathol 2003;30(1):37–40.

12. Powell J, Robson A, Cranston D, et al. High incidence of lichen sclerosus in patients with squamous cell carcinoma of the penis. Br J Dermatol 2001; 145(1):85–9.

13. Das S, Tunuguntla HS. Balanitis xerotica obliterans–a review. World J Urol 2000;18(6):382–7.

14. Bhojwani A, Biyani CS, Nicol A, et al. Bowenoid papulosis of the penis. Br J Urol 1997;80(3):508.

15. Hama N, Ohtsuka T, Yamazaki S. Detection of mucosal human papilloma virus DNA in bowenoid papulosis, Bowen's disease and squamous cell carcinoma of the skin. J Dermatol 2006;33(5):331–7.

16. Auepemkiate S, Thongsuksai P, Boonyaphiphat P. P16(INK4A) expression in Bowen's disease and Bowenoid papulosis. J Med Assoc Thai 2006; 89(9):1460–5.

17. Rogozinski TT, Janniger CK. Bowenoid papulosis. Am Fam Physician 1988;38(1):161–4.

18. Banon Perez VJ, Nicolas Torralba JA, Valdelvira Nadal P, et al. Squamous carcinoma of the penis. Arch Esp Urol 2000;53(8):693–9.

19. Pow-Saug MR, Benavente V, Pow-Saug JE, et al. Cancer of the penis. Cancer Control 2002;9(4): 305–14.

20. Velazquez EF, Cubilla AL. Penile squamous cell carcinoma: anatomic, pathologic and viral studies in Paraguay (1993–2007). Anal Quant Cytol Histol 2007;29(4):185–98.

21. Banon Perez VJ, Nicolas Torralba JA, Valdelvira Nadal P, et al. Malignant neoplasms of the penis. Actas Urol Esp 2000;24(8):652–8.

22. Pietrzak P, Hadway P, Corbishley CM, et al. Is the association between balanitis xerotica obliterans and penile carcinoma underestimated? BJU Int 2006; 98(1):74–6.

23. Daling JR, Madeleine MM, Johnson LG, et al. Penile cancer: importance of circumcision, human papillomavirus and smoking in in situ and invasive disease. Int J Cancer 2005;116(4):606–16.

24. Velazquez EF, Bock A, Soskin A, et al. Preputial variability and preferential association of long phimotic foreskins with penile cancer: an anatomic comparative study of types of foreskin in a general population and cancer patients. Am J Surg Pathol 2003;27(7): 994–8.

25. Bezerra AL, Lopes A, Landman G, et al. Clinicopathologic features and human papillomavirus dna prevalance of warty and squamous cell carcinoma of the penis. Am J Surg Pathol 2001;25(5): 673–8.

26. Cubilla AL, Barreto JE, Caballero C, et al. Pathologic features of epidermoid carcinoma of the penis. A prospective study of 66 cases. Am J Surg Pathol 1993;17(8):753–63.

27. Cubilla AL, Reuter V, Velazquez EF, et al. Histologic classification of penile carcinoma and its relation to outcome in 61 patients with primary resection. Int J Surg Pathol 2001;9(2):111–20.

28. Laskin WB, Fetsch JF, Davis CJ, et al. Granular cell tumor of the penis: clinicopathologic evaluation of 9 cases. Hum Pathol 2005;36(3):291–8.

29. Cubilla AL, Velazquez EF, Young RH. Pseudohyperplastic squamous cell carcinoma of the penis associated with lichen sclerosus. An extremely well differentiated, nonverruciform neoplasm that preferentially affects the foreskin and is frequently misdiagnosed: a report of 10 cases of a distinct clinicopathologic entity. Am J Surg Pathol 2004; 28(7):895–900.

30. Velazquez EF, Barreto JE, Rodriguez I, et al. Limitations in the interpretation of biopsies in patients with penile squamous cell carcinoma. Int J Surg Pathol 2004;12(2):139–46.

31. Guimaraes GC, Lopes A, Campos RS, et al. Front pattern of invasion in squamous cell carcinoma of the penis: new prognostic factor for predicting risk of lymph node metastases. Urology 2006;68(1):148–53.

32. Lopes A, Hidalgo GS, Kowalski LP, et al. Prognostic factors in carcinoma of the penis: multivariate analysis of 145 patients treated with amputation and lymphadenectomy. J Urol 1996;156(5):1637–42.

33. Cubilla AL, Caballero C, Piris A, et al. A novel method to predict mortality in squamous carcinoma of the penis. Lab Invest 2000;80:97A.

34. Campos RS, Lopes A, Guimaraes GC, et al. E-cadherin, MMP-2, and MMP-9 as prognostic markers in penile cancer: analysis of 125 patients. Urology 2006;67(4):797–802.

35. Lopes A, Bezerra AL, Pinto CA, et al. p53 as a new prognostic factor for lymph node metastasis in penile carcinoma: analysis of 82 patients treated with amputation and bilateral lymphadenectomy. J Urol 2002;168(1):81–6.

36. Lowe D, Fletcher CD. Eosinophilia in squamous cell carcinoma of the oral cavity, external genitalia and anus clinical correlations. Histopathology 1984; 8(4):627–32.

37. Bissida NK, Yakout HH, Fahmy WE, et al. Multi-institutional long-term experience with conservative surgery for invasive penile carcinoma. J Urol 2003; 169(2):500–2.

38. Korets R, Koppie TM, Snyder ME, et al. Partial penectomy for patients with squamous cell carcinoma of the penis: the memorial Sloan-Kettering experience. Ann Surg Oncol 2007;14(12):3614–9.

39. Velazquez EF, Soskin A, Bock A, et al. Positive resection margins in partial penectomies: sites of involvement and proposal of local routes of spread of penile squamous cell carcinoma. Am J Surg Pathol 2004;28(3):384–9.

40. Banon Perez VJ, Nicolas Torralba JA, Valdelvira Nadal P, et al. Penile verrucous carcinoma. Arch Esp Urol 1999;52(9):937–40.

41. Seixas AL, Ornellas AA, Marota A, et al. Verrucous carcinoma of the penis: retrospective analysis of 32 cases. J Urol 1994;152(5 Pt 1):1476–8.

42. Masih AS, Stoler MH, Farrow GM, et al. Penile verrucous carcinoma: a clinicopathologic, human papillomavirus typing and flow cytometric analysis. Mod Pathol 1992;5(1):48–55.

43. Barreto JE, Velazquez EF, Ayala E, et al. Carcinoma cuniculatum: a distinctive variant of penile squamous cell carcinoma: report of 7 cases. Am J Surg Pathol 2007;31(1):71–5.

44. Cubilla AL, Velazquez EF, Reuter VE, et al. Warty (condylomatous) squamous cell carcinoma of the

penis: a report of 11 cases and proposed classification of 'verruciform' penile tumors. Am J Surg Pathol 2000;24(4):505–12.

45. Fukunaga M, Yokoi K, Miyazawa Y, et al. Penile verrucous carcinoma with anaplastic transformation following radiotherapy. A case report with human papillomavirus typing and flow cytometric DNA studies. Am J Surg Pathol 1994;18(5):501–5.

46. Cubilla AL, Reuter VE, Gregoire L, et al. Basaloid squamous cell carcinoma: a distinctive human papilloma virus-related penile neoplasm: a report of 20 cases. Am J Surg Pathol 1998;22(6):755–61.

47. Velazquez EF, Melamed J, Barreto JE, et al. Sarcomatoid carcinoma of the penis: a clinicopathologic study of 15 cases. Am J Surg Pathol 2005;29(9): 1152–8.

48. Manglani KS, Manaligod JR, Ray B. Spindle cell carcinoma of the glans penis: a light and electron microscopic study. Cancer 1980;46(10):2266–72.

49. Masera A, Ovcak Z, Volavsek M, et al. Adenosquamous carcinoma of the penis. J Urol 1997;157(6): 2261.

50. Cubilla AL, Ayala MT, Barreto JE, et al. Surface adenosquamous carcinoma of the penis. A report of three cases. Am J Surg Pathol 1996;20(2):156–60.

51. Liegl B, Regauer S. Penile clear cell carcinoma: a report of 5 cases of a distinct entity. Am J Surg Pathol 2004;28(11):1513–7.

52. Banon Perez VJ, Martinez Barba E, Rigabert Montiel M, et al. Basal cell carcinoma of the penis. Arch Esp Urol 2000;53(9):841–3.

53. Kim ED, Kroft S, Dalton DP. Basal cell carcinoma of the penis: case report and review of the literature. J Urol 1994;152(5 Pt 1):1557–9.

54. Macedo AJ, Fichtner J, Hohenfellner R. Extramammary Paget's disease of the penis. Eur Urol 1997; 31(3):382–4.

55. Salamanca J, Benito A, Garcia-Penalver C, et al. Paget's disease of the glans penis secondary to transitional cell carcinoma of the bladder: a report of two cases and review of the literature. J Cutan Pathol 2004;31(4):341–5.

56. Park S, Grossfield GD, McAninch JW, et al. Extramammary Paget's disease of the penis and scrotum: excision, reconstruction and evaluation of occult malignancy. J Urol 2001;166(6):2112–6.

57. Suzuki T, Togo Y, Yasuda K, et al. Prostatic duct adenocarcinoma with pagetoid spread on the glans penis: a case report. Hinyokika Kiyo 2006;52(11): 887–90.

58. Fang AW, Whittaker MA, Theaker JM. Mucinous metaplasia of the penis. Histopathology 2002; 40(2):177–9.

59. Val-Bernal JF, Garijo MF. Pagetoid dyskeratosis of the prepuce. An incidental histologic finding resembling extramammary Paget's disease. J Cutan Pathol 2000;27(8):387–91.

60. Yang WJ, Kim DS, Im YJ, et al. Extramammary Paget's disease of the penis and scrotum. Urology 2005;65(5):972–5.

61. Sanchez-Ortiz R, Huang SF, Tamboli P, et al. Melanoma of the penis, scrotum and male urethra: a 40-year single institution experience. J Urol 2005;173(6):1958–65.

62. Tomic S, Warner TF, Messing E, et al. Penile Merkel cell carcinoma. Urology 1995;45(6):1062–5.

63. Oppenheim AR. Sebaceous carcinoma of the penis. Arch Dermatol 1981;117(5):306–7.

64. Khan MA, Tao W, Mathews P, et al. Penile metastasis arising from transitional cell carcinoma of the urinary bladder. Urol Int 2001;66(3):162–3.

65. Fujimoto N, Hiraki N, Ueoka H, et al. Metastasis to the penis in a patient with squamous cell carcinoma of the lung with a review of reported cases. Lung Cancer 2001;34(1):149–52.

66. Davies SW. Giant condyloma acuminata: Incidence among cases diagnosed as carcinoma of the penis. J Clin Pathol 1965;18:142–9.

67. Cortes JR, Arratia J, Martinez R, et al. Extensive condyloma acuminata of the penis successfully treated with 5% imiquimod cream. Actas Urol Esp 2007; 31(3):276–8.

68. Geiss DF, Del Rosso JQ, Murphy J. Verruciform xanthoma of the glans penis: a benign clinical simulant of genital malignancy. Cutis 1993;51(5): 369–72.

69. Ersahin C, Szpaderska AM, Foreman K, et al. Verruciform xanthoma of the penis not associated with human papillomavirus infection. Arch Pathol Lab Med 2005;129(3):e62–4.

70. Agrawal SK, Bhattacharya SN, Singh N. Pearly penile papules: a review. Int J Dermatol 2004;43(3): 199–201.

71. Leis-Dosil VM, Alijo-Serrano F, Aviles-Izquierdo JA, et al. Angiokeratoma of the glans penis: clinical, histopathological and dermoscopic correlation. Dermatol Online J 2007;13(2):19.

72. Perimenis P, Athanasopoulos A, Gyftopoulos K, et al. Peyronie's disease: epidemiology and clinical presentation of 134 cases. Int Urol Nephrol 2001;32(4): 691–4.

73. Kadioglu A, Tefekli A, Erol B, et al. A retrospective review of 307 men with Peyronie's disease. J Urol 2002;168(3):1075–9.

74. Taylor FL, Levine LA. Peyronie's disease. Urol Clin North Am 2007;34(4):517–34.

75. Arena F, Peracchia G, di Stefano C, et al. Peyronie's disease-incision and dorsal vein grafting combined with contralateral plication in straightening the penis. Scand J Urol Nephrol 1999;33(3): 181–5.

76. Bussey LA, Norman RW, Gupta R. Sclerosing lipogranuloma: an unusual scrotal mass. Can J Urol 2002;9(1):1464–9.

77. Oertel YC, Johnson FB. Sclerosing lipogranuloma of male genitalia. Review of 23 cases. Arch Pathol Lab Med 1977;101(6):321–6.

78. Fetsch JF, Brinsko RW, Davis CJ, et al. A distinctive myointimal proliferation ('myointimoma') involving the corpus spongiosum of the glans penis: a clinicopathologic and immunohistochemical analysis of 10 cases. Am J Surg Pathol 2000;24(11):1524–30.

79. McKenney JK, Collins MH, Carretero AP, et al. Penile myointimoma in children and adolescents: a clinicopathologic study of 5 cases supporting a distinct entity. Am J Surg Pathol 2007;31(10):1622–6.

80. Fetsch JF, Sesterhenn IA, Miettinen M, et al. Epithelioid hemangioma of the penis: a clinicopathologic and immunohistochemical analysis of 19 cases, with special reference to exuberant examples often confused with epithelioid hemangioendothelioma and epithelioid angiosarcoma. Am J Surg Pathol 2004;28(4):523–33.

81. Kumar A, Goyal NK, Trivedi S, et al. Primary cavernous hemangioma of the glans penis: rare case report with a review of the literature. Aesthetic Plast Surg 2008;32(2):386–8.

82. Akyol I, Jayanthi VR, Luquette MH. Verrucous hemangioma of the glans penis. Urology 2008;72(1):230.e15–6.

83. Fetsch JF, Davis CJ, Hallman JR, et al. Lymphedematous fibroepithelial polyps of the glans penis and prepuce: a clinicopathologic study of 7 cases demonstrating a strong association with chronic condom catheter use. Hum Pathol 2004;35(2):190–5.

84. Bartoletti R, Gacci M, Nesi G, et al. Leiomyoma of the corona glans penis. Urology 2002;59(3):445.

85. Park DS, Cho TW, Kang H. Glomus tumor of the glans penis. Urology 2004;64(5):1031.

86. Kumar GP, Sukumar S, Bhat SH, et al. Schwannoma of the penis: a common tumour at a rare site. Scand J Urol Nephrol 2006;40(2):166–7.

87. Fetsch JF, Davis CJ, Miettinen M, et al. Leiomyosarcoma of the penis: a clinicopathologic study of 14 cases with review of the literature and discussion of the differential diagnosis. Am J Surg Pathol 2004;28(1):115–25.

88. Pacifico A, Piccolo D, Fargnoli MC, et al. Kaposi's sarcoma of the glans penis in an immunocompetent patient. Eur J Dermatol 2003;13(6):582–3.

MOLECULAR PATHOLOGY OF THE GENITOURINARY TRACT: MOLECULAR PATHOLOGY OF KIDNEY AND TESTES

S. Joseph Sirintrapun, MD[a], Anil V. Parwani, MD, PhD[b],*

KEYWORDS
- Molecular pathology • Testicular tumors • Renal neoplasms

ABSTRACT

With the advent of newer molecular technologies, our knowledge of cellular mechanisms with tumors of the kidney and testis has grown exponentially. Molecular technologies have led to better understanding of interplay between the von Hippel-Lindau gene and angiogenic cytokines in renal cancer and isochromosome 12p in testicular neoplasms. The result has been development of antiangiogenic-targeted therapy within recent years that has become the mainstay treatment for metastatic renal cell cancer. In the near future, classification and diagnosis of renal and testicular tumors through morphologic analysis will be supplemented by molecular information correlating to prognosis and targeted therapy. This article outlines tumor molecular pathology of the kidney and testis encompassing current genomic, epigenomic, and proteonomic findings.

MOLECULAR PATHOLOGY OF RENAL TUMOR

RENAL TUMORS: ASSOCIATED GENETIC ALTERATIONS

Renal cell carcinomas (RCCs) can be classified morphologically into clear-cell (75%), papillary (10%), chromophobe (5%), and oncocytoma (5%). Each subtype has distinct and well-described molecular abnormalities.[1,2] Sporadic papillary RCCs show trisomy 7 and 17 (**Fig. 1**) and loss of Y.[3,4] Additional chromosomal aberrations of (+8, +12, +16, +20, −9p) are seen with aggressive papillary RCCs.[5] Chromophobe RCCs have multiple losses of chromosomes 1, 2, 6, 10, and 17, but sarcomatoid transformation is found with frequent polysomy of these same chromosomes.[6] The World Health Organization now recognizes rare tumors, such as collecting ducts of Bellini, renal medullary carcinoma, Xp11.2 translocation carcinoma, and mucinous tubular spindle cell carcinoma. Many of these newer tumors incorporate morphology with specific genetic aberrations for classification.[2] These advancements in our understanding of the molecular biology of renal tumors have led to molecular therapeutic targeting, which is the most advanced of all the genitourinary cancers.

MOLECULAR PATHOLOGY OF CLASSIC TUMORS

THE VON HIPPEL-LINDAU GENE AND CLEAR CELL RCC: MOLECULAR PATHOLOGY

Von-Hippel Lindau (VHL) disease predisposes patients to hemangioblastomas of the central nervous system (CNS), pheochromocytomas, endocrine pancreatic tumors, papillary cystadenomas of the pancreas, epididymis, and adnexal organs, in addition to RCCs (**Box 1**).[7] Tumors are

[a] Pathology Informatics, University of Pittsburgh Medical Center, Pittsburgh, PA 15232, USA
[b] Department of Pathology, University of Pittsburgh Medical Center Shadyside Hospital, Room WG 07, 5230 Centre Avenue, Pittsburgh, PA 15232, USA
* Corresponding author.
E-mail address: parwaniav@upmc.edu (A.V. Parwani).

Surgical Pathology 2 (2009) 199–223
doi:10.1016/j.path.2008.08.003

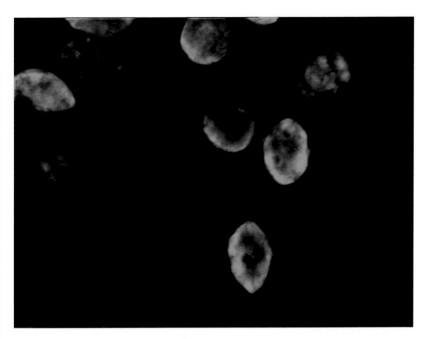

Fig. 1. Trisomy 17 in papillary RCC. Fluorescence in situ hybridization (FISH) displays three signals (*red*) for the chromosome 17 centromeric probe consistent with trisomy 17, a classic finding in papillary RCC. (*Courtesy of* K. Cieply, BS, Pittsburgh, PA).

classically clear cell and tumor presentation can be multifocal and occur simultaneously or in succession.[8] The gene maps to chromosome 3p24-25[9,10] with loss of function with VHL products being the most common genetic defect in sporadic clear cell RCCs.[11] Besides those families with VHL disease, rare familial clear cell RCCs

---

Box 1
Molecular Pathology of Clear Cell RCCs

- Loss of function of the VHL gene (3p24-25) and its products

  Not seen in other sporadic RCC subtypes (ie, papillary, chromophobe)

  Solely a molecular property of clear cell RCCs

- Sporadic clear cell RCCs

  Both copies of the VHL gene inactivated in approximately 60% to 70%

  Most common genetic defect

- VHL disease

  Germline inactivation in one VHL allele with inactivation of a second allele occurring as an early, initiating event in tumor formation

- Rare familial clear cell RCCs

  Constitutional chromosome 3 translocations

  Mapped to various breakpoints distinct from the VHL locus

---

arise from constitutional chromosome 3 translocations mapped to various breakpoints distinct from the VHL locus.[12]

Patients with VHL disease harbor a germline inactivation in one VHL allele, with an inactivation of a second allele occurring as an early, initiating event in tumor formation.[13–15] Patients with sporadic clear cell RCCs have both copies of the VHL gene inactivated in approximately 60% to 70% of cases.[16,17] With other sporadic RCC subtypes, there have been no other mutations of the VHL gene found, implying that VHL mutation is solely a molecular property of clear cell RCCs.[16,17]

VHL AND HYPOXIA-INDUCIBLE FACTOR IN CLEAR CELL RCC TUMORIGENESIS

The VHL protein is a component of an intracellular ubiquitin complex.[18–20] Hypoxia-inducible factor (HIF) is a heterodimeric (HIFα/β) transcription factor whose α subunit is normally targeted by VHL protein for ubiquitination and proteasome degradation under abundant oxygen conditions. When oxygen pressure falls, this targeting is disrupted and the α subunit of HIF stabilizes, moves to the nucleus, and binds to promoter genes (hypoxia response elements), leading to expression of hypoxia-inducible genes.[21–24] As opposed to normal cells, VHL-deficient cells accumulate HIFα under normal oxygen pressure conditions, which eventually lead to the increased expression of these hypoxia-inducible genes, which include genes encoding for angiogenic factors such as vascular endothelial growth factor (VEGF). The up-regulation of HIF in VHL-deficient cells plays a key role in clear cell RCC tumorigenesis (**Fig. 2**).[9,10,25–29]

HIF, besides activating hypoxia response elements, also targets platelet-derived growth factor β (PDGFβ), which can oncogenically transform fibroblasts, promote vascular pericytes, and contribute to tumor vessel maturation.[30–32] HIF targets enzymes that degrade extracellular matrix-like metalloproteinases and lysyl-oxidase, an enzyme that regulates cell-matrix interactions.[33] Transforming growth factor alpha (TGF-α) is transactivated by HIF, which then activates renal cell epidermal growth factor receptor (EGFR).[34] HIF transactivates CXCR4 and stromal-derived factor receptor/CXCR12, and down-regulates E-cadherin.[35,36] Thus, HIF may play a role in metastatic behavior not only with promotion of angiogenesis but its role with epithelial and mesenchymal interactions (**Table 1**).[37]

PI3K/mTOR PATHWAY—ALTERNATIVE REGULATOR OF HIF

HIFα activity is not only regulated by VHL but also through activation of the PI3 kinase (PI3K) pathway. It is this activation of PI3K that leads through a chain of events, namely activation of a phosphorylating mediator AKT. AKT phosphorylates a myriad of proteins, which result in increased cellular survival, proliferation, growth, and metabolism. One downstream phosphorylation target in particular is mTOR, whereby the result is promotion of mTOR-dependent translation of HIFα.[38,39] Amplification of Her2/neu interacts with PI3K to increase HIF activity downstream.[40] mTOR is strategically placed a the intersection of multiple growth factor (ie, insulin, insulin-like growth factor, and PDGF) and nutrient-signaling networks regulating growth, metabolism, and proliferation. The tuberous sclerosis complex 1 or 2 inhibits Rheb activity, which promotes mTOR phosphorylation and activation, eventually leading to increase HIF levels.[39,41–49] The tumor suppressor phosphatase and tensin homolog (PTEN) is also postulated to be a proximal negative regulator of mTOR.[50] Thus, inactivation of PTEN leads to abnormal activation of mTOR and thus increased HIF activity.

VHL DISEASE: MOLECULAR PATHOLOGY

VHL patients are classified as type I and II, mainly on their predisposition to developing pheochromocytoma. Type 1 patients have numerous other

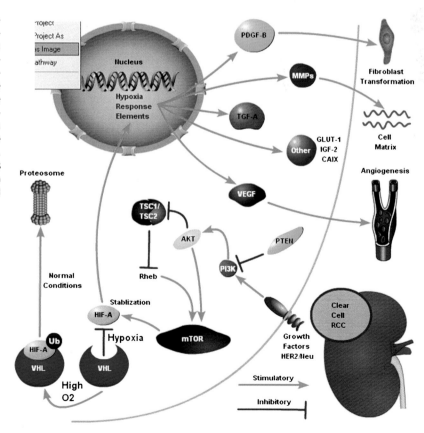

Fig. 2. Molecular pathways in RCC under conditions of high oxygen tensions. HIF is sequestered by VHL for ubiquitination and proteosome degradation. The release of HIF-A begins the signaling cascade by which hypoxia response-gene elements are transcribed. This eventually facilitates tumorigenesis through angiogenic factors and metalloproteinases.

Table 1
Molecular pathology features of the VHL disease types

VHL Type	VHL Affinity for HIF	Risk for Clear Cell RCC Development
I	Total loss of VHL activity	Very high
IIA	High	Low
IIB	Low	High
IIC	Very high	None

For patients with VHL germline mutations, there is an inverse correlation with VHL mutations in their ability to bind HIF and the risk of RCC.

tumors but no pheochromocytomas, while type II patients can develop pheochromocytomas. RCCs are seen in either type I and II, but certain subtypes of II appear to have varying degrees of association.[51,52] Type I VHL mutations generally produce proteins with total functional loss. Thus, there is no regulation of HIF, with eventual over-expression of HIF with the risk of RCC formation being very high. In type II, which is subtyped into A, B, and C, the risk of RCC inversely correlates to affinity of binding to HIF. In IIB, the affinity for HIF is the least, with the risk for RCC being the highest. In IIC, the affinity for HIF is the highest, with the risk for RCC being nil. The subtype IIA is in-between affinity of HIF binding and risk for RCC.[53–57]

The loss of VHL activity is most likely the initiating step in tumorigenesis of clear cell RCCs, but these tumors harbor additional nonrandom genetic events. VHL patients often develop multiple RCC tumors; some remain dormant while others grow quickly and metastasize. This is consistent with a multistep process but leads to hypotheses that the severity of familial or sporadic disease is dictated by these additional genetic defects in the VHL-HIF or parallel pathways.[1,40]

OTHER VHL/HIF DOWNSTREAM TARGETS

Besides angiogenic targets, the VHL/HIF cascade activates other downstream mediators. VHL interacts with RNA polymerase II because of the structural similarities to HIF-binding domains. The binding results in ubiquitination and decreased transcriptional activity for the polymerase.[58,59] Mutant VHL products also have been shown to fail to assemble fibronectin, implying an influence of VHL on extracellular matrix.[60] VHL proteins bind to p53, inhibit its MDM2-mediated ubiquitination, suppress p53 nuclear export, and promote its acetylation by p300 and overall p53 transcriptional activity. Thus, VHL appears to facilitate p53 mediated G1 arrest and promote the apoptotic response.[61,62] Jade-1 is a short-lived, kidney-enriched transcription factor stabilized by VHL

and is believed to suppress tumorigenesis by also increasing apoptosis. This tumor suppressor may act as a proapoptotic barrier but is overcome when VHL is inactivated.[63]

HEREDITARY PAPILLARY AND ONCOCYTIC RENAL TUMORS: MOLECULAR PATHOLOGY

A subset of patients with Hereditary papillary RCC (HPRCC) type 1 is the result of germline activating mutations in the c-MET gene on 7q31.[64,65] The ligand to the c-MET receptor is hepatocyte growth factor/scatter factor (HGF/SF). The binding leads to phosphorylation. HGF stimulation and c-MET autophosphorylation result in promotion of cell proliferation via RAS activation, inhibition of apoptosis through direct activation of PI3K, increased motility by GRB2-associated binding protein 1 (GAB1)-mediated PI3K activation, and tubular structure formation.[66–69] The branching or tubular formation needs coordinated activation of the signal transducer and activator of transcription and GAB1-PLCg signaling pathways.[67] The transmembrane/intracellular beta chain of c-MET has interactions with extracellular signal transduction molecules, such as CD44, plexin, and integrin a6b4, implying that these cytoskeletal changes may lead to metastatic potential.[70,71] VHL and c-MET actually do interact with HIF stabilization through hypoxia, or loss of VHL function results in transcriptional up-regulation and promotion of transforming potential of the c-MET receptor.[72] This interaction may explain why certain RCCs have both clear cell and papillary histologies (**Boxes 2** and **3**).

HLPRCC type II patients do not have the multifocality and bilateral pattern, which characterizes those other familial diseases that predispose to RCC. However, in addition to the obvious leiomyomas characteristic of this syndrome, the RCCs that do develop are of papillary type 2 histology and usually more aggressive, as opposed to tumors of HPRCC type 1.[2,73,74] The gene

---

Box 2
Molecular pathology features of sporadic papillary and oncocytic RCCs

- Papillary RCC

  Trisomy 7 and 7

  Loss of Y

  Aberrations of (+8, +12, +16, +20, −9p)

  Associated with aggressive behavior

- Chromophobe RCC

  Multiple losses of chromosomes 1, 2, 6, 10, and 17

  Polysomy of 1, 2, 6, 10, and 17

  Associated with sarcomatoid transformation

---

responsible, Krebs cycle's enzyme fumarase hydratase (FH), maps to chromosome 1q42.1. FH is most likely a tumor-suppressor gene with loss of the wild-type alleles in HLPRCC-associated tumors.[74–78] FH, being part of the Kreb's cycle, when inhibited leads to accumulation of fumarate precursors, most notably succinate within the cytoplasm. The increased succinate competitively inhibits the enzyme EGLN, which regulates HIF through hydroxylation of proline residues leading to eventual stabilization of HIF.[79,80]

Birt-Hogg-Dube disease is a curious disease where patients develop fibrofolliculomas, trichodiscomas, pleural cysts with spontaneous pneumothoraxes, and multiple and bilateral RCCs of mainly oncocytic morphology, namely oncocytomas, hybrid oncocytic tumors, and chromophobes.[78,81–83] Microscopic oncocytosis is often seen. The gene responsible is folliculin, which

---

Box 3
Molecular pathology features of hereditary papillary and oncocytic RCCs

- Hereditary papillary RCC type 1

  Germline activating mutations of c-MET gene on 7q31

- Hereditary leiomyomatosis apillary RCC (HLPRCC) type II

  Loss of wild-type alleles for the Krebs cycle's enzyme fumarase hydratase on 1q42.1

- Birt-Hogg-Dube disease

  Folliculin on 17p11.2

---

maps to chromosome 17p11.2 and behaves like a tumor suppressor gene.[82,84,85]

MOLECULAR BIOLOGY OF RARER RENAL TUMORS

Molecular pathology features of rare renal tumors are shown in **Box 4**.

TRANSLOCATION-ASSOCIATED RCCS

A newly defined type of RCC are the translocation-associated RCCs. Xp11 translocation carcinoma primarily occurs in children and young adults, with a strong female predominance and with behaviors similar to aggressive adult RCCs presenting often at advanced stages. These tumors comprise one-third of all pediatric RCCs and include ASPL-TFE3 and PRCC-TFE3 gene fusions, TFE3 being a member of the MiTF/TFE transcription factor family. This gene fusion is identical to that found in alveolar soft part sarcoma. Another distinctive type of translocation carcinoma has the t(6,11) (p21;q12) translocation. Cloning of the gene links this entity to the Xp11 translocation carcinomas.[2,85–89]

MUCINOUS TUBULAR AND SPINDLE CELL CARCINOMA: MOLECULAR PATHOLOGY

MTSCC is an unusual tumor characterized by tubules, variable spindled component, low-grade cytology, and mucinous or myxoid stroma. Cytogenetics and comparative genomic hybridization (CGH) show loss of chromosomes 1, 4, 6, 8, 13, 14, 15, and 22.[2,85,90]

ANGIOMYOLIPOMA: MOLECULAR PATHOLOGY

AML is the most common adult mesenchymal tumor. AMLs are usually benign and can occur sporadically or in association with tuberous sclerosis, an autosomal dominant disorder caused by loss of function mutations of TSC1 or TSC2 tumor suppressor genes on chromosomes 9q34 and 16p13, respectively.[2] There are frequent allelic losses of chromosome 16p. These tumors rarely malignantly transform and metastasize. Limited data have shown that the metastases may also have the same loss of chromosome 16p.[85,91]

MIXED EPITHELIAL AND STROMAL TUMOR OF THE KIDNEY: MOLECULAR PATHOLOGY

MESTK is a rare and also newly defined entity. It has similarities to cystic hamartoma of the renal

Box 4
Molecular pathology features of rare renal tumors

- Xp11 translocation carcinomas

    ASPL-TFE3 and PRCC-TFE3 gene fusions

    t(6,11) (p21;q12) translocation

    Represents another subset of tumors

    Nuclear staining for TFE3

    Focal or weak MiTF

Focal or weak pan-cytokeratin

    Positive for vimentin, RCC antigen, and CD10

- Mucinous tubular and spindle cell carcinoma (MTSCC)

    Loss of chromosomes 1, 4, 6, 8, 13, 14, 15, and 22

    Positive for AMACR, CK18, CK19, and EMA

    Variable for markers of proximal tubular derivation - RCC, CD10, and CD15

- Angiomyolipomas (AML)

    Frequent allelic losses of chromosome 16p

    Positive for melanoma markers: HMB-45 and Melan-A

    Positive for smooth muscle actin, desmin, and CD68

    Negative for S100, cytokeratin, and EMA

- Mixed epithelial and stromal tumor of the kidney (MESTK)

    t(1;19)?: 1 reported case

    Positive for estrogen and progesterone receptors

    Positive for desmin and smooth muscle actin in the spindle celled component

    Negative for HMB-45 and CD34

- Primary renal synovial sarcoma

    Classic SYT-SSX fusion gene that results from the translocation of the SYT gene on chromosome 18 with the SSX gene on the X chromosome

- Primary neuroectodermal tumor/Ewing sarcoma (PNET)

    Fusion transcript EWS-FLI1 resulting from t(11;22) (q24;q12)

    Other possibilities are variant translocation of EWS with other ETS-related oncogenes

    Positive for CD99 and vimentin

pelvis, adult type of mesoblastic nephroma, and cystic nephroma. The spindle cell component has a notorious ovarian or solitary fibrous tumor-like stroma. Much more common in women, particularly those of middle age, the tumor marks consistently with estrogen and progesterone receptors, implying that hormones play a role in the tumorigenesis. Translocation t(1;19) has been reported, but only in one case, and the histogenesis is still unknown.[85]

SYNOVIAL SARCOMA AND PNET: MOLECULAR PATHOLOGY

Other rare tumors include primary renal synovial sarcoma and primary neuroectodermal tumor/Ewing sarcoma. Primary renal synovial sarcomas have the classic SYT-SSX fusion gene that results from the translocation of the SYT gene on chromosome 18, with the SSX gene on the X chromosome. PNETs have similar fusion transcript EWS-FLI1 resulting from t(11;22) (q24;q12), but variant translocation of EWS with other ETS-related oncogenes are possible.[85,92]

MOLECULAR BIOLOGY OF PEDIATRIC RENAL TUMORS

Pediatric renal tumors provide significant diagnostic challenges with approximately 25% inaccurately classified by the local institution (**Box 5**). Wilm's tumor is the most common malignant tumor in this age group, comprising 85% of cases. However, the difficulty in diagnosing arises in evaluating the sarcomas that arise in the kidney versus undifferentiated Wilm's tumors whose blastemal or stromal elements can easily be mistaken for these sarcomas. The sarcomas are cellular mesoblastic nephroma (CMN), rhabdoid tumor of the kidney (RTK), and clear cell sarcoma of the kidney (CCSK).[93]

CELLULAR MESOBLASTIC NEPHROMA: MOLECULAR BIOLOGY

CMN, considered intrarenal infantile fibrosarcoma, are round or spindle-cell lesions and occur less than 2 years of age. Greater than 90% of CMNs have t(12;15) (p13;q25), which fuses the ETV6 gene from 12p13 with the NTRK3 receptor gene on 15q25. Hierarchical clustering of gene expression patterns is closer between CMN and RTK than with the other pediatric tumors, but there are genes that distinguish CMN. The genes that are up-regulated are HLX1, SPRY4, ANGPTL2,

Box 5
Molecular pathology features of pediatric renal tumors

- Cellular mesoblastic nephroma

    t(12;15) (p13;q25)

        Fuses the ETV6 gene from 12p13 with the neurotrophin-3 (NTRK3) receptor gene on 15q25

- Rhabdoid tumor of the kidney

    Mutations or deletions which inactivate hSNF5/INI1 gene

        Functions to alter conformation of the DNA-histone complex so that transcription factors have access to target gene

        INI-1 immunohistochemistry

            Negative for RTK

            Positive for other histologies in differential

    Severe up-regulation of the glucagon gene

- Clear cell sarcoma of the kidney

    No consistent immunohistochemical markers or recurrent genetic patterns

    Prominent expression of neural markers and genes involving related Akt and Sonic Hedgehog pathways

- Wilm's Tumor

    WT-1 and WT-2 genes on 11p

        10% of tumors

        Develop in association with syndromes

    PAX6 gene on 11p

        Responsible for aniridia

    Genetic loci for FWT1 on 17q and FWT2 on 19q

        Another familial Wilm's tumor predisposition

        Located outside of chromosome 11

    p53

        Adverse outcome with high expression

    Loss of heterozygosity (LOH) at chromosomes 1p and 16q

        Adverse outcome

    HER

        Critical role in the branching morphogenesis of renal tubules

        Extent of expression associated with level of epithelial differentiation

    Genes associated with progression

        TRIM22

        CENPF

        MYCN

        CTGF

        RARRES3

        EZH2

SRPUL, PTHLH, ADAM12, EGR3, and PDLIM2. The SPRY4 and EGR3 genes are seen in adult cancers, while ADAM12 is seen in related pediatric fibroblastic myofibroblastic tumors, such as aggressive fibromatosis.[93–98]

RHABDOID TUMOR OF THE KIDNEY: MOLECULAR BIOLOGY

RTK are round-cell tumors that are highly aggressive and not only seen in the kidney, but also in the CNS and soft tissues in young children, with survival of 25% of cases. All rhabdoid tumors have mutations or deletions that inactivate the hSNF5/INI1 gene, which functions to alter conformation of the DNA-histone complex so that transcription factors have access to target gene. INI-1 immunohistochemistry can be used to distinguish this entity with negative staining for RTK, seen as opposed to other histologies that are positive. A surprising finding is that the glucagon gene is 40-fold increased over other genes, with some studies reporting that up-regulation of genes in the glycolysis/glucogenesis pathway portend a poor and aggressive prognosis. Other genes up-regulated in RTK are NQO1, RSU1, PLP2, FLJ22662, APLP1, CBX6, AND NIT2.[93,99–104]

CLEAR CELL SARCOMA OF THE KIDNEY: MOLECULAR BIOLOGY

CCSKs are round and spindled lesions of infancy seen only in the kidney, with survival of all stages at 75%. It is the most frequently misdiagnosed pediatric renal tumor because of the various mimicking morphologies. No consistent immunohistochemical markers or recurrent genetic patterns have been described to aid in the diagnosis.[105–107] However, gene expression data show prominent expression of neural markers and genes involving related Akt and Sonic Hedgehog pathways. FOXF1 is a Sonic Hedgehog-dependent forkhead transcription factor, while neuronal pentraxin 1 (NPTX1) and its receptor (NPTXR), engrailed homolog2 (EN2), and DNA segment chromosome 4 (D4S234E) are genes involved in neural activities. All of these increased-expression of neural markers suggest that this tumor is neural or neuroectodermal in histogenesis. Other genes up-regulated are HLXB9, FOXF2, PCDH11.[93,108,109]

WILM'S TUMOR: MOLECULAR BIOLOGY

Wilm's tumor (nephroblastoma) replicates the histology of the developing kidney. Approximately 10% of tumors develop in association with the syndromes associated with WT-1 and WT-2 genes on chromosome 11p.[110,111] Genes such as PAX2 and EYA1 are essential for survival and differentiation in early metanephric development. TMEFF1 is over-expressed and contains structural domains that play a role in growth factor signaling, but may function as a tumor suppressor.[112,113] Additional genetic events are needed for tumorigenesis. PAX6, the gene responsible for aniridia, is found in the region of 11p. Two genetic loci located outside of chromosome 11 that have been associated are familial Wilm's tumor predisposition at FWT1 (17q) and FWT2 (19q). Tumor-suppressor gene mutations with p53 have been seen in Wilm's tumor. High expression of p53 and LOH at chromosomes 1p and 16q are associated with adverse outcome.[114,115] HER plays a critical role in the branching morphogenesis of renal tubules, and its extent of expression may be associated with level of epithelial differentiation.[116] Other genes up-regulated are SCHIP1, MYCN, desmoplakin (DSP), GPR64, and WASF3.[93] Wilm's tumor progression was associated with genes TRIM22, CENPF, MYCN, CTGF, RARRES3, and EZH2.[117]

MOLECULAR TECHNIQUES FOR RENAL CELL CARCINOMA

RENAL CELL CARCINOMA: GENE EXPRESSION PROFILING

To date, gene expression profiling has impacted in the discovery of immunohistochemical markers for diagnosis in the renal tumor subtypes. For instance, vimentin and CD10, which immunohistochemically mark for clear cell RCCs, were discovered by gene expression profiling.[118–122] However, lesser known markers discovered by these means are adipophilin[123] which functions in cell differentiation; glutathione S-transferase alpha, which functions for cell detoxification;[124,125] and CD74, which plays a role in immune response.[118,126] The stem cell factor receptor that functions in

cell differentiation, c-kit, was also discovered by gene profiling and immunohistochemical marks chromophobe RCCs.[127,128]

However, it is reassuring that data from these recent gene expression studies confirm distinct and biologically sensible correlations with morphologic subtypes. Clear cell RCCs over-express immune response and angiogenesis genes corresponding to the characteristic tumor vascular seen with that subtype.[2,119] Chromophobe RCCs and oncocytomas, with their accumulation of mitochondria, over-express energy pathway genes, many associated with mitochondrial biology.[119,129] Microarray studies verified by quantitative RT-PCR and immunohistochemistry correlate well with current models of renal tumor histogenesis. Clear cell RCCs over-express proximal nephron markers megalin and cubilin. The glucose transporter 1 is also expressed immunohistochemically on clear cell RCCs. Papillary RCCs strongly over-express alpha methylacyl CoA racemase.[124,130,131] Chromophobe RCCs and oncocytomas over-express distal nephron markers defensin-1[118,120] parvalbumin[120,132] chloride channel Kb, claudin-7, claudin-8, and EGFR.[118,133–135]

With better knowledge of the clear cell RCC tumorigenesis, several molecular correlates have been discovered to aide in prognostication. Loss of PTEN was increased in all RCCs when compared with normal tissues, but the greatest loss was seen in clear cell (25%) and RCCs with sarcomatoid features (34%). Phosphorylated AKT had the highest frequency in collecting duct (89%), followed by clear cell (58%), suggesting activation pathways other than PTEN loss.[39] P21 is a cell cycle and apoptosis regulating protein, which happens to be stabilized by downstream products of PI3K activation. Nuclear p21 staining was highest in collecting duct carcinomas and lowest in oncocytoma, while cytosolic p21 staining was the opposite: highest in oncocytoma and lowest in clear cell RCC.[39] Where p21 potentially holds the highest prognostic value is determining prognosis of patients with localized or metastatic disease at diagnosis. In localized disease, higher levels of nuclear p21 were associated with a better prognosis, but in patients with metastatic disease at diagnosis higher levels of nuclear and cytosolic p21 were associated with worse survival.[136] Because of its interaction with VHL, p53 expression can potentially predict survival in clear cell RCCs.[137,138] The Mayo Clinic has used high Ki-67 levels as poor independent predictors of clear cell RCCs.[139] There is some evidence that angiogenic activities using various molecular techniques and markers, such as carbonic anhydrase IX (CAIX), HIFα, and VEGF correlate with grade with higher grade clear cell RCCs, showing higher angiogenic activity.[140]

RENAL CELL CARCINOMA: EPIGENETIC PROFILING

Epigenetic investigations into RCC tumorigenesis are still in their infancy. Some data show that promoter methylation of the VHL gene can occur in up to 20% of cases, with rest of the cases being because of LOH and mutation.[141–143] Loss of the tumor-suppressor secreted frizzled-related protein 1 occurs by promoter methylation, resulting in aberrant Wnt signaling. This oncogenic Wnt signaling is involved in tumorigenesis of many solid tumors, including RCCs.[144] Levels of methylation at certain loci can correlate with subtype. Methylation of the promoter for RASSF1A is highest for papillary and clear cell RCCs versus oncocytomas, which are completely unmethylated.[145]

RENAL CELL CARCINOMA: THERAPEUTIC AND PROGNOSTIC TARGETING

Clinical behavior of RCC is often variable, but considerable prognostic information can be determined by histologic subtype and TNM pathologic staging system correlating tumor size and local extension. With histologic subtypes, clear cell RCCs have the highest rate of extrarenal growth, metastasis, and mortality.[2] Papillary and chromophobe carcinomas are generally indolent, but can metastasize or convert to high grade sarcomatoid variants. Both papillary and chromophobe RCCs have peculiar metastatic patterns, with propensity to have regional lymph node spread and liver metastases.[146] Papillary RCCs have the highest rate of multifocality (especially type I) and association with end-stage renal disease.[147,148] Oncocytomas, by strict definition, are benign. Collecting duct carcinomas are very aggressive with the highest tendency to metastasize of all renal epithelial subtypes.[2,147] Hereditary tumors often occur at earlier ages with multifocal presentation.[149]

There are several models from the University of California Los Angeles (UCLA) with the UCLA integrated staging system, Memorial Sloan Kettering with their normogram, and the Mayo Clinic with their stage, size, grade, and necrosis score, which combine clinical parameters and staging, pathologic findings, performance status, and laboratory studies to better determine clinical behavior.[150–154] Laboratory values that are taken into account are erythrocyte sedimentation rate (ESR), C-reactive protein, and thrombocytosis shown to be negative prognostic indicators.[155–158] Lesser known laboratory values include absence of Bcl-2 and FAS (apoptotic related markers) as a positive predictor

for immunotherapy response, and intratumoral neutrophils with low intratumoral CD57 natural killer cells as poor prognostic predictor (**Box 6**).[158]

RCC is among the most chemotherapy and hormonal therapy resistant tumors. For nonmetastatic localized disease, surgery is the gold standard for therapy. Where molecular treatments play a role is with recurrent and metastatic disease. Until recently, the only a treatments in metastatic disease were of high-dose interleukin (IL)-2 and interferon-alpha, with dismal response rates of less than 10% survival.[159–161] These cytokines appear the most effective with clear cell histology.[162] Systemic therapy is currently nonstandard for metastatic RCCs with nonclear histology.[163] With our better understanding of tumor molecular biology, there has been more precise targeting of therapy. Angiogenesis genes are clearly over-expressed in clear cell RCCs, namely because of VHL and HIFα dysregulation. This distinct expression profile implies responsiveness to various antiangiogenic therapies.[164] There is inhibition of downstream HIF targets, such as the receptor tyrosine kinases or their ligands, in single or in combination. There are clinical trials with anti-VEGF antibodies (bevacizumab)[165,166] or small molecular inhibitors of the VEGF receptor 2, PDGFβ, and related receptor tyrosine kinases (sunitinib, sorafenib, axitinib).[166–170]

Box 6
Key molecular prognostic markers for renal tumors

- Positive

   High staining: more than 85% carbonic anhydrase staining (clear cell RCCs)

   Absence of apoptotic-related markers: bcl-2 and FAS (predictor for immunotherapy)

   Nuclear staining of p21 (for localized disease)

- Negative

   Low staining: less than 85% carbonic anhydrase staining (clear cell RCCs)

   Elevated ESR and C-reactive protein

   Thrombocytosis

   Intratumoral neutrophils with low intratumoral CD57 NK cells

   Loss of PTEN

   Phosphorylated AKT

   Nuclear and cytosolic staining for p21 (for metastatic disease)

   High ki-67

There are strategies to target the VHL and HIF proteins in terms of protein synthesis, stability, or transcriptional activity, as well as their regulators. Interestingly, inhibitors of TGFα and EGFR have not currently been as successful.[50] Chemical or small moleculars that inhibit PI3K, AKT, or mTOR can be expected to restrict HIF activity.[40] The kinase inhibitor temsirolimus, an analog of sirolimus, inhibits mTOR.[50,166] It has been proposed that markers like PTEN and AKT would be useful in selection of patients amenable to mTOR targeted therapy (**Fig. 3**).[171] Sunitinib, sorafenib, and temsirolimus down-regulate angiogenesis, but also affect other processes and can inhibit cell proliferation in vitro, meaning that these agents act via more than one mechanism (**Box 7**).[50]

Clear cell RCCs over-express immune response genes, and this expression profile may be important for response to immunotherapy.[118,134,162,172] There is microarray evidence that expression of lymphocyte activator antigen CD70 mediated sensitivity of RCC cells to anti-CD70.[173] RCCs expressing B7-H1, which participates in T-cell costimulation, are significantly associated with cancer progression and death.[158] Angiogenic and immune-response regulators both increase

CAIX, which has been used as a prognostic marker. For nonmetastatic RCC, low CAIX predicted a worse outcome similar to patients with metastatic disease and overall CAIX expression decreased with development of metastasis. CAIX may be used to predict clinical outcome and identify high-risk patients for adjuvant-targeted therapies. CAIX expression has been shown to predict patient outcome in response to IL-2 based immunotherapy. The increase expression of CAIX can also be the target of G250 monoclonal antibody therapy for RCC.[39,164,166,174–176] In distinguishing clear cell RCCs from other subtypes, there have been proposals to use over-expression of angiogenesis genes and coregulation of VEGF and CAIX.[175] Finally, there is recent data that the toll-like receptor 3 (TLR3) pathway may provide a novel therapeutic target for clear cell RCC. TLR3, which has limited expression in normal tissue, was shown to be highly expressed in clear cell RCCs.[177]

With HPRCC type 1, because there is over-expression of c-MET, small inhibitor molecules of c-MET are being pursued.[178,179] Monoclonal antibodies against the beta chain of HGF/SF have been shown to disrupt the ligand-receptor

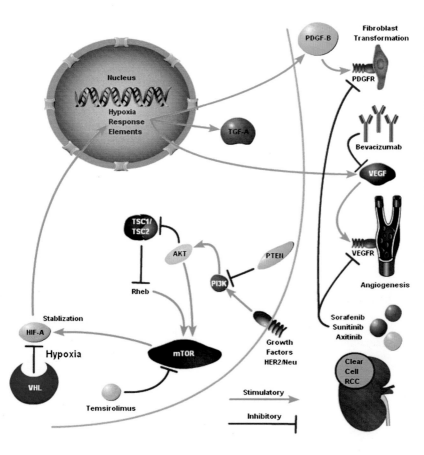

Fig. 3. Molecular therapeutic targeting in RCC. Current molecular-targeted therapy involves tyrosine kinase inhibitors, which can inhibit earlier in tumorigenic signaling at mTOR with temsirolimus, or near the end at VDGFR and PDGFR with sorafenib, sunitinib, and axitinib. Bevacizumab is unique because it is an antibody targeting VEGF.

Box 7
Key molecular therapeutic targets for renal tumors

- Angiogenesis targeting

    Anti-VEGF antibodies—bevacizumab

    Small molecular kinase inhibitors of the VEGF receptor 2, PDGFβ, and related receptor tyrosine kinases

    Sunitinib

    Sorafenib

    Axitinib

- mTOR targeting

    mTOR inhibitor

    Temsirolimus—analog of sirolimus

Box 8
Molecular pathology features of pediatric and adult germ cell tumors

- Pediatric

    Teratoma—diploid, no chromosomal abnormalities

    Yolk sac tumors—aneuploid; gains of 1q and 3; losses of 1 p and 6q

- Adult

    Seminoma/ITGCN—hypertriploidy; isochromosome/abnormalities 12p

    NSGCTs—hypotriploid or hyperdiploid; isochromosome/abnormalities 12p

---

interaction and inhibit growth.[180] Hsp90 inhibition with geldanamycin inhibits c-MET activation but mechanisms are yet delineated.[181] Clinical trials are underway with c-MET-driven tumors in general with single or combination of c-MET signaling, with obvious implications for HPRCC type 1 patients.[181] With HLPRCC, the targeting of HIF and HIF downstream targets in clear-cell RCCs may also work as well.

MOLECULAR PATHOLOGY OF TESTICULAR TUMORS

TESTICULAR TUMORS: OVERVIEW

Associated Genetic Alterations

Genetic conditions, such as Down's syndrome, Klinefelter's, and XY dysgenesis, predispose to germ cell tumors (GCTs). Predisposition is also seen with family history. Brothers of affected patients have an 8- to 10-fold relative risk and fathers and sons have a 4- to 6- fold risk. There have been several investigations into discovery of susceptibility alleles, and these have pointed to chromosome Xq27, polymorphisms of the gene XRCC1, and deletions in chromosome Y.[182–189]

MOLECULAR PATHOLOGY OF GERM CELL TUMORS

CONTRASTS BETWEEN PEDIATRIC AND ADULT GERM CELL TUMORS: MOLECULAR PATHOLOGY

With testicular GCTs, the clinical behavior differs, depending on whether the presentation is during childhood (pre-puberty) or adulthood (**Box 8**). In childhood, GCTs, which are basically teratomas

or yolk sac tumors, generally have benign behaviors. It is those GCTs of adulthood where the behavior is clearly malignant. Unlike adult GCTs, the origin of childhood testicular GCTs is poorly understood. In adolescents and adults, the classical seminomas and nonseminomas originate from intratubular germ cell neoplasia (ITGCN) of the testis, which can usually be seen in seminiferous tubules adjacent to the tumors. The totipotent germ cells in ITGCN are believed to have the unique potential to activate molecular pathways, thus mimicking those occurring during gametogenesis and normal human development. ITGCN is characteristically absent in prepubertal GCTs. These differences in clinical behavior and morphology point to fundamental etiologic differences between childhood GCTs and adult GCTs.[188,190]

In prepuberty, infantile teratomas are usually benign, diploid, and exhibit no chromosomal abnormalities. Infantile yolk sac tumors may be aneuploid and show gains of 1q, 2, 3 p, 9q, 12, 17, 19, 20q, 22, and Y, and losses of 1p, 4, 5 p, 6q, 8q, and Xp, with gains of 1q and 3 and losses of 1p and 6q being the most notable.[191–195] Adolescent testicular GCTs have cytogenetics that reflect adult GCTs with near-triploidy; loss of 11, 13, and 18 and gain of 7, 8, X, and isochromosome 12p.[194]

With adult GCTs, both seminomas and nonseminomatous germ cell tumors (NSGCTs) can be characterized by changes in DNA ploidy.[196,197] Pure seminomas and ITGCN are associated with hypertriploidy.[191,196–201] NSGCTs are often hypotriploid or hyperdiploid.[191,202] With classical cytogenetic karyotyping and comparative genomic hybridization, numerous and more specific chromosomal imbalances and structural abnormalities have been identified.[188,191,203–209] However, few have been consistently demonstrated except for isochromosome 12p.[210,211]

ISOCHROMOSOME 12P IN TESTICULAR GERM CELL TUMORS

Isochromosome 12p is the most consistent and specific chromosomal change found in testicular GCTs with approximately 80% of adult NSGCTs and 50% or greater of pure seminomas possessing at least one i(12p) (**Box 9**; **Figs. 4** and **5**).[211–214] When i(12p) is not found, then there is usually some aberration of 12p with over-representation or rearrangement of that portion of chromosome 12.[215–217] Chromosome 12p gains are felt to be an early change associated with GCTs; however, its finding in ITGCN is sporadic and thus implies that gain of 12p may reflect invasive potential.[211,218–221]

Approximately 400 genes are located in the entire short arm of chromosome 12, and to date specific genes on 12p associated with GCTs have yet to be identified. A specific region 12p11.2 to p12.1 is often amplified, with SOX5, JAW1, and K-RAS genes located in this region (**Fig. 6**).[188,195,222,223] However, over-amplifications of these specific genes, RAS in particular, have yet to predict response to therapy and survival.[216] Expression of cyclin D2, the product of the CCDN2 gene on 12p13, is seen in ITGCN, seminomas, and NSGCTs. With activation of cyclin D2, germ cells re-enter the cell cycle and then genomic instability leads to loss of other tumor suppressor genes, eventually leading to neoplastic progression. More potential candidate genes include the glucose transporter GLUT3, glycolytic enzymes GAPDH and TPI1, and self-renewal and pluripotency genes NANOG, DPPA3, and GDF3.[188] Despite the clear association of 12p with adult GCTs, correlations with clinical behavior, use for

diagnosis, and prognostic information have yet to be demonstrated.[209,224–226] One rare diagnostic use is with FISH of i(12p) in distinguishing the rare testicular epidermoid cyst from teratoma.[227]

MOLECULAR TECHNIQUES FOR TESTICULAR GERM CELL TUMORS

Molecular pathology features of GCTs are shown in **Box 10**.

TESTICULAR GERM CELL TUMORS: GENOMIC EXPRESSION PROFILING

Genomic investigations have shown some differences between seminomas and NSGCTs; however, there is rarely good consistency in findings from study to study. Seminomas have demonstrated expression signatures of spermatogenesis-associated genes (PRAME, MAGEA4, SPAG1,

---

Box 9
Molecular pathology features of isochromosome 12p

- Candidate Genes

  SOX5

  JAW1

  K-RAS

  Cyclin D2

  Glucose transporter GLUT3

  Glycolytic enzymes GAPDH and TPI1

  Self-renewal and pluripotency genes NANOG, DPPA3, AND GDF3

Box 10
Molecular pathology features of GCTs

- Intratubular germ cell neoplasia

  WNT signaling cascade pathways

- Seminoma

  ETV4—progression to seminoma

  POU5F1 (Oct 3/4)—high in seminomas

  Spermatogenesis-associated genes (PRAME, MAGEA4, SPAG1, and HPX)

- Nonseminomatous GCT

  Regulatory genes (DNMT3B and SOX2)

  Small molecular weight keratins (KRT8 and KRT18)

  POU5F1 (Oct 3/4)—high in ECC; low in teratoma

  Telomerase—high in ECC; low in teratoma

  CGB—high in choriocarcinomas

  BMP2—high in YST

  LCN2—high in teratomas

- Spermatocytic seminoma

  Polyploidy

  Chromosome 9 gains

  Preserved telomerase activity

  Placental-like alkaline phosphatase (PLAP)—negative

  c-kit—less positive than other GCTs

Fig. *4.* Isochromosome 12p Isochromosome. 12p is the most consistent and specific chromosomal change found in testicular GCTs, with approximately 80% of adult NSGCTs and 50% or greater of pure seminomas possessing at least one i(12p). Isochromosome 12p occurs when it has lost the q arm and replaced it with a copy of its p arm.

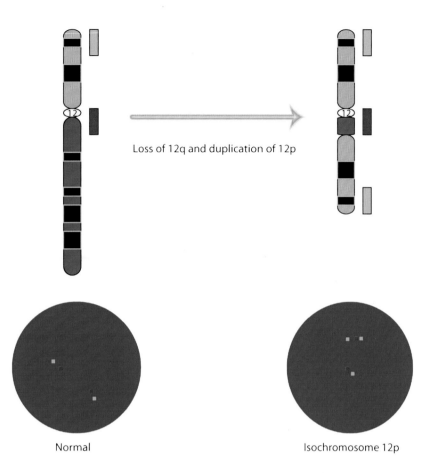

Loss of 12q and duplication of 12p

Normal   Isochromosome 12p

and HPX). Embryonal carcinomas have shown expression signatures of regulatory genes DNMT3B and SOX2, as well as small molecular weight keratins (KRT8 and KRT18).[228,229] Other work has potentially shown that seminomas can be divided or clustered into two groups: seminomas with a totally separate molecular profile and seminomas with a molecular profile similar to embryonal carcinomas.[230] With help of newer bioinformatics tools with databases, such as Ingenuity, WNT signaling cascade pathways have been implicated in the pathogenesis of ITGCN, along with ETV4 in the progression to seminoma.[231,232] Choriocarcinomas are associated with high expression of CGB. Yolk sac tumors show high BMP2, teratomas show high LCN2, and embryonal carcinomas show high POU5F1 (Oct3/4).[233]

Telomerase activity appears to be associated with certain histologic differentiation of GCTs. Highest expression is seen in embryonal carcinomas, with none seen in mature teratomas, postulating that its presence contributes to proliferative capacity.[234,235] Clinical relevance is still undetermined and evidence for telomere length differences in seminomas and NSGCTs

have yet to show relation with telomerase activity.[236]

Other molecular markers used often in immunohistochemistry are the c-kit tyrosine kinase receptor and Oct 3/4. Mutations of c-kit are seen in seminomas, while over-expression is seen in some NSGCTs and ITGCN.[237–241] The clinical significance is uncertain and even blockage of the pathway with imatinib has proven ineffective.[242,243] POU5F1 (Oct 3/4) is a very interesting marker that serves as a transcription factor, is expressed in pluripotent embryonic stem cells, and is down-regulated during differentiation.[195]

Malignant transformation of teratomas is an interesting morphologic finding. This is seen even in teratomas where the GCT component has clonal origin confirmed by presence of i(12p). The transformed malignancy contains abnormalities characteristic of the differentiated malignant phenotype, but studies—partially because the phenomenon is rare—are few.[188]

Spermatocytic seminomas, classically described as a variant of seminoma, appear to be a completely different from the other GCTs. Clinically, these tumors happen in older men and are

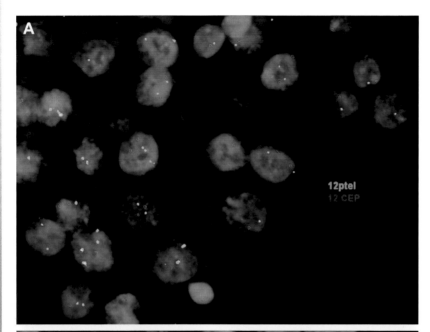

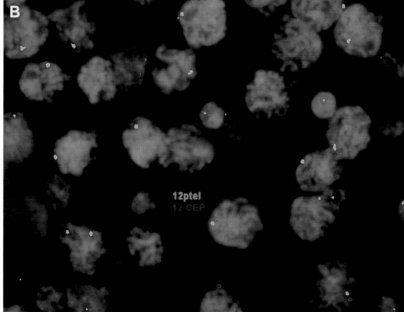

Fig. 5. In normal cells, FISH shows two centromeric (*red*) signals and two subtelomeric (*green*) signals for the p arm (*A*). When isochromosome 12p is present, there will be two green signals in close proximity to a red signal indicating the presence of a duplicate of the 12p arm (*B*) (*Courtesy of* K. Cieply, BS, Pittsburgh, PA).

associated with neither ITGCN nor loss of imprinting.[192,193] Moreover, immunohistochemical evidence supports this difference with these tumors showing negative PLAP and less c-kit positivity.[244,245] Cytogenetically, spermatocytic seminomas tend to be polyploid rather than aneuploid, as with GCTs. The only other consistent molecular profiles with these tumors are gain of chromosome 9 and preserved telomerase activity.[191,195,214,235,245–247]

NON-GERM CELL TUMORS: GENOMIC EXPRESSION PROFILING

There is little information on molecular biology of non-GCTs (**Box 11**). CGH and immunohistochemical analysis of Sertoli cell tumors show gains of entire chromosome X and over-expression of AMACR/P504S.[248–250] For Leydig cell tumors, the most frequent findings were gain of chromosome X, 19, or 19p, and loss of chromosome 8

Fig. 6. Amplification of 12p. When i(12p) is not found in GCTs, then there is usually some aberration of 12p with over-representation or rearrangement of that portion of chromosome 12. FISH shows amplification of the centromeric (*red*) signals and subtelomeric (*green*) signals; however, the number of the green signals is considerably more, indicating that there amplification of 12p (*Courtesy of* K. Cieply, BS, Pittsburgh, PA).

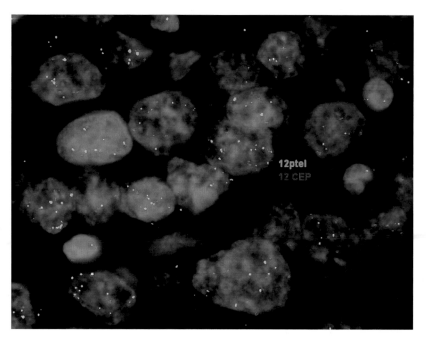

and 16.[248] Testis-specific protein Y-encoded gene (TSPY), a tandem repeat gene located on the Y chromosome, seems to play a role in predisposing dysgenetic gonads of intersex individuals to oncogenesis.[251] With diffuse large B-cell lymphoma in the testis, deletions of 6q are seen.[252]

TESTICULAR GERM CELL TUMORS:
EPIGENETICS PROFILING

There is considerable evidence that epigenetics and genomic imprinting are important pathogenetic determinants of GCTs. Epigenetic modifications are intimately involved in the regulation of expression of genes during normal development, but also represent a means by which expression of genes can be silenced during transformation. Epigenetic changes disturbing gene expression regulation may result in cancer development. Seminomas appear to be devoid of methylation, and nonseminomas have methylation levels comparable to other tumors. With NSGCT, DNA methylation seems to

---

Box 11
Molecular pathology features of non-GCTs

- Sertoli cell tumors—gain X, over-expression AMACR

- Leydig cell tumors—gain X, 19, or 19p; loss 8 and 16

- Intersex dysgenetic gonads—TSPY

- Diffuse large B-cell lymphoma—6q

---

increase with differentiation, with embryonal carcinomas harboring the lowest levels of DNA promoter hypermethylation, whereas well-differentiated teratomas display the highest.[253–255] Promoter methylation of tumor-suppressor genes is seen with testisin, a serine protease expressed in normal testis, and p53.[256] Other genes with aberrant promoter hypermethylation include genes PRSS21, MGMT, and RASSF1A aiding in malignant transformation.[188,257] Even POU5F1 (Oct 3/4) has been noted to have differential methylation in an upstream region.[258] As opposed to hypermethylation, hypomethylation with up-regulation of DNA-methyltransferase 3A expression has shown to modulate tumorigenesis.[259] A recent development is with the polycomb repressive complex responsible for the global control of gene expression and maintenance of pluripotency when brought to a genomic site, epigenetically modifying chromatin, usually via histone H3K27 methylation. The effect is repression of transcription across nonrepeat portions of the genome.[188] With genomic imprinting, testicular GCTs show a consistent expression of both parental alleles of the H19 and IGF2 genes, meaning that testicular GCTs of adults may develop from precursor cells in which the imprinting has been either erased or subjected to a consistent relaxation of its effect.[192,193,260]

TESTICULAR GERM CELL TUMORS:
MIRNA PROFILING

Some of the most novel work involves the role of nonprotein-encoding RNAs, such as miRNAs in

GCTs. It has been demonstrated that miRNAs are present in regulating differentiation of stem cells and are further retained in GCTs.[261,262] Because miRNAs target and interfere with the expression of mRNA, this also explains the discrepancies seen between high expression levels in genomic analysis and absent proteins seen in proteonomic analysis.[263] Interference by miRNA has been shown with the numbing of the p53 pathways in GCTs.[264,265]

TESTICULAR GERM CELL TUMORS: PROGNOSTIC MOLECULAR PROFILING

Much research is now focused on understanding the genetic basis of chemotherapy resistance. Most testicular GCTs are highly sensitive to cisplatin-based chemotherapy, with cure rates greater than 80%. It is those patients with lower likelihood of complete remission with chemotherapy that now pose a therapeutic dilemma. Clinically, the patients most likely to fail include high serum tumors markers and extrapulmonary metastases. The DNA damage response (DDR) is the concept of a physiologic anti-cancer barrier in early stages of cancer development. It is the unique lack of DDR activation in GCTs that reflects the biology of the gonocyte. Lack of DDR activation avoids the pressure to select for mutations in DDR genes, such as p53 or ATM.[266] Differentiated histology, such as teratomas, has notorious resistance to cisplatin-based chemotherapy. There is some belief that these tumors harbor p53 mutations; however, evidence for common inactivation of p53 in the development of cisplatin resistance is lacking.[267–269] Other genes implicated are multidrug resistance protein 1, a membrane glycoprotein drug efflux pump.[270] There is also some evidence that gene amplifications of 1q, 2p, 7q, 9q, 15q, and 20q, rather than 12p, may have an association with chemotherapy resistance.[271] Unfortunately, at this time with immunohistochemistry, there are no markers or panel of markers for cell proliferation or susceptibility to apoptosis and resistance that will predict response to treatment.[188] With gene expression profiling, new insights in the early pathogenetic events of GCT formation and therapy resistance will potentially identify better biomarkers for such difficult cases.

REFERENCES

1. Motzer RJ, Bander NH, Nanus DM. Renal-cell carcinoma. N Engl J Med 1996;335(12):865–75.
2. Eble JN, Sauter G, Epstein JI, et al. Tumours of the urinary system and male genital organs. WHO classification of tumours. Lyon (France): IARC Press; 2004.
3. Moch H, et al. Genetic aberrations detected by comparative genomic hybridization are associated with clinical outcome in renal cell carcinoma. Cancer Res 1996;56(1):27–30.
4. Lau LC, et al. Cytogenetic alterations in renal tumors: a study of 38 Southeast Asian patients. Cancer Genet Cytogenet 2007;175(1):1–7.
5. Gunawan B, et al. Cytogenetic and morphologic typing of 58 papillary renal cell carcinomas: evidence for a cytogenetic evolution of type 2 from type 1 tumors. Cancer Res 2003;63(19):6200–5.
6. Brunelli M, et al. Chromosomal gains in the sarcomatoid transformation of chromophobe renal cell carcinoma. Mod Pathol 2007;20(3):303–9.
7. Lonser RR, et al. von Hippel-Lindau disease. Lancet 2003;361(9374):2059–67.
8. Maher ER, et al. Clinical features and natural history of von Hippel-Lindau disease. Q J Med 1990; 77(283):1151–63.
9. Latif F, et al. Identification of the von Hippel-Lindau disease tumor suppressor gene. Science 1993; 260(5112):1317–20.
10. Iliopoulos O, et al. Tumour suppression by the human von Hippel-Lindau gene product. Nat Med 1995;1(8):822–6.
11. Na X, et al. Overproduction of vascular endothelial growth factor related to von Hippel-Lindau tumor suppressor gene mutations and hypoxia-inducible factor-1 alpha expression in renal cell carcinomas. J Urol 2003;170(2 Pt 1):588–92.
12. Van Erp F, et al. Chromosome 3 translocations and the risk to develop renal cell cancer: a Dutch intergroup study. Genet Couns 2003;14(2):149–54.
13. Stolle C, et al. Improved detection of germline mutations in the von Hippel-Lindau disease tumor suppressor gene. Hum Mutat 1998;12(6): 417–23.
14. Prowse AH, et al. Somatic inactivation of the VHL gene in Von Hippel-Lindau disease tumors. Am J Hum Genet 1997;60(4):765–71.
15. Lubensky IA, et al. Allelic deletions of the VHL gene detected in multiple microscopic clear cell renal lesions in von Hippel-Lindau disease patients. Am J Pathol 1996;149(6):2089–94.
16. Gnarra JR, et al. Post-transcriptional regulation of vascular endothelial growth factor mRNA by the product of the VHL tumor suppressor gene. Proc Natl Acad Sci U S A 1996;93(20):10589–94.
17. Shuin T, et al. Frequent somatic mutations and loss of heterozygosity of the von Hippel-Lindau tumor suppressor gene in primary human renal cell carcinomas. Cancer Res 1994;54(11):2852–5.
18. Conaway JW, Kamura T, Conaway RC. The Elongin BC complex and the von Hippel-Lindau tumor suppressor protein. Biochim Biophys Acta 1998; 1377(2):M49–54.

19. Duan DR, et al. Inhibition of transcription elongation by the VHL tumor suppressor protein. Science 1995;269(5229):1402–6.

20. Kibel A, et al. Binding of the von Hippel-Lindau tumor suppressor protein to Elongin B and C. Science 1995;269(5229):1444–6.

21. Maxwell PH, et al. The tumour suppressor protein VHL targets hypoxia-inducible factors for oxygen-dependent proteolysis. Nature 1999;399(6733):271–5.

22. Ohh M, et al. Ubiquitination of hypoxia-inducible factor requires direct binding to the beta-domain of the von Hippel-Lindau protein. Nat Cell Biol 2000;2(7):423–7.

23. Semenza GL. HIF-1 and mechanisms of hypoxia sensing. Curr Opin Cell Biol 2001;13(2):167–71.

24. Kaelin WG Jr. The von Hippel-Lindau tumor suppressor protein and clear cell renal carcinoma. Clin Cancer Res 2007;13(2 Pt 2):680s–4s.

25. Giaccia AJ, Simon MC, Johnson R. The biology of hypoxia: the role of oxygen sensing in development, normal function, and disease. Genes Dev 2004;18(18):2183–94.

26. Hanahan D, Folkman J. Patterns and emerging mechanisms of the angiogenic switch during tumorigenesis. Cell 1996;86(3):353–64.

27. Harris AL. Hypoxia—a key regulatory factor in tumour growth. Nat Rev Cancer 2002;2(1):38–47.

28. Saaristo A, Karpanen T, Alitalo K. Mechanisms of angiogenesis and their use in the inhibition of tumor growth and metastasis. Oncogene 2000;19(53):6122–9.

29. Veikkola T, Alitalo K. VEGFs, receptors and angiogenesis. Semin Cancer Biol 1999;9(3):211–20.

30. Dibb NJ, Dilworth SM, Mol CD. Switching on kinases: oncogenic activation of BRAF and the PDGFR family. Nat Rev Cancer 2004;4(9):718–27.

31. Bjarnegard M, et al. Endothelium-specific ablation of PDGFB leads to pericyte loss and glomerular, cardiac and placental abnormalities. Development 2004;131(8):1847–57.

32. Lindblom P, et al. Endothelial PDGF-B retention is required for proper investment of pericytes in the microvessel wall. Genes Dev 2003;17(15):1835–40.

33. Erler JT, et al. Lysyl oxidase is essential for hypoxia-induced metastasis. Nature 2006;440(7088):1222–6.

34. Ananth S, et al. Transforming growth factor beta1 is a target for the von Hippel-Lindau tumor suppressor and a critical growth factor for clear cell renal carcinoma. Cancer Res 1999;59(9):2210–6.

35. Esteban MA, et al. Regulation of E-cadherin expression by VHL and hypoxia-inducible factor. Cancer Res 2006;66(7):3567–75.

36. Staller P, et al. Chemokine receptor CXCR4 down-regulated by von Hippel-Lindau tumour suppressor pVHL. Nature 2003;425(6955):307–11.

37. Thiery JP. Epithelial-mesenchymal transitions in tumour progression. Nat Rev Cancer 2002;2(6):442–54.

38. Hay N. The Akt-mTOR tango and its relevance to cancer. Cancer Cell 2005;8(3):179–83.

39. Lam JS, et al. Protein expression profiles in renal cell carcinoma: staging, prognosis, and patient selection for clinical trials. Clin Cancer Res 2007;13(2 Pt 2):703s–8s.

40. Iliopoulos O. Molecular biology of renal cell cancer and the identification of therapeutic targets. J Clin Oncol 2006;24(35):5593–600.

41. Brugarolas J, et al. Regulation of mTOR function in response to hypoxia by REDD1 and the TSC1/TSC2 tumor suppressor complex. Genes Dev 2004;18(23):2893–904.

42. Brugarolas JB, et al. TSC2 regulates VEGF through mTOR-dependent and -independent pathways. Cancer Cell 2003;4(2):147–58.

43. Gao X, et al. Tsc tumour suppressor proteins antagonize amino-acid-TOR signaling. Nat Cell Biol 2002;4(9):699–704.

44. Inoki K, et al. TSC2 is phosphorylated and inhibited by Akt and suppresses mTOR signaling. Nat Cell Biol 2002;4(9):648–57.

45. Ito N, Rubin GM. Gigas, a Drosophila homolog of tuberous sclerosis gene product-2, regulates the cell cycle. Cell 1999;96(4):529–39.

46. Potter CJ, Pedraza LG, Xu T. Akt regulates growth by directly phosphorylating Tsc2. Nat Cell Biol 2002;4(9):658–65.

47. Tapon N, et al. The Drosophila tuberous sclerosis complex gene homologs restrict cell growth and cell proliferation. Cell 2001;105(3):345–55.

48. Hudson CC, et al. Regulation of hypoxia-inducible factor 1alpha expression and function by the mammalian target of rapamycin. Mol Cell Biol 2002;22(20):7004–14.

49. Majumder PK, et al. mTOR inhibition reverses Akt-dependent prostate intraepithelial neoplasia through regulation of apoptotic and HIF-1-dependent pathways. Nat Med 2004;10(6):594–601.

50. Brugarolas J. Renal-cell carcinoma—molecular pathways and therapies. N Engl J Med 2007;356(2):185–7.

51. Chen YT, et al. Messenger RNA expression ratios among four genes predict subtypes of renal cell carcinoma and distinguish oncocytoma from carcinoma. Clin Cancer Res 2005;11(18):6558–66.

52. Crossey PA, et al. Identification of intragenic mutations in the von Hippel-Lindau disease tumour suppressor gene and correlation with disease phenotype. Hum Mol Genet 1994;3(8):1303–8.

53. Clifford SC, et al. Contrasting effects on HIF-1alpha regulation by disease-causing pVHL mutations correlate with patterns of tumourigenesis in von

Hippel-Lindau disease. Hum Mol Genet 2001; 10(10):1029–38.

54. Hoffman MA, et al. von Hippel-Lindau protein mutants linked to type 2C VHL disease preserve the ability to downregulate HIF. Hum Mol Genet 2001; 10(10):1019–27.

55. Knauth K, et al. Renal cell carcinoma risk in type 2 von Hippel-Lindau disease correlates with defects in pVHL stability and HIF-1alpha interactions. Oncogene 2006;25(3):370–7.

56. Kondo K, et al. Inhibition of HIF2alpha is sufficient to suppress pVHL-defective tumor growth. PLoS Biol 2003;1(3):E83.

57. Maranchie JK, et al. The contribution of VHL substrate binding and HIF1-alpha to the phenotype of VHL loss in renal cell carcinoma. Cancer Cell 2002;1(3):247–55.

58. Kuznetsova AV, et al. von Hippel-Lindau protein binds hyperphosphorylated large subunit of RNA polymerase II through a proline hydroxylation motif and targets it for ubiquitination. Proc Natl Acad Sci U S A 2003;100(5):2706–11.

59. Na X, et al. Identification of the RNA polymerase II subunit hsRPB7 as a novel target of the von Hippel-Lindau protein. EMBO J 2003;22(16): 4249–59.

60. Ohh M, et al. The von Hippel-Lindau tumor suppressor protein is required for proper assembly of an extracellular fibronectin matrix. Mol Cell 1998; 1(7):959–68.

61. Roe JS, et al. p53 stabilization and transactivation by a von Hippel-Lindau protein. Mol Cell 2006; 22(3):395–405.

62. Tang N, et al. pVHL function is essential for endothelial extracellular matrix deposition. Mol Cell Biol 2006;26(7):2519–30.

63. Zhou MI, et al. Jade-1, a candidate renal tumor suppressor that promotes apoptosis. Proc Natl Acad Sci U S A 2005;102(31):11035–40.

64. Duh FM, et al. Gene structure of the human MET proto-oncogene. Oncogene 1997;15(13):1583–6.

65. Lubensky IA, et al. Hereditary and sporadic papillary renal carcinomas with c-met mutations share a distinct morphological phenotype. Am J Pathol 1999;155(2):517–26.

66. Boccaccio C, Comoglio PM. Invasive growth: a MET-driven genetic programme for cancer and stem cells. Nat Rev Cancer 2006;6(8):637–45.

67. Giordano S, et al. Transfer of motogenic and invasive response to scatter factor/hepatocyte growth factor by transfection of human MET protooncogene. Proc Natl Acad Sci U S A 1993;90(2): 649–53.

68. Ponzetto C, et al. A multifunctional docking site mediates signaling and transformation by the hepatocyte growth factor/scatter factor receptor family. Cell 1994;77(2):261–71.

69. Furge KA, et al. Identification of deregulated oncogenic pathways in renal cell carcinoma: an integrated oncogenomic approach based on gene expression profiling. Oncogene 2007;26(9):1346–50.

70. Comoglio PM. Pathway specificity for Met signalling. Nat Cell Biol 2001;3(7):E161–2.

71. Giordano S, et al. The semaphorin 4D receptor controls invasive growth by coupling with Met. Nat Cell Biol 2002;4(9):720–4.

72. Pennacchietti S, et al. Hypoxia promotes invasive growth by transcriptional activation of the met protooncogene. Cancer Cell 2003;3(4):347–61.

73. Launonen V, et al. Inherited susceptibility to uterine leiomyomas and renal cell cancer. Proc Natl Acad Sci U S A 2001;98(6):3387–92.

74. Merino MJ, et al. The morphologic spectrum of kidney tumors in hereditary leiomyomatosis and renal cell carcinoma (HLRCC) syndrome. Am J Surg Pathol 2007;31(10):1578–85.

75. Alam NA, Olpin S, Leigh IM. Fumarate hydratase mutations and predisposition to cutaneous leiomyomas, uterine leiomyomas and renal cancer. Br J Dermatol 2005;153(1):11–7.

76. Lehtonen R, et al. Biallelic inactivation of fumarate hydratase (FH) occurs in nonsyndromic uterine leiomyomas but is rare in other tumors. Am J Pathol 2004;164(1):17–22.

77. Morris MR, et al. Molecular genetic analysis of FIH-1, FH, and SDHB candidate tumour suppressor genes in renal cell carcinoma. J Clin Pathol 2004;57(7): 706–11.

78. Toro JR, et al. Birt-Hogg-Dube syndrome: a novel marker of kidney neoplasia. Arch Dermatol 1999; 135(10):1195–202.

79. Isaacs JS, et al. HIF overexpression correlates with biallelic loss of fumarate hydratase in renal cancer: novel role of fumarate in regulation of HIF stability. Cancer Cell 2005;8(2):143–53.

80. Selak MA, et al. Succinate links TCA cycle dysfunction to oncogenesis by inhibiting HIF-alpha prolyl hydroxylase. Cancer Cell 2005;7(1):77–85.

81. Birt AR, Hogg GR, Dube WJ. Hereditary multiple fibrofolliculomas with trichodiscomas and acrochordons. Arch Dermatol 1977;113(12):1674–7.

82. Nickerson ML, et al. Mutations in a novel gene lead to kidney tumors, lung wall defects, and benign tumors of the hair follicle in patients with the Birt-Hogg-Dube syndrome. Cancer Cell 2002;2(2): 157–64.

83. Roth JS, et al. Bilateral renal cell carcinoma in the Birt-Hogg-Dube syndrome. J Am Acad Dermatol 1993;29(6):1055–6.

84. Schmidt LS, et al. Birt-Hogg-Dube syndrome, a genodermatosis associated with spontaneous pneumothorax and kidney neoplasia, maps to chromosome 17p11.2. Am J Hum Genet 2001; 69(4):876–82.

85. Shen SS, et al. Recently described and emphasized entities of renal neoplasms. Arch Pathol Lab Med 2007;131(8):1234–43.

86. Argani P, et al. Xp11 translocation renal cell carcinoma in adults: expanded clinical, pathologic, and genetic spectrum. Am J Surg Pathol 2007; 31(8):1149–60.

87. Ramphal R, et al. Pediatric renal cell carcinoma: clinical, pathologic, and molecular abnormalities associated with the members of the mit transcription factor family. Am J Clin Pathol 2006;126(3): 349–64.

88. Bruder E, et al. Morphologic and molecular characterization of renal cell carcinoma in children and young adults. Am J Surg Pathol 2004;28(9):1117–32.

89. Argani P, Ladanyi M. Recent advances in pediatric renal neoplasia. Adv Anat Pathol 2003;10(5): 243–60.

90. Shen SS, et al. Mucinous tubular and spindle cell carcinoma of kidney is probably a variant of papillary renal cell carcinoma with spindle cell features. Ann Diagn Pathol 2007;11(1):13–21.

91. Martignoni G, et al. Renal angiomyolipoma with epithelioid sarcomatous transformation and metastases: demonstration of the same genetic defects in the primary and metastatic lesions. Am J Surg Pathol 2000;24(6):889–94.

92. Argani P, et al. Primary renal synovial sarcoma: molecular and morphologic delineation of an entity previously included among embryonal sarcomas of the kidney. Am J Surg Pathol 2000;24(8): 1087–96.

93. Huang CC, et al. Classification of malignant pediatric renal tumors by gene expression. Pediatr Blood Cancer 2006;46(7):728–38.

94. Knezevich SR, et al. ETV6-NTRK3 gene fusions and trisomy 11 establish a histogenetic link between mesoblastic nephroma and congenital fibrosarcoma. Cancer Res 1998;58(22):5046–8.

95. Knezevich SR, et al. A novel ETV6-NTRK3 gene fusion in congenital fibrosarcoma. Nat Genet 1998;18(2):184–7.

96. Cabrita MA, Christofori G. Sprouty proteins: antagonists of endothelial cell signaling and more. Thromb Haemost 2003;90(4):586–90.

97. Inoue A, et al. Transcription factor EGR3 is involved in the estrogen-signaling pathway in breast cancer cells. J Mol Endocrinol 2004;32(3):649–61.

98. Skubitz KM, et al. Gene expression in giant-cell tumors. J Lab Clin Med 2004;144(4):193–200.

99. Bonnin JM, et al. The association of embryonal tumors originating in the kidney and in the brain. A report of seven cases. Cancer 1984;54(10): 2137–46.

100. Vujanic GM, et al. Rhabdoid tumour of the kidney: a clinicopathological study of 22 patients from the International Society of Paediatric Oncology (SIOP) nephroblastoma file. Histopathology 1996; 28(4):333–40.

101. Weeks DA, et al. Renal neoplasms mimicking rhabdoid tumor of kidney. A report from the National Wilms' Tumor Study Pathology Center. Am J Surg Pathol 1991;15(11):1042–54.

102. Versteege I, et al. Truncating mutations of hSNF5/INI1 in aggressive paediatric cancer. Nature 1998;394(6689):203–6.

103. Hoot AC, et al. Immunohistochemical analysis of hSNF5/INI1 distinguishes renal and extra-renal malignant rhabdoid tumors from other pediatric soft tissue tumors. Am J Surg Pathol 2004;28(11): 1485–91.

104. Pomeroy SL, et al. Prediction of central nervous system embryonal tumour outcome based on gene expression. Nature 2002;415(6870):436–42.

105. Argani P, et al. Clear cell sarcoma of the kidney: a review of 351 cases from the National Wilms Tumor Study Group Pathology Center. Am J Surg Pathol 2000;24(1):4–18.

106. Seibel NL, et al. Effect of duration of treatment on treatment outcome for patients with clear-cell sarcoma of the kidney: a report from the National Wilms' Tumor Study Group. J Clin Oncol 2004; 22(3):468–73.

107. Argani P, et al. Detection of the ETV6-NTRK3 chimeric RNA of infantile fibrosarcoma/cellular congenital mesoblastic nephroma in paraffin-embedded tissue: application to challenging pediatric renal stromal tumors. Mod Pathol 2000;13(1): 29–36.

108. Cutcliffe C, et al. Clear cell sarcoma of the kidney: up-regulation of neural markers with activation of the sonic hedgehog and Akt pathways. Clin Cancer Res 2005;11(22):7986–94.

109. Mahlapuu M, Enerback S, Carlsson P. Haploinsufficiency of the forkhead gene Foxf1, a target for Sonic Hedgehog signaling, causes lung and foregut malformations. Development 2001;128(12): 2397–406.

110. Coppes MJ, Haber DA, Grundy PE. Genetic events in the development of Wilms' tumor. N Engl J Med 1994;331(9):586–90.

111. Green DM, et al. Screening of children with hemihypertrophy, aniridia, and Beckwith-Wiedemann syndrome in patients with Wilms tumor: a report from the National Wilms Tumor Study. Med Pediatr Oncol 1993;21(3):188–92.

112. Li CM, et al. Gene expression in Wilms' tumor mimics the earliest committed stage in the metanephric mesenchymal-epithelial transition. Am J Pathol 2002;160(6):2181–90.

113. Gery S, et al. TMEFF1 and brain tumors. Oncogene 2003;22(18):2723–7.

114. Kim S, Chung DH. Pediatric solid malignancies: neuroblastoma and Wilms' tumor. Surg Clin North Am 2006;86(2):469–87, xi.

115. Sredni ST, et al. Immunohistochemical detection of p53 protein expression as a prognostic indicator in Wilms tumor. Med Pediatr Oncol 2001;37(5):455–8.

116. Salem M, et al. Association between the HER2 expression and histological differentiation in Wilms tumor. Pediatr Surg Int 2006;22(11):891–6.

117. Zirn B, et al. Expression profiling of Wilms tumors reveals new candidate genes for different clinical parameters. Int J Cancer 2006;118(8):1954–62.

118. Young AN, et al. Expression profiling of renal epithelial neoplasms: a method for tumor classification and discovery of diagnostic molecular markers. Am J Pathol 2001;158(5):1639–51.

119. Higgins JP, et al. Gene expression patterns in renal cell carcinoma assessed by complementary DNA microarray. Am J Pathol 2003;162(3):925–32.

120. Young AN, et al. Beta defensin-1, parvalbumin, and vimentin: a panel of diagnostic immunohistochemical markers for renal tumors derived from gene expression profiling studies using cDNA microarrays. Am J Surg Pathol 2003;27(2):199–205.

121. Moch H, et al. High-throughput tissue microarray analysis to evaluate genes uncovered by cDNA microarray screening in renal cell carcinoma. Am J Pathol 1999;154(4):981–6.

122. Avery AK, et al. Use of antibodies to RCC and CD10 in the differential diagnosis of renal neoplasms. Am J Surg Pathol 2000;24(2):203–10.

123. Yao M, et al. Gene expression analysis of renal carcinoma: adipose differentiation-related protein as a potential diagnostic and prognostic biomarker for clear-cell renal carcinoma. J Pathol 2005; 205(3):377–87.

124. Takahashi M, et al. Molecular subclassification of kidney tumors and the discovery of new diagnostic markers. Oncogene 2003;22(43):6810–8.

125. Chuang ST, et al. Overexpression of glutathione s-transferase alpha in clear cell renal cell carcinoma. Am J Clin Pathol 2005;123(3):421–9.

126. Saito T, et al. MHC class II antigen-associated invariant chain on renal cell cancer may contribute to the anti-tumor immune response of the host. Cancer Lett 1997;115(1):121–7.

127. Yamazaki K, et al. Overexpression of KIT in chromophobe renal cell carcinoma. Oncogene 2003; 22(6):847–52.

128. Petit A, et al. KIT expression in chromophobe renal cell carcinoma: comparative immunohistochemical analysis of KIT expression in different renal cell neoplasms. Am J Surg Pathol 2004;28(5):676–8.

129. Tickoo SK, et al. Ultrastructural observations on mitochondria and microvesicles in renal oncocytoma, chromophobe renal cell carcinoma, and eosinophilic variant of conventional (clear cell) renal cell carcinoma. Am J Surg Pathol 2000;24(9):1247–56.

130. Tretiakova MS, et al. Expression of alpha-methylacyl-CoA racemase in papillary renal cell carcinoma. Am J Surg Pathol 2004;28(1):69–76.

131. Ozcan A, et al. Expression of GLUT1 in primary renal tumors: morphologic and biologic implications. Am J Clin Pathol 2007;128(2):245–54.

132. Martignoni G, et al. Parvalbumin is constantly expressed in chromophobe renal carcinoma. Mod Pathol 2001;14(8):760–7.

133. Rohan S, et al. Gene expression profiling separates chromophobe renal cell carcinoma from oncocytoma and identifies vesicular transport and cell junction proteins as differentially expressed genes. Clin Cancer Res 2006;12(23):6937–45.

134. Schuetz AN, et al. Molecular classification of renal tumors by gene expression profiling. J Mol Diagn 2005;7(2):206–18.

135. Young AN, et al. Renal epithelial neoplasms: diagnostic applications of gene expression profiling. Adv Anat Pathol 2008;15(1):28–38.

136. Weiss RH, et al. p21 is a prognostic marker for renal cell carcinoma: implications for novel therapeutic approaches. J Urol 2007;177(1):63–8 [discussion: 68–9].

137. Phuoc NB, et al. Immunohistochemical analysis with multiple antibodies in search of prognostic markers for clear cell renal cell carcinoma. Urology 2007;69(5):843–8.

138. Zigeuner R, et al. Value of p53 as a prognostic marker in histologic subtypes of renal cell carcinoma: a systematic analysis of primary and metastatic tumor tissue. Urology 2004;63(4):651–5.

139. Tollefson MK, et al. Ki-67 and coagulative tumor necrosis are independent predictors of poor outcome for patients with clear cell renal cell carcinoma and not surrogates for each other. Cancer 2007;110(4): 783–90.

140. Baldewijns MM, et al. High-grade clear cell renal cell carcinoma has a higher angiogenic activity than low-grade renal cell carcinoma based on histomorphological quantification and qRT-PCR mRNA expression profile. Br J Cancer 2007;96(12):1888–95.

141. Banks RE, et al. Genetic and epigenetic analysis of von Hippel-Lindau (VHL) gene alterations and relationship with clinical variables in sporadic renal cancer. Cancer Res 2006;66(4):2000–11.

142. Kondo K, et al. Comprehensive mutational analysis of the VHL gene in sporadic renal cell carcinoma: relationship to clinicopathological parameters. Genes Chromosomes Cancer 2002;34(1):58–68.

143. Brauch H, et al. VHL alterations in human clear cell renal cell carcinoma: association with advanced tumor stage and a novel hot spot mutation. Cancer Res 2000;60(7):1942–8.

144. Dahl E, et al. Frequent loss of SFRP1 expression in multiple human solid tumours: association with aberrant promoter methylation in renal cell carcinoma. Oncogene 2007;26(38):5680–91.

145. Gonzalgo ML, et al. Molecular profiling and classification of sporadic renal cell carcinoma by quantitative methylation analysis. Clin Cancer Res 2004; 10(21):7276–83.

146. Renshaw AA, Richie JP. Subtypes of renal cell carcinoma. Different onset and sites of metastatic disease. Am J Clin Pathol 1999;111(4):539–43.

147. Amin MB, et al. Prognostic impact of histologic subtyping of adult renal epithelial neoplasms: an experience of 405 cases. Am J Surg Pathol 2002; 26(3):281–91.

148. Takahashi S, et al. Renal cell adenomas and carcinomas in hemodialysis patients: relationship between hemodialysis period and development of lesions. Acta Pathol Jpn 1993;43(11):674–82.

149. Cohen D, Zhou M. Molecular genetics of familial renal cell carcinoma syndromes. Clin Lab Med 2005;25(2):259–77.

150. Zisman A, et al. Improved prognostication of renal cell carcinoma using an integrated staging system. J Clin Oncol 2001;19(6):1649–57.

151. Kattan MW, et al. A postoperative prognostic nomogram for renal cell carcinoma. J Urol 2001; 166(1):63–7.

152. Ficarra V, et al. External validation of the Mayo Clinic Stage, Size, Grade and Necrosis (SSIGN) score to predict cancer specific survival using a European series of conventional renal cell carcinoma. J Urol 2006;175(4):1235–9.

153. Motzer RJ, et al. Survival and prognostic stratification of 670 patients with advanced renal cell carcinoma. J Clin Oncol 1999;17(8):2530–40.

154. Tsui KH, et al. Prognostic indicators for renal cell carcinoma: a multivariate analysis of 643 patients using the revised 1997 TNM staging criteria. J Urol 2000;163(4):1090–5, quiz 1295.

155. Sengupta S, et al. The preoperative erythrocyte sedimentation rate is an independent prognostic factor in renal cell carcinoma. Cancer 2006; 106(2):304–12.

156. Lamb GW, et al. The relationship between the preoperative systemic inflammatory response and cancer-specific survival in patients undergoing potentially curative resection for renal clear cell cancer. Br J Cancer 2006;94(6):781–4.

157. O'Keefe SC, et al. Thrombocytosis is associated with a significant increase in the cancer specific death rate after radical nephrectomy. J Urol 2002; 168(4 Pt 1):1378–80.

158. Ljungberg B. Prognostic markers in renal cell carcinoma. Curr Opin Urol 2007;17(5):303–8.

159. Fyfe G, et al. Results of treatment of 255 patients with metastatic renal cell carcinoma who received high-dose recombinant interleukin-2 therapy. J Clin Oncol 1995;13(3):688–96.

160. Atkins MB, Regan M, McDermott D. Update on the role of interleukin 2 and other cytokines in the treatment of patients with stage IV renal carcinoma. Clin Cancer Res 2004;10(18 Pt 2):6342.

161. Atkins MB, et al. Innovations and challenges in renal cancer: consensus statement from the first International Conference. Clin Cancer Res 2004; 10(18 Pt 2):6277S–81S.

162. Motzer RJ, et al. Treatment outcome and survival associated with metastatic renal cell carcinoma of non-clear-cell histology. J Clin Oncol 2002;20(9):2376–81.

163. Stadler WM. Therapeutic options for variant renal cancer: a true orphan disease. Clin Cancer Res 2004;10(18 Pt 2):6393S–6S.

164. Gordon MS. Novel antiangiogenic therapies for renal cell cancer. Clin Cancer Res 2004;10(18 Pt 2): 6377S–81S.

165. Yang JC, et al. A randomized trial of bevacizumab, an anti-vascular endothelial growth factor antibody, for metastatic renal cancer. N Engl J Med 2003; 349(5):427–34.

166. Larkin JM, Chowdhury S, Gore ME. Drug insight: advances in renal cell carcinoma and the role of targeted therapies. Nat Clin Pract Oncol 2007; 4(8):470–9.

167. Escudier B, et al. Sorafenib in advanced clear-cell renal-cell carcinoma. N Engl J Med 2007;356(2): 125–34.

168. Fabian MA, et al. A small molecule-kinase interaction map for clinical kinase inhibitors. Nat Biotechnol 2005;23(3):329–36.

169. Motzer RJ, et al. Sunitinib versus interferon alfa in metastatic renal-cell carcinoma. N Engl J Med 2007;356(2):115–24.

170. Motzer RJ, et al. Sunitinib in patients with metastatic renal cell carcinoma. JAMA 2006;295(21): 2516–24.

171. Pantuck AJ, et al. Prognostic relevance of the mTOR pathway in renal cell carcinoma: implications for molecular patient selection for targeted therapy. Cancer 2007;109(11):2257–67.

172. Thompson RH, et al. Tumor B7-H1 is associated with poor prognosis in renal cell carcinoma patients with long-term follow-up. Cancer Res 2006; 66(7):3381–5.

173. Law CL, et al. Lymphocyte activation antigen CD70 expressed by renal cell carcinoma is a potential therapeutic target for anti-CD70 antibody-drug conjugates. Cancer Res 2006;66(4):2328–37.

174. Said J. Biomarker discovery in urogenital cancer. Biomarkers 2005;10(Suppl 1):S83–6.

175. Amatschek S, et al. Tissue-wide expression profiling using cDNA subtraction and microarrays to identify tumor-specific genes. Cancer Res 2004; 64(3):844–56.

176. Kopper L, Timar J. Genomics of renal cell cancer—does it provide breakthrough? Pathol Oncol Res 2006;12(1):5–11.

177. Morikawa T, et al. Identification of Toll-like receptor 3 as a potential therapeutic target in clear cell renal cell carcinoma. Clin Cancer Res 2007;13(19):5703–9.

178. Christensen JG, et al. A selective small molecule inhibitor of c-Met kinase inhibits c-Met-dependent phenotypes in vitro and exhibits cytoreductive anti-tumor activity in vivo. Cancer Res 2003;63(21):7345–55.

179. Sattler M, et al. A novel small molecule met inhibitor induces apoptosis in cells transformed by the oncogenic TPR-MET tyrosine kinase. Cancer Res 2003;63(17):5462–9.

180. Burgess T, et al. Fully human monoclonal antibodies to hepatocyte growth factor with therapeutic potential against hepatocyte growth factor/c-Met-dependent human tumors. Cancer Res 2006;66(3):1721–9.

181. Bottaro DP, et al. Identification of the hepatocyte growth factor receptor as the c-met proto-oncogene product. Science 1991;251(4995):802–4.

182. Bor P, et al. Screening for Y microdeletions in men with testicular cancer and undescended testis. J Assist Reprod Genet 2006;23(1):41–5.

183. Rapley E. Susceptibility alleles for testicular germ cell tumour: a review. Int J Androl 2007;30(4):242–50 [discussion: 250].

184. Bianchi NO, Richard SM, Pavicic W. Y chromosome instability in testicular cancer. Mutat Res 2006;612(3):172–88.

185. Tsuchiya N, et al. Association of XRCC1 gene polymorphisms with the susceptibility and chromosomal aberration of testicular germ cell tumors. Int J Oncol 2006;28(5):1217–23.

186. Crockford GP, et al. Genome-wide linkage screen for testicular germ cell tumour susceptibility loci. Hum Mol Genet 2006;15(3):443–51.

187. Nathanson KL, et al. The Y deletion gr/gr and susceptibility to testicular germ cell tumor. Am J Hum Genet 2005;77(6):1034–43.

188. Houldsworth J, et al. Biology and genetics of adult male germ cell tumors. J Clin Oncol 2006;24(35):5512–8.

189. Giwercman A, et al. Testicular cancer and molecular genetics. Andrologia 2005;37(6):224–5.

190. Jorgensen N, et al. DNA content and expression of tumour markers in germ cells adjacent to germ cell tumours in childhood: probably a different origin for infantile and adolescent germ cell tumours. J Pathol 1995;176(3):269–78.

191. Looijenga LH, de Munnik H, Oosterhuis JW. A molecular model for the development of germ cell cancer. Int J Cancer 1999;83(6):809–14.

192. van Gurp RJ, et al. Biallelic expression of the H19 and IGF2 genes in human testicular germ cell tumors. J Natl Cancer Inst 1994;86(14):1070–5.

193. Verkerk AJ, et al. Unique expression patterns of H19 in human testicular cancers of different etiology. Oncogene 1997;14(1):95–107.

194. Bussey KJ, et al. Chromosome abnormalities of eighty-one pediatric germ cell tumors: sex-, age-, site-, and histopathology-related differences—a Children's Cancer Group study. Genes Chromosomes Cancer 1999;25(2):134–46.

195. Reuter VE. Origins and molecular biology of testicular germ cell tumors. Mod Pathol 2005;18(Suppl 2):S51–60.

196. Hittmair A, et al. Testicular seminomas are aneuploid tumors. Lab Invest 1995;72(1):70–4.

197. Rosenberg C, et al. Chromosomal gains and losses in testicular germ cell tumors of adolescents and adults investigated by a modified comparative genomic hybridization approach. Lab Invest 1999;79(12):1447–51.

198. Baretton G, et al. Deoxyribonucleic acid ploidy in seminomas with and without syncytiotrophoblastic cells. J Urol 1994;151(1):67–71.

199. de Graaff WE, et al. Ploidy of testicular carcinoma in situ. Lab Invest 1992;66(2):166–8.

200. el-Naggar AK, et al. DNA ploidy in testicular germ cell neoplasms. Histogenetic and clinical implications. Am J Surg Pathol 1992;16(6):611–8.

201. Skotheim RI, et al. Novel genomic aberrations in testicular germ cell tumors by array-CGH, and associated gene expression changes. Cell Oncol 2006;28(5–6):315–26.

202. Rosenberg C, et al. Comparative genomic hybridization in hypotriploid/hyperdiploid tumors. Cytometry 1997;29(2):113–21.

203. Looijenga LH, et al. Testicular germ cell tumors of adults show deletions of chromosomal bands 11p13 and 11p15.5, but no abnormalities within the zinc-finger regions and exons 2 and 6 of the Wilms' tumor 1 gene. Genes Chromosomes Cancer 1994;9(3):153–60.

204. de Jong B, et al. Pathogenesis of adult testicular germ cell tumors. A cytogenetic model. Cancer Genet Cytogenet 1990;48(2):143–67.

205. Mayer F, et al. Aneuploidy of human testicular germ cell tumors is associated with amplification of centrosomes. Oncogene 2003;22(25):3859–66.

206. Oosterhuis JW, et al. Chromosomal constitution and developmental potential of human germ cell tumors and teratomas. Cancer Genet Cytogenet 1997;95(1):96–102.

207. Bergthorsson JT, et al. A genome-wide study of allelic imbalance in human testicular germ cell tumors using microsatellite markers. Cancer Genet Cytogenet 2006;164(1):1–9.

208. McIntyre A, et al. Defining minimum genomic regions of imbalance involved in testicular germ cell tumors of adolescents and adults through genome wide microarray analysis of cDNA clones. Oncogene 2004;23(56):9142–7.

209. Skotheim RI, et al. Candidate genes for testicular cancer evaluated by in situ protein expression analyses on tissue microarrays. Neoplasia 2003; 5(5):397–404.

210. Henegariu O, et al. Characterization of gains, losses, and regional amplification in testicular germ cell tumor cell lines by comparative genomic hybridization. Cancer Genet Cytogenet 2004;148(1): 14–20.

211. van Echten J, et al. No recurrent structural abnormalities apart from i(12 p) in primary germ cell tumors of the adult testis. Genes Chromosomes Cancer 1995;14(2):133–44.

212. Atkin NB, Baker MC. i(12 p): specific chromosomal marker in seminoma and malignant teratoma of the testis? Cancer Genet Cytogenet 1983;10(2): 199–204.

213. Bosl GJ, et al. Clinical relevance of the i(12 p) marker chromosome in germ cell tumors. J Natl Cancer Inst 1994;86(5):349–55.

214. McIntyre A, et al. Genomic copy number and expression patterns in testicular germ cell tumours. Br J Cancer 2007;97(12):1707–12.

215. Rodriguez E, et al. Molecular cytogenetic analysis of i(12 p)-negative human male germ cell tumors. Genes Chromosomes Cancer 1993;8(4):230–6.

216. Roelofs H, et al. Restricted 12 p amplification and RAS mutation in human germ cell tumors of the adult testis. Am J Pathol 2000;157(4):1155–66.

217. Suijkerbuijk RF, et al. Overrepresentation of chromosome 12 p sequences and karyotypic evolution in i(12 p)-negative testicular germ-cell tumors revealed by fluorescence in situ hybridization. Cancer Genet Cytogenet 1993;70(2):85–93.

218. Chaganti RS, Rodriguez E, Bosl GJ. Cytogenetics of male germ-cell tumors. Urol Clin North Am 1993;20(1):55–66.

219. Rosenberg C, et al. Overrepresentation of the short arm of chromosome 12 is related to invasive growth of human testicular seminomas and nonseminomas. Oncogene 2000;19(51):5858–62.

220. Sandberg AA, Meloni AM, Suijkerbuijk RF. Reviews of chromosome studies in urological tumors. III. Cytogenetics and genes in testicular tumors. J Urol 1996;155(5):1531–56.

221. Vos A, et al. Cytogenetics of carcinoma in situ of the testis. Cancer Genet Cytogenet 1990;46(1):75–81.

222. Mostert MC, et al. Identification of the critical region of 12 p over-representation in testicular germ cell tumors of adolescents and adults. Oncogene 1998;16(20):2617–27.

223. Suijkerbuijk RF, et al. Amplification of chromosome subregion 12p11.2-p12.1 in a metastasis of an i(12 p)-negative seminoma: relationship to tumor progression? Cancer Genet Cytogenet 1994; 78(2):145–52.

224. Schmidt BA, et al. Up-regulation of cyclin-dependent kinase 4/cyclin D2 expression but down-regulation of cyclin-dependent kinase 2/cyclin E in testicular germ cell tumors. Cancer Res 2001; 61(10):4214–21.

225. Sherr CJ. Mammalian G1 cyclins. Cell 1993;73(6): 1059–65.

226. Sicinski P, et al. Cyclin D2 is an FSH-responsive gene involved in gonadal cell proliferation and oncogenesis. Nature 1996;384(6608):470–4.

227. Cheng L, et al. Interphase fluorescence in situ hybridization analysis of chromosome 12 p abnormalities is useful for distinguishing epidermoid cysts of the testis from pure mature teratoma. Clin Cancer Res 2006;12(19):5668–72.

228. Biermann K, et al. Genome-wide expression profiling reveals new insights into pathogenesis and progression of testicular germ cell tumors. Cancer Genomics Proteomics 2007;4(5):359–67.

229. Biermann K, et al. Gene expression profiling identifies new biological markers of neoplastic germ cells. Anticancer Res 2007;27(5A):3091–100.

230. Hofer MD, et al. Identification of two molecular groups of seminomas by using expression and tissue microarrays. Clin Cancer Res 2005;11(16): 5722–9.

231. Almstrup K, et al. Improved gene expression signature of testicular carcinoma in situ. Int J Androl 2007;30(4):292–302 [discussion: 303].

232. Gashaw I, et al. Gene signatures of testicular seminoma with emphasis on expression of ets variant gene 4. Cell Mol Life Sci 2005;62(19–20):2359–68.

233. Korkola JE, et al. Gene expression-based classification of nonseminomatous male germ cell tumors. Oncogene 2005;24(32):5101–7.

234. Albanell J, et al. Telomerase activity in germ cell cancers and mature teratomas. J Natl Cancer Inst 1999;91(15):1321–6.

235. Delgado R, et al. Expression of the RNA component of human telomerase in adult testicular germ cell neoplasia. Cancer 1999;86(9):1802–11.

236. Nowak R, et al. Germ cell-like telomeric length homeostasis in nonseminomatous testicular germ cell tumors. Oncogene 2000;19(35):4075–8.

237. Jacobsen GK, Norgaard-Pedersen B. Placental alkaline phosphatase in testicular germ cell tumours and in carcinoma-in-situ of the testis. An immunohistochemical study. Acta Pathol Microbiol Immunol Scand [A] 1984;92(5):323–9.

238. Jorgensen N, et al. Expression of immunohistochemical markers for testicular carcinoma in situ

by normal human fetal germ cells. Lab Invest 1995; 72(2):223–31.

239. Tian Q, et al. Activating c-kit gene mutations in human germ cell tumors. Am J Pathol 1999; 154(6):1643–7.

240. Izquierdo MA, et al. Differential expression of the c-kit proto-oncogene in germ cell tumours. J Pathol 1995;177(3):253–8.

241. Rajpert-De Meyts E, Skakkebaek NE. Expression of the c-kit protein product in carcinoma-in-situ and invasive testicular germ cell tumours. Int J Androl 1994;17(2):85–92.

242. Einhorn LH, et al. Phase II study of imatinib mesylate in chemotherapy refractory germ cell tumors expressing KIT. Am J Clin Oncol 2006;29(1):12–3.

243. McIntyre A, et al. Amplification and overexpression of the KIT gene is associated with progression in the seminoma subtype of testicular germ cell tumors of adolescents and adults. Cancer Res 2005;65(18):8085–9.

244. Kraggerud SM, et al. Spermatocytic seminoma as compared to classical seminoma: an immunohistochemical and DNA flow cytometric study. APMIS 1999;107(3):297–302.

245. Rosenberg C, et al. Chromosomal constitution of human spermatocytic seminomas: comparative genomic hybridization supported by conventional and interphase cytogenetics. Genes Chromosomes Cancer 1998;23(4):286–91.

246. Looijenga LH, et al. Genomic and expression profiling of human spermatocytic seminomas: primary spermatocyte as tumorigenic precursor and DMRT1 as candidate chromosome 9 gene. Cancer Res 2006;66(1):290–302.

247. Verdorfer I, et al. Molecular cytogenetic analysis of human spermatocytic seminomas. J Pathol 2004; 204(3):277–81.

248. Verdorfer I, et al. Leydig cell tumors of the testis: a molecular-cytogenetic study based on a large series of patients. Oncol Rep 2007;17(3):585–9.

249. Sato K, et al. Sertoli cell tumor of the testis, not otherwise specified, presenting extensive hemorrhage and overexpression of alpha-methylacyl-CoA racemase (AMACR/P504S). Virchows Arch 2007; 450(3):361–3.

250. Verdorfer I, et al. Sertoli-Leydig cell tumours of the ovary and testis: a CGH and FISH study. Virchows Arch 2007;450(3):267–71.

251. Li Y, et al. Testis-specific protein Y-encoded gene is expressed in early and late stages of gonadoblastoma and testicular carcinoma in situ. Urol Oncol 2007;25(2):141–6.

252. Bosga-Bouwer AG, et al. Array comparative genomic hybridization reveals a very high frequency of deletions of the long arm of chromosome 6 in testicular lymphoma. Genes Chromosomes Cancer 2006;45(10):976–81.

253. Lind GE, Skotheim RI, Lothe RA. The epigenome of testicular germ cell tumors. APMIS 2007;115(10): 1147–60.

254. Schulz WA, Hoffmann MJ. Transcription factor networks in embryonic stem cells and testicular cancer and the definition of epigenetics. Epigenetics 2007;2(1):37–42.

255. Okamoto K, Kawakami T. Epigenetic profile of testicular germ cell tumours. Int J Androl 2007;30(4): 385–92 [discussion: 392].

256. Kempkensteffen C, et al. Epigenetic silencing of the putative tumor suppressor gene testisin in testicular germ cell tumors. J Cancer Res Clin Oncol 2006;132(12):765–70.

257. Honorio S, et al. Frequent epigenetic inactivation of the RASSF1A tumour suppressor gene in testicular tumours and distinct methylation profiles of seminoma and nonseminoma testicular germ cell tumours. Oncogene 2003;22(3):461–6.

258. De Jong J, et al. Differential methylation of the OCT3/4 upstream region in primary human testicular germ cell tumors. Oncol Rep 2007;18(1): 127–32.

259. Ishii T, et al. Up-regulation of DNA-methyltransferase 3A expression is associated with hypomethylation of intron 25 in human testicular germ cell tumors. Tohoku J Exp Med 2007;212(2):177–90.

260. Kawakami T, et al. Erasure of methylation imprint at the promoter and CTCF-binding site upstream of H19 in human testicular germ cell tumors of adolescents indicate their fetal germ cell origin. Oncogene 2006;25(23):3225–36.

261. Gillis AJ, et al. High-throughput microRNAome analysis in human germ cell tumours. J Pathol 2007;213(3):319–28.

262. Looijenga LH, et al. Relevance of microRNAs in normal and malignant development, including human testicular germ cell tumours. Int J Androl 2007;30(4):304–14 [discussion: 314–5].

263. Novotny GW, et al. Analysis of gene expression in normal and neoplastic human testis: new roles of RNA. Int J Androl 2007;30(4):316–26 [discussion: 326–7].

264. Voorhoeve PM, et al. A genetic screen implicates miRNA-372 and miRNA-373 as oncogenes in testicular germ cell tumors. Adv Exp Med Biol 2007; 604:17–46.

265. Voorhoeve PM, et al. A genetic screen implicates miRNA-372 and miRNA-373 as oncogenes in testicular germ cell tumors. Cell 2006;124(6):1169–81.

266. Bartkova J, et al. DNA damage response in human testes and testicular germ cell tumours: biology and implications for therapy. Int J Androl 2007; 30(4):282–91 [discussion: 291].

267. Houldsworth J, et al. Human male germ cell tumor resistance to cisplatin is linked to TP53 gene mutation. Oncogene 1998;16(18):2345–9.

268. Kersemaekers AM, et al. Role of P53 and MDM2 in treatment response of human germ cell tumors. J Clin Oncol 2002;20(6):1551–61.

269. Kerley-Hamilton JS, et al. A p53-dominant transcriptional response to cisplatin in testicular germ cell tumor-derived human embryonal carcinoma. Oncogene 2005;24(40):6090–100.

270. Schrader AJ, et al. Clinical impact of MDR1-expression in testicular germ cell cancer. Exp Oncol 2007;29(3):212–6.

271. Rao PH, et al. Chromosomal amplification is associated with cisplatin resistance of human male germ cell tumors. Cancer Res 1998;58(19):4260–3.

Index

Note: Page numbers of article titles are in **boldface** type.

Surgical Pathology 2 (2009) 225–234
doi:10.1016/S1875-9181(08)00048-2

surgpath.theclinics.com